Health Services for Cancer Survivors

Michael Feuerstein · Patricia A. Ganz
Editors

# Health Services for Cancer Survivors

## Practice, Policy and Research

Springer

*Editors*
Michael Feuerstein, Ph.D., M.P.H.
Professor
Departments of Medical/Clinical
Psychology and Preventive
Medicine/ Biometrics
Uniformed Services University
of the Health Sciences
Bethesda, MD
USA
mfeuerstein@usuhs.mil

Patricia A. Ganz, M.D.
American Cancer Society Clinical
Research Professorship
Comprehensive Cancer Center
Jonsson Comprehensive Cancer Center
University of California
Los Angeles, CA
USA
pganz@mednet.ucla.edu

ISBN 978-1-4419-1347-0 e-ISBN 978-1-4419-1348-7
DOI 10.1007/978-1-4419-1348-7
Springer New York Dordrecht Heidelberg London

Library of Congress Control Number: 2011926001



Printed on acid-free paper

Springer is part of Springer Science+Business Media (www.springer.com)

# Preface

## Introduction

### *Now What?*

The question many cancer patients have when primary treatment for their cancer is over is … now what? They often ask, "Do I just try to cope with a 'new normal' that my doctors and nurses talk about? Do I deal with each problem that I now confront on my own so I can move forward in my recovery? Do I need some type of different health care now that I have been diagnosed and treated for cancer? How can I stay healthy even with my new medical history?" Over the past decade, efforts to improve the health of cancer survivors have moved at lightning speed. This book was conceptualized and assembled to provide a comprehensive review of this progress, as well as to lay the foundation for future improvements in survivorship care.

This book follows the complementary publications of *Cancer Survivorship: Today and Tomorrow* [1] and *The Handbook of Cancer Survivorship* [2] both published in 2007. Those two volumes, edited by Drs. Ganz and Feuerstein respectively, were published to provide those involved in the daily care of cancer survivors, health care researchers, and survivors themselves, timely information on specific long-term and late effects associated with cancer survivorship. They also informed readers of the recent knowledge regarding research and practice in both the medical and nonmedical dimensions of cancer survivorship. However, an important question that was not addressed by either of those volumes is how do we translate the information on cancer survivorship into efforts to provide "quality care" for cancer survivors?

Conventional wisdom is that health care for the cancer survivor is really not very different than for any other chronic illnesses. The survivor needs to receive surveillance for cancer recurrence usually by oncology, routine physical exams and preventive services from primary care, as well as health promotion advice focused on physical activity, weight, and stress management. There is an assumption that all of these things will fall into place during the posttreatment period, and that everyone on the health care team as well as the survivor knows the drill. However, this is not always the case, and what is more problematic, the chaotic way in which posttreatment care occurs raises the question, should delivery of the cancer survivor's long-term health care be more pro-active and comprehensive with a more personalized prescription?

The increasing number of cancer survivors populating the practices of many oncology specialists and primary care providers is raising practical questions about how to provide the best quality care in our still fragmented health care system. Although guidelines are emerging, currently high-quality evidence for many recommendations of care is limited, with wide use of consensus and expert opinion.

This book was written to help fill the current gap in knowledge dissemination related to quality care for cancer survivors. For example, a recent survey of primary care providers indicated that they want to provide meaningful care to patients who are survivors of cancer, but because of a lack of training expressed concern with doing so [3]. As the number of cancer survivors in the USA and around the world increases exponentially and as the world population ages at the current rate, there is every reason to predict a major upsurge in both the incidence and prevalence of all types of cancers [4]. To respond to this major public health challenge, bold steps to improve the breadth and depth of knowledge and skills of those who can provide quality health care to cancer survivors across their lifespan must be a priority. This book represents an effort to help achieve that.

To put this into perspective, let us reflect on the personal experience of one of us (MF). MF has lived through the flurry of aggressive cancer treatments. Understandably at the time of diagnosis, neither concerned nor aware of long-term or late effects, survival was the priority. It was only after M completion of radiation treatment and a few months of chemotherapy that his RI indicated that the primary brain tumor was not visible that his focus shifted to the persistent symptoms resulting from treatment, new health concerns, functional loss, and distress. The cancer diagnosis was anaplastic astrocytoma, an inoperable cancer of the glial cells in the brain. The prognosis was not good. He was 52. Following resection to confirm the neuropathology, 59 Gy of cranial radiation and 12 months of chemotherapy, he was informed by the neuro-oncology group that things looked good for now and that there was nothing else to do with the exception of routine surveillance. These visits were critical to detect when or if the brain tumor returned. With a very genuine and positive intent, he was told to "Go and enjoy life." He was on his own now with his wife, family, and friends. His primary care physician, while very competent, commented that the best way to manage his health now is to proceed just as we would without a history of cancer.

Dr. Feuerstein describes his experience, which is not unique, as follows:

At the prime of life I was confronted with this new challenge. I wanted to return to my life as it was prior to diagnosis. After all, I was only 52. I began searching for solutions to various problems that I now experienced … unimaginable fatigue, memory and organizational difficulties, weight gain, hearing loss, low levels of activity, problems at work because of the diagnosis of cancer, and an intense fear that the aggressive tumor would return as a stage four glioblastoma multiforme (GBM), which I was told can frequently happen. The last thing I wanted was to be the manager of my own care. For some reason, even I thought that after a diagnosis of such a serious illness that there would be someone like Dr. Marcus Welby (the well-known television character who in his fatherly way knew just how to manage all his patients' health and emotional problems) who would doctor me back to health and help me forever! Well, of course, this did not happen nor was it realistic. I did think there must be a better way.

A few years after my treatment, I ran across the report by the Institute of Medicine (IOM), *From Cancer Patient to Cancer Survivor* [5] that indeed laid out a better solution! The recommendations in this book, consistent with the IOM's position on quality health published a few years earlier [6], indicated that my experience was not that unusual. In the IOM report on adult cancer survivors, whose committee includes many of the authors of chapters in this book, the problems in transitioning from a cancer patient to a cancer survivor were described with provision of some simple but profound solutions. Over the 5 years since that report, many researchers and clinicians have been busy developing additional knowledge and potential solutions regarding the long-term and late effects of cancer treatment, and detection and management of these problems from a biopsychosocial perspective [7]. Their focus has been on creating and implementing new approaches to address the many challenges cancer survivors and the health care system face. This was very consistent with how I as a clinical psychologist learned to treat patients with chronic pain, disability, and chronic illness in general, with a focus on chronic disease and functional restoration. My work as Director of Behavioral Medicine Services at the University of Rochester Medical Center, Division of Behavioral and Psychosocial Medicine (created by Dr. George Engel), along with my interactions with George Engel, Bob Ader, and many pioneers of the emerging research and practice of biopsychosocial medicine gave me a greater appreciation of the role of psychosocial factors in all types of diseases. This experience provided me with the necessary knowledge to begin my efforts to improve the quality of my cancer survivorship care [8].

I met Dr. Patricia Ganz after the publication of the IOM report in 2007. Dr. Ganz, a pioneer in providing quality care for cancer survivors, and her staff at UCLA were kind enough to complete a Cancer Survivor Care Plan for me. I am not a fan of anecdotes or testimonials so let us call this a case study! The bottom line is that this approach helped me to manage and "palliate" symptoms that I thought by this time after treatment I just needed to accept. It provided the comprehensive perspective as a cancer survivor that I knew I needed. While we cannot overstate the potential of just having a personalized "plan" completed, at this point in the evolution of cancer survivor care it is an important element for setting the stage to receive quality health care in a coordinated and comprehensive manner. Although it awaits empirical support [9], it was a systematic process that helped me recalibrate my trajectory forward. As my challenges become more evident to me, it has been clear to me that I needed something like this [10]. Since that time, Dr. Ganz and I have developed a professional relationship and this book has evolved from that experience.

Dr. Ganz comments, reflecting on her more than 30 years as a medical oncologist and as a founding member of the National Coalition for Cancer Survivorship (NCCS) in 1986: I began my first academic appointment in 1978 on the faculty at UCLA at an affiliated VA hospital where I was given an opportunity to establish an oncology ward that would serve the rehabilitation and palliative care needs of our patients. This was a blessing in disguise, for while the world of medicine was just beginning to embrace the earliest British versions of hospice and Elizabeth Kubler

Ross's treatise on death and dying, I had an opportunity to realize that palliative care was something valuable to all patients with cancer from the time of diagnosis until death. Unfortunately, many of the veterans whom I treated suffered from advanced forms of cancer that were not curable, but for some, we achieved long-term durable remissions, and we included a focus on rehabilitation, pain and symptom control, nutrition, and psychosocial support as an integral part of their care. Because patients were often hospitalized for the 6-week duration of radiation at that time, the support staff and nurses all got to know the patients and their families well and were attentive to a robust set of rehabilitation needs.

I was also fortunate in these early years to begin working with a psychiatrist and psychologist (Dr. Coscarelli continues to collaborate with me clinically and contributes an important chapter to this book) on a research project that focused on understanding the day-to-day needs of cancer patients and took a behaviorally based approach to potential intervention. If we did not understand the problems facing the patient, how could we help them cope? This early work formed the basis of a decade or more of research that we conducted developing tools and interventions to measure patient-reported quality of life, as well as the testing of rehabilitation interventions to improve the outcomes for newly diagnosed cancer patients who were expected to have good long-term survival. When I was contacted by Dr. Fitzhugh Mullan to join a small group of people in Albuquerque, New Mexico, in 1986, to discuss issues related to cancer survivorship, I was ready and able to join the adventure, investing my $100 towards the birth of a new organization, The National Coalition for Cancer Survivorship (NCCS).

Over the years, working as a clinician, but more recently largely focused on research, I have had an incredible opportunity to see the mission and vision of the NCCS realized and to have played an active part in that evolution of events. Participating as a member of the IOM committee that prepared the 2005 report on adult cancer survivors, as well as working very hard these past 5 years to implement its recommendations, has given me pause to realize how challenging it is to produce change in the health care system. Even when we have an evidence-based therapy – something like beta blockers that were found to be life saving after heart attacks – dissemination and institutionalization of such therapies may take one to two decades. Implementing survivorship care and survivorship care plans is still in the steep part of the dissemination curve.

In 2006, with funding from the Lance Armstrong Foundation, we were fortunate to be able to establish a Survivorship Center of Excellence at UCLA's Jonsson Comprehensive Cancer Center, where I have worked for the past two decades. This infrastructure grant has allowed us to develop several models for delivery of survivorship care in the Los Angeles region and to work to serve the patients who come for care either at UCLA or our affiliated community sites. We focus on improving the quality of care for cancer survivors – a major goal of this book – and are serving as a laboratory to develop and refine strategies that will work and can be used in other communities. Using a palliative care approach has served us well in these settings and continues to remind me that I have not strayed very far from the medical practice I engaged in early in my career, expect now the vast majority of patients we treat are long-term survivors, and the need to organize high-quality care for these individuals is even greater. Our cancer therapies are more complex, longer in duration, and sometimes more toxic, and we still do not have all the evidence for definitive guidelines for survivorship care. However, this should not stop us from moving forward with a focus on improving the quality of care for survivors, but this is a work in progress.

## Organization of Book

*Quality Health Care for Cancer Survivors* is divided into four broad parts. In Part I of the book, authors provide systematic discussions of the problems faced by cancer survivors in the search for quality care and just what quality care for cancer survivors might look like. Following these introductory chapters, Part II covers areas that if present in a cancer survivor need to be targeted in a coordinated effort to improve a number of outcomes related to health, function, and well-being. The identification of current and potential future problems represents an important aspect of quality care. This procedure referred to as the Cancer Survivorship Care Plan (CSCP) provides an opportunity to do just that and has the potential to integrate care for cancer survivors and serve as a first step. The challenge of managing the many symptoms and problem areas identified in the CSCP, which can present barriers to recovery over time, is discussed along with the need to initiate and maintain healthy lifestyles, optimize function and well-being, and the need to identify and respond to disparities in health care and outcomes.

Part III provides examples of current efforts in primary care, oncology, medical center, and community settings. A chapter that covers Survivorship Clinics, a recently developed approach to survivorship health care that provides innovative clinical practice and research on its outcomes [11], is also included. The final chapter in this section covers end-of-life care, a topic that is often not considered within the context of cancer survivorship. It is cogently argued that despite this lack of attention in the cancer survivorship literature, quality care demands better integration of end-of-life care into comprehensive survivorship care. More research and clinical efforts to better understand and attend to this element of survivorship are critical. It is time that this area of care is more seriously considered.

Part IV provides reviews of basic areas in health services and operations research and development that the editors think may prove important to attend to when working toward creating and implementing innovative approaches to quality health care in cancer survivors. Quality efforts must be sensitive to the epidemiology of cancer survivorship, especially as it relates to major events such as recurrent and new cancers and comorbidities. Health economics enters into all decisions impacting quality care, and a primer of topics in this area is provided to better understand the various approaches used to consider whether or not a new treatment is broadly effective and justifies implementation. A professor of health services in a course one of us took years ago quotes the following when discussing quality care: "We are all looking for Mercedes Benz care with a Ford price tag."

Even if the new health care reform in the USA impacts disparities related to access and outcomes, the chapter on health disparities is an important reminder that quality cancer survivor care is something we need to achieve for us all. Design and redesign of systems are also often very complicated to achieve. The editors thought that readers could benefit from a consideration of the field of human factors not well known by those involved in cancer research and practice, but a viable field to improve the performance of complex systems. It is hoped that an introduction to its unique "operational engineering" perspective within the context of humans working in complex health care environments may provide innovative technology and insights to help generate improvements in systems of care for cancer survivors.

This book represents the expertise and wisdom of a wide range of specialists. The comprehensive coverage provides the reader with the clear message that quality of care in cancer survivorship is needed now and involves many different specialties. Medicine, nursing, and other health providers and colleagues in many related fields can provide the perspective and knowledge to create an integrative approach to care. Many practice models from the academic medical centers to community hospitals to solo or group practices must be involved.

The chapters in this book highlight challenges as well as identify potential solutions that will require a stronger evidence base to substantiate. However, waiting for these data is not an option. Action must be taken. The day-to-day lives of millions are very much impacted by our actions in this area. As these chapters indicate, additional evidence must be accumulated to better inform the quality of our efforts. However, at present there are hundreds of thousands of experienced providers whose expertise can be brought to bear on this problem. These resources should be set into play NOW.

All authors of this book are active and authoritative researchers and/or practitioners in the areas they write about. They were selected to provide a firsthand perspective on the relevant literature and the application of this knowledge to elements of quality cancer survivorship care. While this book is structured to move through chapters serially, each chapter can stand on its own as a reference for that given area. Although there is some redundancy of references and themes in certain chapters, this overlap was intentional because at this point in time many of these references are seminal in setting the stage for innovation in a number of areas of quality long-term care (e.g., the 2005 IOM report on cancer survivors).

This book also contains a timely chapter on the newly created health care reform in the USA in 2010 and considers its implications for cancer survivors. This in-depth analysis provides a window into opportunities for improving the quality of care cancer survivors now receive in the USA. It should also be of interest to our international colleagues who are working to improve the health care of cancer survivors in their respective countries. In the final chapter, Drs. Feuerstein and Ganz provide some thoughts regarding lessons learned from approaches to chronic illnesses in areas other than cancer that appear to be applicable to cancer survivorship care over the long run. These elements of chronic care need to be tailored to individual cancer survivors. Over two decades of research and practice related to non cancer chronic illness can provide us with useful information for guiding integration of elements of cancer survivorship health care within primary care.

It is abundantly clear that cancer survivor health care needs reform. Many cancer survivors go along with "care as usual" and do the best they can. Given the current and expected numbers of cases, it is essential that cancer survivors receive a level of quality health care that provides the necessary elements to optimize health, function, and well-being over the long term and is fiscally responsive. This care should be comprehensive, integrated, evidence-based, and tailored to cancer survivors with their unique history of exposures and resultant long-term and late effects.

Bethesda, Maryland — Michael Feuerstein, Ph.D., M.P.H.
Los Angeles. California — Patricia A. Ganz, M.D.

## References

1. Ganz P, editor. Cancer survivorship: today and tomorrow. New York: Springer; 2007.
2. Feuerstein M, editor. The handbook of cancer survivorship. New York: Springer; 2007.
3. Bober S, Recklitis C, Campbell E, Park E, Kutner J, Najita J, et al. Caring for cancer survivors: a survey of primary care physicians. Cancer. 2009;115(18 Suppl):4409–18.
4. Garcia M , Jemal A, Ward EM, Center MM, Hao Y, Siegel RL, et al. Global cancer facts and figures. Atlanta, GA: American Cancer Society; 2007.
5. Hewitt M, Greenfield S, Stovall E, editors. From cancer patient to cancer survivor: lost in transition. Washington, DC: National Academy Press; 2006.
6. Kohn L, Corrigan J, Donaldson M, editors. Crossing the quality chasm: a new health system for the 21st century. Washington, DC: National Academy Press; 2001.
7. Engel G. The need for a new medical model: a challenge for biomedicine. Science. 1977;196(4286):129–36.
8. Feuerstein M, Findley P. The cancer survivor's guide: the essential handbook to life after cancer. New York: Marlowe & Company; 2006.
9. Earle C. Long term care planning for cancer survivors: a health services research agenda. J Cancer Survivorship. 2007;1(1):64–74.
10. Feuerstein M. The cancer survivorship care plan: health care in the context of cancer. J Oncol Pract. 2009;5(3):113–5.
11. Shapiro C, McCabe M, Syrjala K, Friedman D, Jacobs L, Ganz P, et al. The LIVESTRONG Survivorship Center of Excellence Network. J Cancer Survivorship. 2009;3(1):4–11.

# Acknowledgments

The first people I want to acknowledge are the health care providers that have helped me (MF) along the way as a cancer survivor: Drs. Gary Fisher, Henry Brem, Alessandro Olivi, and Howard A. Fine. Clearly, without their quality care this book would not be a reality. I also must acknowledge my coeditor Dr. Patti Ganz who is a great caring physician, who I also saw as a cancer survivor. I received my very own cancer survivor evaluation and care plan about 3 years posttreatment. It helped me move forward as a cancer survivor managing fatigue, hearing loss, and weight gain to mention a few areas. Patti has also been a colleague and friend. She is a bright light in cancer survivorship care and I am honored to have edited this book with her.

We also would like to thank all the authors of the chapters in *Quality Care for Cancer Survivors*. Their names are in the list of contributors. Each author worked very hard to get this project done within a year despite their busy clinical and research schedules. For this effort of kindness we are all grateful. We have pulled together the best and brightest in their respective areas to provide a thoughtful and scientifically sound perspective on quality health care for cancer survivors. This information will be invaluable to transform health care for cancer survivors to the level that we all expect as providers, cancer survivors, families, caregivers, health care administrators, and policy makers.

I also want to thank my family for providing me with the love and support to complete projects such as this. My wife Shelly; children Sara, Andrew, and Erica; son-in-law Umang; my grandchildren Kiran, Maya,and Zain; brother David; and mother Shirley have all been a major source of energy and inspiration for me to just "keep on ticking." My father Irving S. Feuerstein will always be a guiding light.

I must also thank all of the other cancer survivors who have discussed with me the many challenges that they have had day in and day out following primary treatment. This, above all, gives me the drive to keep focused in any way I can to improve the health care we access in order to optimize function and well-being.

Also, I want to thank Bill Tucker and Janice Stern, editors at Springer, who have supported my efforts in cancer survivorship over the last 6 years. They helped launch the *Journal of Cancer Survivorship: Research and Practice* and the books related to various aspects of cancer survivorship that were generated in the last few years, including this one. Both Bill and Janice have become strong advocates for cancer survivors, and we all owe them a debt of gratitude for keeping this effort going.

I also want to recognize the assistance we have received from Gina L. Bruns, Briana L. Todd, and Michal C. Moskowitz throughout this project. Their thoughtful input and practical help on many aspects of this project provided the support that is so essential when creating such a volume. Thank you.

Michael Feuerstein, Ph.D., M.P.H.

Mike Feuerstein is a hard act to follow! I cannot imagine what he must have been like before cancer entered his life. He is the consummate multitasker who has made this book happen, with me coming along for the ride. So, I am grateful for having had the opportunity to develop this close professional relationship with him through coediting this book. He is an exceptional cancer survivor who is really making a difference. His drive and creativity are woven throughout the book, especially in the chapters in which he threw people together to work on a topic, where they had differing points of view and would not have considered working together. I think the product is quite novel.

As for me, I am grateful for all of the people in my life who have been so supportive over the years, helping me to carve out an atypical career as an oncology professional and researcher, and allowing me to work towards a vision of better quality care for cancer patients and survivors. This includes my husband Tom, and children David and Rebecca. They were hearing dinner table conversations about cancer survivors in the early 1980s and must have thought I was nuts. But my colleague Anne Coscarelli (coauthor of the chapter on Psychosocial Care for Survivors) and I plugged away developing tools to measure the impact of cancer and its treatments on patients' lives, focusing on the development of rehabilitation interventions for cancer patients and survivors, and trying to persuade the funding agencies that there was merit in our cause. Now after more than 25 years, it is great to be acknowledged for my work and being able to provide leadership in this important aspect of cancer care.

I also want to thank my parents for providing me with the practical and financial support to pursue a career in medicine. Completing college in the late 1960s, with growing awareness of politics and social injustice, as well as being one of only three women in my medical school class, gave me a pioneering and individualistic spirit as I pursued medicine and postgraduate training. I knew I had to work hard to keep up with the guys, but also knew I was a lot smarter than most of them. So taking the time to look at the whole patient and figure out what was going on was a real challenge. Although this was often considered "soft" and "touchy-feely," my early work in quality of life assessment was the prelude to what ultimately became my focus on understanding and treating the late effects of cancer and its treatment. To my current research colleagues and collaborators – Julie Bower, Annette Stanton, Julia Rowland, Steve Cole, Michael Irwin, Tom Belin, and Steve Castellon – I am most grateful to you all for teaching me about the fields of psychology, psychiatry, biostatistics, psychoneuroimmunology, and neuropsychology, as I try to learn your disciplines and apply them to the problems of cancer survivors. Understanding the biology of cancer's late effects is now my passion, and devising targeted interventions (whether behavioral or pharmacologic) to address these late effects will hopefully be realized before I end my career.

This book must also be dedicated to my friends and colleagues who served on the IOM committee with me to write the 2005 report on cancer survivors – *From Cancer Patient to Cancer Survivor: Lost in Transition* – which is extensively cited throughout this book. Special thanks to Maria Hewitt, Ellen Stovall, Craig Earle, John Ayanian, and Betty Ferrell, who have all continued to work so hard to disseminate the messages in that report. We were full of excitement then about the results of our committee deliberations. But we were naive to think that our recommendations would be rapidly adopted – especially recommendation 2 regarding the treatment summary and survivorship care plan.

We are all looking forward to the time when there will no longer be a need for specialized cancer survivorship programs, and that such care will be a routine component of oncology care. To this end, this book works hard to rationalize the need for survivorship care as an essential part of high-quality medical care.

Patricia A. Ganz, M.D.

# Contents

# Contributors

**Kauser Ahmed**
Jonsson Comprehensive Cancer Center, University of California,
Los Angeles, CA, USA
kahmed@mednet.ucla.edu

**John Z. Ayanian**
Brigham and Women's Hospital, Harvard Medical School,
Harvard School of Public Health, Boston, MA, USA
ayanian@hcp.med.harvard.edu

**K. Scott Baker**
Fred Hutchinson Cancer Research Center,
Seattle, WA, USA
ksbaker@fhcrc.org

**Jacqueline Casillas**
Jonsson Comprehensive Cancer Center, University of California,
Los Angeles, CA, USA
jcasillas@mednet.ucla.edu

**Mandi Pratt Chapman**
Office of Cancer Survivorship, The George Washington
University Cancer Institute, Washington, DC, USA

**Anne Coscarelli**
University of California, Los Angeles, CA, USA
acoscarelli@mednet.ucla.edu

**Denice Economou**
Nursing Research and Education, Jonsson Comprehensive Cancer Center,
City of Hope National Medical Center, Duarte, CA, USA
deconomou@coh.org

**Betty Ferrell**
Division of Nursing Research and Education,
Department of Population Sciences, City of Hope, Duarte, CA, USA
bferrell@coh.org

**Michael Feuerstein**
Departments of Medical & Clinical Psychology, Preventive Medicine and Biometrics, Uniformed Services University of the Health Sciences, Bethesda, MD, USA
mfeuerstein@usuhs.mil

**Patricia A. Ganz**
Jonsson Comprehensive Cancer Center, UCLA Schools of Medicine and Public Health, Los Angeles, CA, USA
pganz@mednet.ucla.edu

**Laura S. Gilchrist**
St. Catherine University, Children's Hospitals and Clinics, Minneapolis, MN, USA
lsgilchrist@stkate.edu

**Marcia Grant**
Nursing Research and Education, City of Hope National Medical Center, Duarte, CA, USA
mgrant@coh.org

**Eva Grunfeld**
Ontario Institute for Cancer Research and University of Toronto, Toronto, Canada
Eva.Grunfeld@utoronto.ca

**Caroline Huffman**
Lance Armstrong Foundation, Austin, TX, USA
caroline.huffman@laf.org

**Linda A. Jacobs**
Abramson Cancer Center, University of Pennsylvania, Philadelphia, PA, USA
linda.jacobs@uphs.upenn.edu

**Michael Jefford**
Australian Cancer Survivorship Centre, Peter MacCallum Cancer Center, East Melbourne, Victoria, Australia;
Dentistry and Health Sciences, University of Melbourne, Melbourne, Victoria, Australia
Michael.Jefford@petermac.org

**Jennifer Jones**
Princess Margaret Hospital, University Health Network and University of Toronto, Toronto, Canada
jennifer.jones@uhn.on.ca

**Nancy L. Keating**
Department of Health Care Policy, Harvard Medical School, Boston, MA, USA
keating@hcp.med.harvard.edu

**Elena M. Kouri**
Department of Health Care Policy, Harvard Medical School, Boston,
MA, USA
kouri@hcp.med.harvard.edu

**Jennifer Lee**
Emergency Medicine and Health Policy, The George Washington University,
Washington, DC, USA

**Jennifer Lund**
Department of Epidemiology, Gillings School of Global Public Health,
University of North Carolina at Chapel Hill, Chapel Hill, NC, USA
jlund@email.unc.edu

**Jennifer Malin**
Jonsson Comprehensive Cancer Center, University of California,
Los Angeles and Greater Los Angeles Veterans Administration,
Los Angeles, CA, USA
drjmalin@gmail.com

**Jun J. Mao**
Department of Family Medicine,
University of Pennsylvania, Philadelphia, PA, USA

**Mary S. McCabe**
Memorial Sloan-Kettering Cancer Center,
Weill Medical College, Cornell University, New York, NY, USA
mccabem@mskcc.org

**Ken Miller**
Lance Armstrong Foundation Adult Survivorship Program,
Dana-Farber Cancer Institute, Boston, MA, USA
Kenneth_Miller @DFCI.Harvard.edu

**Carla Munévar**
Division of Nursing Research and Education, Department of Population Sciences,
City of Hope, Duarte, CA, USA
cmunevar@coh.org

**Larissa Nekhlyudov**
Harvard Medical School;
Harvard Vanguard Medical Associates,
Boston, MA, USA
Larissa_Nekhlyudov@harvardpilgrim.org

**Kevin C. Oeffinger**
Memorial Sloan-Kettering Cancer Center, New York, USA
oeffingk@mskcc.org

**Robyn Osborn**
Center for Health Disparities, Department Medical and Clinical Psychology,
Uniformed Services University of Health Sciences, Bethesda, MD 20814, USA
rosborn@usuhs.mil

**Steven R. Patierno**
The George Washington University Cancer Institute, Washington, DC, USA

**Tricia L. Psota**
Center for Health Disparities, Department of Medical and Clinical Psychology,
Uniformed Services University of the Health Sciences,
Bethesda, MD, USA

**Christopher Recklitis**
Dana-Farber Cancer Institute, Harvard Medical School, Boston, MA, USA
christopher_recklitis@dfci.harvard.edu

**Sara Rosenbaum**
Department of Health Policy, The George Washington University School of Public
Health and Health Services, Washington, DC, USA
sara.rosenbaum@gwumc.edu

**Julia H. Rowland**
Office of Cancer Survivorship, National Cancer Institute, Bethesda, MD, USA
rowlandj@mail.nih.gov

**Jaesin Sa**
Center for Health Disparities, Department of Medical and Clinical Psychology,
Uniformed Services University of the Health Sciences, Bethesda, MD, USA

**Emma-Jane Sayers**
Australian Cancer Survivorship Centre, Peter MacCallum Cancer Centre,
East Melbourne, Victoria, Australia
Emma-Jane.Sayers@petermac.org

**Tracy Sbrocco**
Center for Health Disparities, Department of Medical and Clinical Psychology,
Uniformed Services University of the Health Sciences,
Bethesda, MD, USA
tsbrocco@usuhs.mil

**Mary E. Sesto**
Division of Physical Therapy, Department of Orthopedics,
Department of Industrial and Systems Engineering, University of Wisconsin,
Madison, WI, USA
msesto@wisc.edu

**Julie K. Silver**
Harvard Medical School, Boston, MA, USA
Julie_silver@hms.harvard.edu

**Virginia Sun**
Division of Nursing Research and Education, Department of Population Sciences, City of Hope, Duarte, CA, USA
vsun@coh.org

**Amye J. Tevaarwerk**
Hematology/Oncology, Wisconsin Institute for Medical Research (WIMR). University of Wisconsin, Madison WI, USA
at4@medicine.wisc.edu

**Emile Tompa**
Institute for Work & Health, Toronto, ON, Canada
etompa@iwh.on.ca

**Douglas A. Wiegmann**
Department of Industrial and Systems Engineering, University of Wisconsin, Madison, WI, USA
dawiegmann@wisc.edu

**Robin Yabroff**
Health Services and Economics Branch, Applied Research Program
Division of Cancer Control and Population Sciences, National Cancer Institute, NIH, Bethesda, MD, USA
yabroffr@mail.nih.gov

**Xinhua Yu**
Division of Epidemiology and Biostatistics, School of Public Health, University of Memphis, Memphis, TN 38152, USA
xyu2@memphis.edu

# Part I
# Quality of Health Care for Cancer Survivors

# Chapter 1
# Specific Challenges in Optimizing Health Care for Cancer Survivors

**Jennifer Jones and Eva Grunfeld**

## Introduction

In this chapter, we briefly describe the epidemiological and clinical factors that have led to the growing interest in cancer survivorship. We then describe the development of the term "cancer survivor", reviewing definitions that have been applied to the term. Finally, we highlight the challenges that cancer survivorship poses to both patients and the health care systems.

## Epidemiological and Clinical Factors

It is estimated that over 40% of individuals born today will receive a diagnosis of cancer within their lifetime [1]. Worldwide over 10 million new cases of cancer are diagnosed every year, and this number will continue to rise due mainly to increase in size and aging of the population as well as early detection methods [2]. The burden and challenges that cancer poses to health care systems as well as on patients, their families, friends, and communities represent a global public health crisis that demands the attention of many. Fortunately, despite the increasing incidence of cancer, mortality rates have dropped significantly over the past three decades among the most prevalent cancer types (e.g., breast, colon, prostate) due to improvements in prevention, such as reduced tobacco use, screening and early detection, and the development of new, more effective treatments for some cancers. On average, two-thirds of cancer patients can now expect long-term survival [3].

There are now well over 12 million individuals living with a personal history of cancer in the USA and more than 25 million worldwide representing a tripling of the number of survivors since the early 1970s [1, 4]. In the next year, the first members

J. Jones (✉)
Princess Margaret Hospital, University Health Network and University of Toronto, Toronto, Canada
e-mail: jennifer.jones@uhn.on.ca

M. Feuerstein and P.A. Ganz (eds.), *Health Services for Cancer Survivors*,
DOI 10.1007/978-1-4419-1348-7_1, © Springer Science+Business Media, LLC 2011

of the baby boom cohort (those born between 1946 and 1964) will turn 65 and over the next 20 years the percentage of persons aged 65 years and older will nearly double in the USA to 20% of the population [5]. This, together with continued advancements in cancer survival rates, is expected to result in a doubling of the number of individuals living with a personal history of cancer by 2050 [6, 7].

## Who Is a Cancer Survivor?

It was not long ago that cancer was considered an incurable disease. At that time, the term "cancer survivor" was used to describe the family members after the death of a loved one to cancer [8]. However, in 1985 an article entitled "Seasons of Survival: Reflections of a Physician with Cancer" appeared in the *New England Journal of Medicine* written by a young pediatrician named Fitzhugh Mullan, who had recently been treated for cancer [9]. In this article, Dr. Mullan reflected on his experience as a cancer patient and on his discussions with other cancer patients and was the first to propose the term "cancer survivor" in relation to the patient experience. In this now celebrated article, Mullan proposed three phases or "seasons" of survival including: (1) *acute survival*, which begins at diagnosis and covers the treatment phase; (2) *extended survival*, which is the period when the patient first finishes treatment and enters into a phase of watchful waiting; and (3) *permanent survival*, which is analogous to being "cured" and a time in which focus turns to long-term physical, psychological, and social effects of cancer treatment [9].

Since that time there has been some debate and much confusion about who a "cancer survivor" is with both broad and narrow definitions being proposed [10, 11]. The broad definition of cancer survivor is most commonly used and encompasses all individuals from the point of cancer diagnoses through the balance of their life including those who are actively dying from the disease and has also been expanded to include family and friends. This definition, or variants of it, has been adopted by numerous organizations including the National Coalition for Cancer Survivors (NCCS), the National Cancer Institute (NCI) Office of Cancer Survivorship, the Centers for Disease Control and Prevention (CDC), the American Cancer Society (ACS), and the Lance Armstrong Foundation (LAF) [8, 9, 12–17].

While an evidence-based definition of cancer survivor has yet to come forward, the period postacute diagnosis and primary treatments (may include recurrence of cancer) has emerged as a distinct phase in the cancer trajectory with its own set of unique and multifaceted challenges, and as such, many have chosen to focus on this specific time period arguing that this phase is distinct and remains poorly understood [18–20]. For example, while the NCI Office of Cancer Survivorship adopted the very broad definition of the survivor from the point of diagnosis, they have chosen to focus their research efforts on those individuals in the posttreatment phase [15]. For the purpose of this chapter, we will be using the narrower definition of cancer survivor and focusing primarily on the issues in the posttreatment phase.

## Challenges Facing Cancer Survivors and Health Systems

Over the last decade, a number of advocacy groups including the NCCS, LAF, and ACS along with expert consensus panels and governmental reports [14, 19, 21] have contributed to an increased awareness of cancer survivorship and have strongly advocated for the need to address the unique medical, psychosocial, and economic challenges that cancer survivors face. Further, they have recommended improvement in the quality of survivorship care to address the unmet needs of cancer survivors, particularly their need for support as they transition from treatment to the follow-up phase of the cancer trajectory [19, 22, 23]. In 2006, a pivotal report entitled *From Cancer Patient to Cancer Survivors: Lost in Transition* very clearly identified survivorship as a distinct phase in the cancer trajectory [19]. The report included very clear consensus-based recommendations in terms of the essential components of survivorship care (see Table 1.1) [19] and outlined ten practical recommendations to improve the care provided to survivors many of which will require coordinated efforts and changes to our health care systems (see Table 1.2).

While the growing numbers of cancer survivors is without doubt a great achievement, the long-term impact of cancer and its treatments on the lives of patients and their families poses emergent and complex problems including: (1) lack of an evidence base to guide the identification, prevention, and treatment of persistent and long-term adverse effects of cancer and cancer treatments; (2) limited cancer health care resources, which are directed primarily toward treatment of new and advanced cancers; (3) the reliance on acute, intermittent care delivery; and (4) limited understanding of how to integrate across health care sectors, cancer-related health care needs with other chronic conditions experienced by many cancer survivors.

Similar to active treatment, the survivorship phase of the cancer trajectory is associated with a number of supportive care needs within the physical, psychosocial, spiritual, informational and practical domains [24–26]. Patients transitioning from primary cancer treatment to follow-up care face a number of significant challenges in order to restore and sustain their health and overall well-being and, for this reason, it is important to recognize that survivors represent a vulnerable and high-risk population. Quality of care for cancer survivors must start with

**Table 1.1** Essential components of survivorship care

| |
|---|
| 1. Prevention of recurrence and new cancers, and of other late effects |
| 2. Surveillance for cancer spread, recurrence, or second cancers; assessment of medical and psychosocial late effects |
| 3. Intervention for the consequences of cancer and its treatment, for example: medical problems such as lymphedema and sexual dysfunction; symptoms, including pain and fatigue; psychological distress experienced by cancer survivors and their caregivers; and concerns related to employment, insurance, and disability and |
| 4. Coordination between specialists and primary care providers to ensure that all of the survivors health needs are met |

Reprinted with permission from the National Academies Press, Copyright 2005, National Academy of Sciences

**Table 1.2** Ten recommendations from the IOM report (From Institute of Medicine and National Research Council [19])

| | |
|---|---|
| 1. | Health care providers, patient advocates, and other stakeholders should work to raise awareness of the needs of cancer survivors, establish cancer survivorship as a distinct phase of cancer care, and act to ensure the delivery of appropriate survivorship care |
| 2. | Patients completing primary treatment should be provided with a comprehensive care summary and follow-up plan that is clearly and effectively explained. This "Survivorship Care Plan" should be written by the principal provider(s) that coordinated oncology treatment. This service should be reimbursed by third-party payers of health care |
| 3. | Health care providers should use systematically developed clinical practice guidelines, assessment tools, and screening instruments to help identify and manage late effects of cancer and its treatment. Existing guidelines should be refined, and new evidence-based guidelines should be developed through public and private sector efforts |
| 4. | Quality of survivorship care measures should be developed through public/private partnerships and quality assurance programs implemented by health systems to monitor and improve the care that all survivors receive |
| 5. | CMS, NCI, AHRQ, VA, and other qualified organizations should support demonstration programs to test models of coordinated, interdisciplinary survivorship care in diverse communities and across systems of care |
| 6. | Congress should support CDC, other collaborating institutions, and the states in developing comprehensive cancer control plans that include consideration of survivorship care and promoting the implementation, evaluation, and refinement of existing state cancer control plans |
| 7. | NCI, professional associations, and voluntary organizations should expand and coordinate their efforts to provide educational opportunities to health care providers to equip them to address the health care and quality of life issues facing cancer survivors |
| 8. | Employers, legal advocates, health care providers, sponsors of support services, and government agencies should act to eliminate discrimination and minimize adverse effects of cancer on employment, while supporting cancer survivors with short-term and long-term limitations in ability to work |
| 9. | Federal and state policymakers should act to ensure that all cancer survivors have access to adequate and affordable health insurance. Insurers and payers of health care should recognize survivorship care as an essential part of cancer care and design benefits, payment policies, and reimbursement mechanisms to facilitate coverage for evidence-based aspects of care |
| 10. | NCI, CDC, AHRQ, CMS, VA, private voluntary organizations such as ACS, and private health insurers and plans should increase their support of survivorship research and expand mechanisms for its conduct. New research initiatives focused on cancer patient follow-up are urgently needed to guide effective survivorship care |

shifting from a disease-focused approach to a wellness-centered approach that provides coordinated, patient-centered, comprehensive care, which includes both surveillance for recurrence and detection and treatment of the late and long-term effects of cancer and its treatment. In addition, care should include increased surveillance for other noncancer health problems and health promotion in order to minimize dysfunction and/or disability and maximize well-being and overall quality of life [19, 27, 28].

Almost all major types of cancer treatment (i.e., surgery, radiotherapy, chemotherapy, endocrine therapy) can result in side effects that can impair well-being, physical, and psychosocial functioning and overall quality of life and may persist after treatment ends (long-term effects). In addition, new late effects may also manifest months or even years after treatment ends. Both long-term and late effects can be further complicated by pre-existing risk factors such as older age, pre-existing comorbidities, genetic risks, as well as behavioral and lifestyle factors [29]. The long-term and late effects experienced by survivors of cancer are common and numerous, but knowledge regarding exact incidence, prevalence, and risk factors remains quite limited [13, 26, 30].

## *Physical Effects and Well-Being*

Cancer treatments can affect almost all body systems and result in long-term and late effects such as cardiac and respiratory dysfunction, cognitive impairments, pain, fatigue, neuropathy, functional limitations, sleep disturbances, sexual dysfunction, and infertility [25, 26, 30–40]. Cancer survivors are at risk of local and distant recurrence of their primary cancer and also at significant risk of second primary cancers [41]. In addition, as they age they are at risk for development of other chronic conditions including coronary heart disease, diabetes, and osteoporosis thus raising the issue of tertiary prevention [42, 43]. Weight gain and obesity after diagnosis is also a common problem [44–46] and has the potential to not only increase risk for cancer recurrence and second primary cancers, but also places them at risk for other chronic conditions related to obesity such as heart disease and diabetes [46, 47]. Further, while data from some large cohorts of cancer survivors suggest that, over time, survivors appear to be functioning well and report few functional limitations, they do report more limitations in their activities of daily living than controls without a cancer history, even after controlling for known risk factors [48].

## *Psychosocial Well-Being*

In addition to the physical effects of cancer and its treatments, patients and their families also face significant psychosocial and economic consequences [19, 23, 49]. Psychosocial concerns such as the fear of cancer recurrence, anxiety, emotional vulnerability, issues related to sexual dysfunction, and altered body image are often common. Feelings of uncertainty, fear, or anger are among the concerns identified by survivors and can have an impact on quality of life and ability to cope [14, 24, 50–54]. Clinical levels of depression and anxiety have been documented in approximately 1/3 of cancer survivors up to 5 years posttreatment [54–56]. In addition, survivors report changes in social outcomes such as relationships, communication, or community involvement [50, 57, 58]. Despite this, the psychosocial and support needs of many survivors and their families are not being met [14, 19]. The Dutch Association of Comprehensive Cancer Centers (DACCC) has developed clinical practice guidelines that recommend survivors should be screened (no time specification) for psychological concerns such as anxiety, worries, and other topics related to quality of life [59]. Other guidelines are more explicit, recommending a high level of vigilance for psychological symptoms, with clinical assessments throughout the recovery period at 6 months, 1 year, and annually thereafter [60].

Cancer survivors often have practical concerns relating to insurance, financial issues, and employment with up to 1/4 unable to work or limiting the amount of work they can do [19, 23, 61–66]. The IOM report (2006) has advocated for the need to eliminate discrimination and minimize effects of cancer on employment, and to support cancer survivors with transitions back to work [19]. Further, they urge policy makers to act in order to ensure that cancer survivors have access to comprehensive yet affordable health insurance [19].

## *Aging and Comorbidity*

While cancer can occur at any age, the risk of cancer increases with age. Individuals over 70 represent roughly 40% of new cancer diagnosis and 60% of cancer deaths [6]. With the aging population, over the next two decades, cancer clinicians will be treating a greater proportion of older patients, many of whom will present with one or more pre-existing comorbid conditions [67, 68]. While aging in itself is a predictor of functional decline and comorbid conditions, elderly cancer survivors report poorer quality of life and poorer self-reported health, more chronic conditions, psychological problems, and functional limitations, and they are at higher risk of functional decline compared to age-matched controls [69]. All of these factors pose significant threats to their ability to live independently [70–72]. Despite constituting the largest faction of the survivor population, survivors over the age of 65 have rarely been included in research [73]. As a result, we know very little about the effect of comorbid conditions on cancer diagnosis, treatment, subsequent health, or quality of life; or about how the adverse effects of one chronic condition can impact on another. Further, it is not clear if interventions developed for younger cancer survivors are relevant and effective for older populations [73].

## *Role of Health Promotion*

Providing meaningful and practical support and education to survivors has the potential to facilitate consequential and impactful changes in behavior and lifestyle, which may not only reduce the risk for recurrence and secondary cancers but reduce the risk for a number of other diseases and conditions [46, 74–78].

Guidelines on lifestyle recommendations have been developed for cancer survivors that recommend healthy foods, with an emphasis on plant sources, and adopting a physically active lifestyle [75, 79]. Unfortunately, while most cancer survivors are meeting recommendations for cancer-specific screening and surveillance [80, 81], a sizeable percentage of cancer survivors continue to engage in unhealthy behaviors. For example, less than half of survivors report meeting the recommendations for daily intake of fruits and vegetables and for daily physical exercise

[82–85]. Likewise, moderate to heavy drinking has been reported by over 30% of cancer survivors [80, 82] and over 50% of cancer survivors who smoked prior to diagnosis continue to smoke [86]. It is estimated that 52–69% of cancer survivors are considered overweight or obese [77, 85], rates that are similar to age-matched controls without cancer.

Encouragingly, for some cancer survivors the impact of a cancer diagnosis can result in the desire to make significant lifestyle changes [85–88], presenting clinicians with an opportunity to target prevention strategies [77]. Consequently, primary care providers and oncologists providing follow-up care for survivors should routinely screen and encourage cancer survivors to maintain a healthy weight and be physically active and should provide counseling for alcohol use or tobacco use [89–92]. Studies have demonstrated that the majority of cancer survivors have a strong interest in making positive lifestyle changes [85, 86], and a sizable minority of survivors report actually making positive changes in their diet, dietary supplement use, physical activity, and quitting smoking [86, 93]. Controlled studies have shown that over time cancer survivors are more likely than population-based controls to adopt multiple healthy behaviors [94].

Practical, effective, and cost-effective behavior change and psychosocial interventions for survivors, including both supervised and distant-based interventions, still need to be developed. However, a number of interventions that target healthy lifestyle changes (such as smoking cessation, healthy diet, and regular exercise) have been shown to have a positive benefit for preventing disease, disability, and reducing the impact of late and long-term effects such as fatigue [76, 95–103]. Interventions based on evidence-based theoretical models such as the trans-theoretical model (TTM), social cognitive theory (SCT), and cognitive behavior theory (CBT) have been shown to be effective at changing lifestyle management behaviors such as diet and exercise and smoking cessation [104]. Unfortunately, adherence and sustainability is a big challenge [105]. Elderly cancer survivors, who are the largest group to benefit from these interventions, are the least likely group to undertake behavior change or maintain it [85, 106–108], suggesting the need to target this high risk group and to develop new and tailored approaches that meet their needs.

It is not yet clear why some cancer survivors are more likely to make changes compared to others and research examining how to engage and activate survivors around their follow-up care is needed [109]. Some research suggests that illness perceptions may play an important role. For example, survivors who believe that unhealthy behaviors contributed to their cancer and could prevent recurrence are more likely to change their behavior [110]. Further, self-efficacy may also play an important role in adherence [111, 112]. Self-efficacy refers to the personal belief in one's competence to carry out the behavior required to successfully deal with difficult or challenging tasks and to cope with adversity to reach a desired goal [113, 114]. Studies, which have incorporated cognitive-behavioral and motivational strategies focusing on increasing self-efficacy, have shown some promise in terms of increasing physical activity adherence [115, 116].

Psychosocial interventions that focus specifically on psychological and social outcomes have not been reported as frequently in the literature. However, preliminary evidence suggests that they have the potential to improve outcomes such as mood [117], feelings of hope [118], uncertainty, knowledge, and social support [119, 120]. Further, recent evidence suggests that interventions that address the return to work of breast cancer survivors may be beneficial [65], but again more research is needed in this area.

## Challenges to Providing Quality Long-Term Survivorship Care

While there has been a call to develop effective treatment models and methods to maximize rehabilitation, the reality remains that many survivorship issues continue to be relatively neglected and poorly understood [121]. There remains wide variation in the clinical care and the organization of services available to address the needs of cancer survivors. The current approach overall to survivorship care remains indistinct, and patients and health care providers are still unclear about who is responsible for addressing ongoing follow-up care. Without the development of organizational standards of care and evidence-based practice guidelines for the care of cancer survivors health and supportive care provision will continue to vary widely in terms of its delivery and quality.

### *Clinical Practice Guidelines*

One key recommendation from the IOM is that survivorship care should be based on evidence-based clinical practice guidelines, assessment tools, and evaluation instruments [19]. The development of evidence-based guidelines have the potential to reduce variations in health care delivery and improve the follow-up care provided to cancer survivors while also improving efficiency and efficacy of care [121]. Unfortunately, due to insufficient data, evidence-based guidelines for cancer survivors are lacking. Consequently, while clinicians are treating increasing numbers of cancer survivors, they must provide care without adequate evidence to guide them. This lack of evidence regarding follow-up care and surveillance for cancer survivors results in substantial variability in terms of the care that cancer survivors receive and likely account for the fact that many cancer survivors continue to receive inadequate and poorly coordinated care [19, 28].

The challenges in obtaining high-quality evidence on which to base comprehensive evidence-based guidelines have been highlighted in the literature [27, 49, 122, 123]. These include the complexity of very heterogeneous survivor populations, many of whom have multiple unrelated comorbid conditions. In addition, although their cumulative burden is significant, many of the outcomes of interest are relatively uncommon and consequently surveillance and interventional studies require the recruitment of very large samples that are followed over long periods of time [27, 49, 122, 123]. Lastly, the lack of guidelines on how to care for survivors leads to large practice variation resulting in difficulties in conducting and interpreting data synthesis and meta-analysis [49, 122]. When possible, guidelines should be developed based on high quality evidence; reliance on consensus should be reserved for those situations where evidence is too limited [124]. However, as Earle has argued, consensus guidelines can play an important role in the "evolution of knowledge" through their ability to raise awareness of the issues faced by survivors and importantly, through the standardization of care [122]. This standardization of care can in turn facilitate the study of the effects of care and lead to the development of the evidence which can then be used to further inform and revise guidelines, until there is enough evidence on which to create evidence-based guidelines [122]. The approach taken by the Children's Oncology Group in developing long-term follow-up guidelines [125] is a good example of how both evidence- and consensus-based approaches can be combined for guideline development. However, there are limitations to this approach whereby guideline recommendations may be influenced by bias or current standard practice, rather than evidence-based practice [126].

Over the past few years, a number of organizations have begun to develop guidelines addressing aspects of organizational care as well as care relating to psychosocial or supportive care needs during the survivorship phase. While some of these are considered to be evidence-based [59, 91, 92, 127], the majority are consensus-based [60, 75, 79, 89, 90, 109, 128, 129]. The American Society for Clinical Oncology has released and updated guidelines for follow-up care of breast and colon cancers which are based on both consensus of experts and the "best available evidence" [130–133]. In addition, the NCCN, which has developed over 100 clinical guidelines for cancer [134], has also incorporated limited consensus-based recommendation for surveillance and management of common problems faced by cancer survivors. However, as with other guidelines, uptake is a problem since many survivors do not receive the basic recommended follow-up [135, 136]. This highlights the need to not only develop clear evidence-based guidelines but to design and evaluate effective and innovative dissemination and knowledge transfer strategies to insure uptake [137, 138].

## *Models of Care*

The IOM report has documented several models for providing survivor follow-up care, which include shared-care model (between an oncologist and a primary care physician [PCP]), a nurse-led model, and a multidisciplinary model of care [19]. Other delivery models have been proposed including risk-based follow-up care, academic institutional based programs and cancer specific clinics [121]. Despite this, due to a lack of empirical evidence, it remains difficult to determine what are best practices or optimal models of care for cancer survivors [19, 27]. While there appears to be consensus that both oncologists and PCP play key roles in the medical care of cancer survivors [139], their responsibilities remain very poorly defined and lack clarity [140], which can lead to deficiencies in the care that is provided [141]. As a result, patients often report that they do not know what to expect once treatment is over; some feel that they are not being cared for and in some cases survivors describe feeling "abandoned" [142]. Clinical practice guidelines developed to date generally recommend the need to clearly designate one specific care provider for the follow-up care of cancer survivors [143]. Traditionally, follow-up care has been provided by oncology specialists which, in part, may be due to the fact that cancer is often treated within the context of clinical trial protocols which require defined treatment and follow-up regimens. Due to improvements in cancer survival rates and cancer outcomes now most survivors have finished cancer treatments and are relatively well. Given the growing incidence and prevalence of cancer, intensive oncology specialist follow-up is likely not sustainable [144] and often unnecessary [145, 146]. Encouragingly, if provided with support and education, PCPs state they are willing to take on the long-term care of cancer survivors [28, 147, 148].

While patients perceive that they receive high quality care from PCPs, some express concern regarding their PCPs knowledge of late effects of cancer therapies and ways to treat symptoms related to their disease or its treatment [149]. Research to date has documented that patients followed exclusively by PCPs undergo fewer screening tests for cancer recurrence compared to those followed by oncology specialists, and conversely patients who are followed by oncologists receive less non-cancer-related care [139, 149–155]. Encouragingly, Grunfeld and colleagues have demonstrated that, when provided with adequate information and support, breast cancer survivors are more satisfied with PCP follow-up compared to follow-up by an oncology specialist [156]. Moreover, breast cancer specific visits are longer in primary care and the costs to survivors and to the health system are lower in those followed by a PCP [150, 157]. In addition, there is no increase in delay in diagnosing recurrence, in reinitiating specialist care, or the rate of serious clinical events associated with recurrence as a result of PCP follow-up (Figs. 1.1, 1.2, and 1.3)

| STUDY | YEARS | METHODS | SUBJECTS |
|---|---|---|---|
| Phase I | 1991-1992 | Focus Groups | Patients (England) |
| | 1992-1993 | Focus Groups | Patients (England) |
| | 1992-1993 | Survey | GPs (England) |
| | 1992-1993 | Survey | Specialists (England) |
| Phase II | 1993-1994 | RCT (n=296) | English Patients |
| Phase III | 1997-2003 | RCT (n=968) | Canadian Patients |
| Phase IV | 2007 + | RCT (n=400) | Canadian Patients |

**Fig. 1.1** Testing a model of PCP-based follow-up of breast cancer patients

| Randomized Trial (18 months follow-up) | Trial Group | | Difference (95%CI) |
|---|---|---|---|
| | PCP n = 148 | Specialist n = 141 | |
| Time to diagnosis of recurrence (days) | 22 days | 21 days | 1.5 (–13 to 22) |
| Total time with the patient (min) | 35.6 | 20.7 | 14.9* (11.3 to18.4) |
| Cost per patient (£s) | 65 | 195 | –130 * (–149 to –112) |
| Time cost to the patient (min) | 53 | 82 | –29 * (–37 to –23) |

- No difference in health-related quality of life over time
- No difference in anxiety or depression over time
- GP patients more satisfied

*p<0.001 *Grunfeld et al BMJ 1996*

**Fig. 1.2** Summary of results of phase II trial

| Randomized Trial (median 3.5 years follow-up) | Trial Group Number of patients (%) | | Risk Difference CC – PCP (95% CI) |
|---|---|---|---|
| | PCP n = 483 | Specialist n = 485 | |
| Rate of serious clinical events (35 SCEs over 3,240 patient years) | 17 (3.5%) | 18 (3.7%) | 0.19% (-2.26; 2.65) |
| Recurrence | 54 (11.2%) | 64 (13.2%) | 2.02% (-2.13; 6.16) |
| Death (all causes) | 29 (6.0%) | 30 (6.2%) | 0.18% (-2.90: 3.26) |

- No difference in health-related quality of life over time
- No difference in anxiety or depression over time
- PCP patients more satisfied

*Grunfeld et al JCO 2006*

**Fig. 1.3** Summary of results of phase III trial

[150, 157]. However, the reality is that, outside of studies where PCP are provided with clear guidelines, when patients are transferred away from oncologists and back to primary care, the PCPs are frequently given little or no information about the treatments or the surveillance required and transfer rates are low [158]. Unfortunately, this finding highlights the fragmentation of care between the primary care and oncology care sectors, and the urgent need for improved coordination of care as

**Table 1.3** Perceived barriers to care

| Barriers to Care |
| --- |
| Lack of standards of care for long-term adult cancer survivors |
| Inadequate preparation/formal training around survivorship issues |
| Limited access to mental health referrals for cancer survivors |
| Lack of time to adequately address cancer survivorship issues |
| Inadequate access to patients' cancer treatment history |
| Patient anxiety or fears about health |
| Lack of practical experience in caring for cancer survivors |
| Limited access to cancer specialists when needed |
| Limited access to non-cancer specialists such as cardiac or endocrine specialists |
| Patient reluctance to discuss previous cancer history |

Adapted from Bober et al, 2009.

patient's transition across health care sectors [135]. Despite being willing to provide follow-up care [28, 147, 148], almost half of PCPs feel that they had not been adequately prepared or trained to deliver care to long-term survivors (see Table 1.3) [140]. These results underscore the pressing need for increased education and training in survivorship care [149, 159–164]. In this regard, both the Association of Comprehensive Cancer Centers (ACCC) and the IOM among others have recommend the expansion and coordination of efforts to provide further education and educational opportunities to health care providers in order to enable them to address the complex needs and issues faced by cancer survivors [19, 23, 128].

## *Survivorship Care Plans*

One of the IOM recommendations which has received increasing attention in the literature is the need for cancer programs to implement Survivorship Care Plans (SCPs) to prepare survivors for transition from the active treatment to the posttreatment survivorship phase [24, 165]. SCPs are a comprehensive and individualized treatment summary and care plan tool comprised of information on the patient's diagnosis, cancer treatments, and the ongoing follow-up care and monitoring required [23]. The goal is to generate a plan that is personalized to the patient's specific disease, treatments, and identified needs. Ideally, the SCP should go beyond the standard follow-up document, which typically focuses on surveillance for recurrence, to address the long-term physical and psychosocial effects of cancer, monitoring for and preventing late effects, and promoting a healthy lifestyle and risk reduction [19, 137]. While data to support their efficacy are still needed, SCPs have the potential to empower and inform both survivors and PCPs on the follow-up care and monitoring required and to be a valuable communication tool to facilitate exchange of information between cancer survivors and other health care providers including PCPs [122, 135, 166].

While there appears to be consensus among cancer experts and advocacy groups on the need for SCPs and their potential to improve the quality of survivorship care – through improved care coordination, patient–physician communication, and efficiency in terms of information flow [19, 137, 151, 167, 168] – this recommendation has yet to be fully realized and there remain a number of significant logistical barriers that need to be addressed in order to develop a sustainable and effective process for implementation [169]. Challenges include workforce and reimbursement issues, lack of guidelines to inform care plans, and lack of training for primary care providers [27]. In its report, the IOM provided an outline of what should be included in an ideal SCP [19]; however, there is a need to tailor this information to be useful to both patients and their health care providers, and there remains considerable debate about what should be included in SCPs and also who should be responsible for developing and populating these plans [27].

A feasible SCP will need to be efficient given the volume of patients in ambulatory cancer treatment centers. Further, it must clearly state who will be responsible for implementing the plan and should provide a standardized way to communicate to both the patient and those involved in their care about what has happened and what needs to happen moving forward. The need for tailoring is clear as "one model (SCP) does not fit all" cancer organizations or even cancer types [169]. Rather a flexible consultative model of delivery, which is appropriate to the setting, should be developed, implemented, and then evaluated for acceptability and impact [170]. In the USA, a number of individual cancer centers as well as advocacy groups have started to develop their own SCP or adopted and adapted others (i.e., ASCO Care Plan, Journey Forward, Prescription for Living, LIVESTRONG) [169]. However, to date, there has been limited formal evaluation of these plans and their implementation among cancer survivors, and consequently there are no data to suggest that they are actually effective. As SCPs continue to be developed, studies that evaluate the different components of the SCP, its impact on coordination of care, patient outcomes, and cost effectiveness will be critical.

## *Challenges for Research Related to Quality of Care*

There currently exists a unique opportunity to learn from the knowledge and experiences of cancer survivors in order to better understand the factors that cause morbidity and mortality and ultimately to improve the quality of their lives while reducing the ongoing cost of survivorship care. Over the past decade, research in cancer survivors has grown and there has been a consequent increase in articles on cancer survivorship appearing in the literature including the development of survivor specific journals such as the *Journal of Cancer Survivorship*: *Practice and Research* established in 2007 (http://www.springer.com/public+health/journal/11764). In addition, research funding opportunities are also slowly growing, although investment for survivorship research remains modest compared to treatment-related research [172].

Up until recently, cancer clinical trials have largely been conducted during primary cancer treatments. Consequently, most of what we know about the late effects of cancer treatments has been learned through the long-term follow-up of participants enrolled in clinical trials of cancer treatments [12, 49, 171]. Relatively few clinical trials have included late effects as primary end points or have evaluated the appropriateness of follow-up strategies for individuals following the completion of primary cancer treatments, and often they only include general measures of quality of life rather than measures which are relevant specifically to cancer survivors [173, 174]. Many of the studies centered on adult survivors have been small, cross-sectional or retrospective and are from single institutions and their focus has primarily been on short-term (less than 5 years) outcomes. The majority of studies have been conducted with breast cancer survivors and there has been very little research on other types of cancers. Outcomes for certain populations of survivors such as those from ethnic or culturally diverse backgrounds, those with lower income and/or lower education, and rural residents have been underrepresented in survivorship research. Survivors over 65 years of age are also poorly represented in the literature despite the fact that they represent two-thirds of cancer survivors. Research that contributes to our knowledge of late and long-term effects, including their prevention, detection, and treatment is needed [12, 49, 123, 171]. In addition, health services research is needed to further identify and understand the concerns and issues faced by cancer survivors and to identify effective, coordinated and sustainable models of survivorship care. Evidence regarding the frequency, intensity, and type of follow-up required for cancer survivors remains sparse, and the development of optimal evidence-based surveillance practices is a research priority [27]. Further the development and evaluation of SCPs, innovative interventions, and strategies to implement quality care using innovative methodologies is needed [12, 19, 27, 171]. The use of health information technology, involving electronic medical records that can be accessed by oncologists, PCPs and patients and electronic decision support tools which can be readily updated as new evidence becomes available are some innovative areas that require more attention [135].

There are many challenges in conducting cancer survivorship research due to the diversity of the population and the large number of confounding variables including age, treatments received and tissue treated, presence of underlying comorbidities, and the difficulties in following survivors over time [12, 27, 122, 172]. These, along with the constant evolution of cancer therapy and the shifting nature of survivor's issues over time, will require the development of new and novel epidemiological methods and substantial, sustained investments of both time and money. Longitudinal studies must include large and diverse populations followed over very long periods of time. This likely require multicenter cohorts and coordinated efforts through population-based registries and larger notional and international research consortiums and networks. Research is also needed to determine what interventions are effective and if interventions that have already been developed and tested during primary cancer treatments with younger populations and other chronic conditions can be translated to cancer survivors and older populations [103, 175]. Analytic study designs, clinical trials, and interventions using innovative hybrid designs such as nested case-control, case-cohort, and pragmatic preference trials are required. It will be important for newly developed and tested interventions to be generalizable to a wide range of settings outside of tertiary care centers. These interventions should take into account preferences of survivors and use a variety of modalities (e.g., telephone, web-based, groups) that can be implemented by different health care providers and even survivors themselves. Finally, the development of survivorship research will likely require more interaction between the scientists and survivorship advocates and "service users" in order to ensure the relevance of cancer survivorship research. It will be important for researchers to include survivors on their research teams in order to inform the development of methods and interpretation of findings. This participatory approach will help to ensure "translational relevance" and may help to improve dissemination of the findings [172]. Further, while training and guidance is required, survivors have the potential to play a key role on funding review panels.

## Summary

The large and growing prevalence of individuals with a personal history of cancer has created new challenges for cancer patients, their families, the cancer system, and the broader health care system. This is a happy challenge in that, for a large part, it stems from the successes of early diagnosis and treatment. As a result, for most people diagnosed with cancer today, it is a chronic condition rather than a life limiting condition. The challenge to provide quality health care to cancer survivors pertains to their physical and psychosocial well-being, as well as to general health promotion. This requires new and creative approaches to tools (such as clinical practice guidelines and survivorship care plans) as well as models of care. In addition, there is an urgent need to develop and support survivorship education and research.

## References

1. Ries LAG, Melbert D, Krapcho M, Mariotto A, Miller BA, Feuer EJ, et al. SEER Cancer Statistics Review, 1975–2005. Bethesda, MD: National Cancer Institute; 2007.
2. Curado MP, Edwards B, Shin HR, Storm H, Ferlay J, Heanue M, et al. Cancer incidence in five continents. Lyon, France: IARC Press; 2007.
3. Jemal A, Ward E, Thun M. Declining death rates reflect progress against cancer. PLoS ONE. 2010;5(3):e9584.
4. World Cancer Research Fund, American Institute for Cancer Research. Food, nutrition, physical activity, and the prevention of cancer: a global perspective. Washington, DC: AICR; 2007.
5. US Census Bureau. Projections of the population by selected age groups and sex for the United States: 2010–2050. Available from: http://www.census.gov/population/www/projections/summarytables.html.

6. Canadian Cancer Society's Steering Committee. Canadian Cancer Statistics 2009. Toronto: Canadian Cancer Society; 2009.
7. Edwards BK, Howe HL, Ries LA, Thun MJ, Rosenberg HM, Yancik R, et al. Annual report to the nation on the status of cancer, 1973–1999, featuring implications of age and aging on U.S. cancer burden. Cancer. 2002;94(10):2766–92.
8. Leigh S. Cancer survivorship: defining our destiny. In: Hoffman B, editor. A cancer survivor's almanac. Hoboken, NJ: Wiley; 2004.
9. Mullan F. Seasons of survival: reflections of a physician with cancer. N Engl J Med. 1985;313(4):270–3.
10. Leigh S. Survivorship. In: Burke CC, editor. Psychosocial dimensions of oncology nursing care. Pittsburgh, PA: Oncology Nursing Society; 1998. p. 129–49.
11. Twombly R. What's in a name: who is a cancer survivor? J Natl Cancer Inst. 2004;96(19): 1414–5.
12. Aziz NM. Cancer survivorship research: challenge and opportunity. J Nutr. 2002;132: S3494–503.
13. Aziz NM, Rowland JH. Trends and advances in cancer survivorship research: challenge and opportunity. Semin Radiat Oncol. 2003;13(3):248–66.
14. President's Cancer Panel. Living beyond cancer: finding a new balance. Bethesda, MD: National Cancer Institute; 2004.
15. National Cancer Institute. About cancer survivorship research: survivorship definitions [internet]. 2010 [cited 2010 Apr 10]. Available from: http://cancercontrol.cancer.gov/ocs/definitions.html.
16. National Coalition for Cancer Survivorship. The organization: national coalition for cancer survivorship [internet]. 2010 [cited 2010 Apr 9]. Available from: http://www.canceradvocacy.org/about/org/.
17. CDC and LAF (Centers for Disease Control and Prevention and the Lance Armstrong Foundation). A National Action Plan for Cancer Survivorship: advancing public health strategies. Atlanta, GA: CDC; 2004.
18. Feuerstein M. Defining cancer survivorship. J Cancer Surviv. 2007;1(1):5–7.
19. Institute of Medicine and National Research Council. In: Hewitt M, Greenfeld S, Stovall E (eds). From patient to cancer survivor: lost in transition. Washington, DC: National Academies Press; 2005.
20. National Cancer Institute (NCI). Cancer Control Continuum [internet]. 2005 [cited 2010 Apr 10]. Available from http://cancercontrol.cancer.gov/od/continuum.html.
21. Institute of Medicine. Meeting psychosocial needs of women with breast cancer. Washington, DC: The National Academies Press; 2004.
22. National Cancer Institute. About cancer survivorship research: survivorship definitions [Internet]. 2004 [cited 2010 Apr 10]. Available from: http://dccps.nci.nih.gov/ocs/definitions.html.
23. Institute of Medicine. Cancer care for the whole patient: meeting psychosocial health needs. Washington, DC: National Academies Press; 2007.
24. Jacobsen PB. Clinical practice guidelines for the psychosocial care of cancer survivors. Cancer. 2009;115(18 Suppl):4419–29.
25. Miller KD, Triano LR. Medical issues in cancer survivors – a review. Cancer J. 2008;14(6):375–87.
26. Ganz PA. Survivorship: adult cancer survivors. Prim Care. 2009;36(4):721–41.
27. Jacobs LA, Palmer SC, Schwartz LA, DeMichele A, Mao JJ, Carver J, et al. Adult cancer survivorship: evolution, research, and planning care. CA Cancer J Clin. 2009;59(6): 391–410.
28. Cheung WY, Neville BA, Cameron DB, Cook EF, Earle CC. Comparisons of patient and physician expectations for cancer survivorship care. J Clin Oncol. 2009;27(15):2489–95.
29. Mao JJ, Armstrong K, Bowman MA, Xie SX, Kadakia R, Farrar JT. Symptom burden among cancer survivors: impact of age and comorbidity. J Am Board Fam Med. 2007;20(5): 434–43.

30. Carver JR, Shapiro CL, Ng A, Jacobs L, Schwartz C, Virgo KS, et al. American Society of Clinical Oncology Clinical Evidence Review on the ongoing care of adult cancer survivors: cardiac and pulmonary late effects. J Clin Oncol. 2007;25(25):3991–4008.
31. Stone PC, Minton O. Cancer-related fatigue. Eur J Cancer. 2008;44(8):1097–104.
32. Lee SJ, Schover LR, Partridge AH, Patrizio P, Wallace WH, Hagerty K, et al. American Society of Clinical Oncology Recommendations on fertility preservation in cancer patients. J Clin Oncol. 2006;24(18):2917–31.
33. Fossa SD, Vassilopoulou-Sellin R, Dahl AA. Long term physical sequelae after adult-onset cancer. J Cancer Surviv. 2008;2(1):3–11.
34. Correa DD, Ahles TA. Neurocognitive changes in cancer survivors. Cancer J. 2008;14(6):396–400.
35. Stewart A, Bielajew C, Collins B, Parkinson M, Tomiak E. A meta-analysis of the neuropsychological effects of adjuvant chemotherapy treatment in women treated for breast cancer. Clin Neuropsychol. 2006;20(1):76–89.
36. Burton AW, Fanciullo GJ, Beasley RD, Fisch MJ. Chronic pain in the cancer survivor: a new frontier. Pain Med. 2007;8(2):189–98.
37. Polomano RC, Farrar JT. Pain and neuropathy in cancer survivors. Cancer Nurs. 2006;29 (2 Suppl):39–47.
38. Roscoe JA, Kaufman ME, Matteson-Rusby SE, Palesh OG, Ryan JL, Kohli S, et al. Cancer-related fatigue and sleep disorders. Oncologist. 2007;12(1 Suppl):35–42.
39. Camp-Sorrell D. Cardiorespiratory effects in cancer survivors. Cancer Nurs. 2006;29 (2 Suppl):55–9.
40. Pelusi J. Sexuality and body image. Research on breast cancer survivors documents altered body image and sexuality. Am J Nurs. 2006;106(3 Suppl):32–8.
41. Ng AK, Kenney LB, Gilbert ES, Travis LB. Secondary malignancies across the age spectrum. Semin Radiat Oncol. 2010;20(1):67–78.
42. Brown BW, Brauner C, Minnotte MC. Non-cancer deaths in white adult cancer patients. J Natl Cancer Inst. 1993;85(12):979–87.
43. Newschaffer CJ, Otani K, McDonald MK, Penberthy LT. Causes of death in elderly prostate cancer patients and in a comparison nonprostate cancer cohort. J Natl Cancer Inst. 2000;92(8):613–21.
44. Goodwin PJ, Ennis M, Pritchard KI, McCready D, Koo J, Sidlofsky S, et al. Adjuvant treatment and onset of menopause predict weight gain after breast cancer diagnosis. J Clin Oncol. 1999;17(1):120–9.
45. Demark-Wahnefried W, Peterson BL, Winer EP, Marks L, Aziz N, Marcom PK, et al. Changes in weight, body composition, and factors influencing energy balance among premenopausal breast cancer patients receiving adjuvant chemotherapy. J Clin Oncol. 2001;19(9):2381–9.
46. Rock CL, Demark-Wahnefried W. Nutrition and survival after the diagnosis of breast cancer: a review of the evidence. J Clin Oncol. 2002;20(15):3302–16.
47. Kroenke CH, Chen WY, Rosner B, Holmes MD. Weight, weight gain, and survival after breast cancer diagnosis. J Clin Oncol. 2005;23(7):1370–80.
48. Sweeney C, Schmitz KH, Lazovich D, Virnig BA, Wallace RB, Folsom AR. Functional limitations in elderly female cancer survivors. J Natl Cancer Inst. 2006;98(8):521–9.
49. Bhatia S, Robison LL. Cancer survivorship research: opportunities and future needs for expanding the research base. Cancer Epidemiol Biomark Prev. 2008;17(7):1551–7.
50. Stanton AL. Psychosocial concerns and interventions for cancer survivors. J Clin Oncol. 2006;24(32):5132–7.
51. Stein KD, Syrjala KL, Andrykowski MA. Physical and psychological long-term and late effects of cancer. Cancer. 2008;112(11 Suppl):2577–92.
52. Andrykowski MA, Lykins E, Floyd A. Psychological health in cancer survivors. Semin Oncol Nurs. 2008;24(3):193–201.
53. Costanzo ES, Ryff CD, Singer BH. Psychosocial adjustment among cancer survivors: findings from a national survey of health and well-being. Health Psychol. 2009;28(2):147–56.

54. Mehnert A, Koch U. Psychological comorbidity and health-related quality of life and its association with awareness, utilization, and need for psychosocial support in a cancer register-based sample of long-term breast cancer survivors. J Psychosom Res. 2008;64(4):383–91.
55. Tsunoda A, Nakao K, Hiratsuka K, Yasuda N, Shibusawa M, Kusano M. Anxiety, depression and quality of life in colorectal cancer patients. Int J Clin Oncol. 2005;10(6):411–7.
56. Kornblith AB, Ligibel J. Psychosocial and sexual functioning of survivors of breast cancer. Semin Oncol. 2003;30(6):779–813.
57. Alfano CM, Rowland JH. Recovery issues in cancer survivorship: a new challenge for supportive care. Cancer J. 2006;12(5):432–43.
58. Meyerowitz BE, Kurita K, D'Orazio LM. The psychological and emotional fallout of cancer and its treatment. Cancer J. 2008;14(6):410–3.
59. Urological Tumours National Working Group. Renal cell carcinoma: nation wide guideline, version 1.1. The Netherlands: Dutch Association of Comprehensive Cancer Centres; 2006.
60. Rizzo JD, Wingard JR, Tichelli A, Lee SJ, Van Lint MT, Burns LJ, et al. Recommended screening and preventive practices for long-term survivors after hematopoietic cell transplantation: joint recommendations of the European Group for Blood and Marrow Transplantation, Center for International Blood and Marrow Transplant Research, and the American Society for Blood and Marrow Transplantation (EBMT/CIBMTR/ASBMT). Bone Marrow Transplant. 2006;37(3):249–61.
61. Earle CC, Chretien Y, Morris C, Ayanian JZ, Keating NL, Polgreen LA, et al. Employment among survivors of lung cancer and colorectal cancer. J Clin Oncol. 2010;28(10):1700–5.
62. de Boer AG, Taskila T, Ojajarvi A, van Dijk FJ, Verbeek JH. Cancer survivors and unemployment: a meta-analysis and meta-regression. JAMA. 2009;301(7):753–62.
63. Ell K, Xie B, Wells A, Nedjat-Haiem F, Lee PJ, Vourlekis B. Economic stress among low-income women with cancer: effects on quality of life. Cancer. 2008;112(3):616–25.
64. Peuckmann V, Ekholm O, Sjogren P, Rasmussen NK, Christiansen P, Moller S, et al. Health care utilization and characteristics of long-term breast cancer survivors: nationwide survey in Denmark. Eur J Cancer. 2009;45(4):625–33.
65. Hoving JL, Broekhuizen ML, Frings-Dresen MH. Return to work of breast cancer survivors: a systematic review of intervention studies. BMC Cancer. 2009;9:117.
66. Longo CJ, Fitch M, Deber RB, Williams AP. Financial and family burden associated with cancer treatment in Ontario, Canada. Support Care Cancer. 2006;14(11):1077–85.
67. SEER. Office of Cancer Survivorship, National Cancer Institute. Prevalence statistics [Internet]. 2002 [cited 2010 Apr 1]. Available from: http://dccps.nci.nih.gov/ocs/prevalence/prevalence.html#age.
68. Yancik R, Ries L. Aging and cancer in America: demographic and epidemiologic perspectives. Hematol Oncol Clin North Am. 2000;14:17–23.
69. Rao AV, Demark-Wahnefried W. The older cancer survivor. Crit Rev Oncol Hematol. 2006;60(2):131–43.
70. Mandelblatt JS, Edge SB, Meropol NJ, Senie R, Tsangaris T, Grey L, et al. Predictors of long-term outcomes in older breast cancer survivors: perceptions versus patterns of care. J Clin Oncol. 2003;21(5):855–63.
71. Chirikos TN, Russell-Jacobs A, Jacobsen PB. Functional impairment and the economic consequences of female breast cancer. Women Health. 2002;36(1):1–20.
72. Hewitt M, Rowland JH, Yancik R. Cancer survivors in the United States: age, health, and disability. J Gerontol A Biol Sci Med Sci. 2003;58(1):82–91.
73. Rowland JH, Yancik R. Cancer survivorship: the interface of aging, comorbidity, and quality care. J Natl Cancer Inst. 2006;98(8):504–5.
74. Pinto BM, Trunzo JJ, Reiss P, Shiu SY. Exercise participation after diagnosis of breast cancer: trends and effects on mood and quality of life. Psychooncology. 2002;11(5):389–400.
75. Brown JK, Byers T, Doyle C, Coumeya KS, Demark-Wahnefried W, Kushi LH, et al. Nutrition and physical activity during and after cancer treatment: an American Cancer Society guide for informed choices. CA Cancer J Clin. 2003;53(5):268–91.

76. Demark-Wahnefried W, Morey MC, Clipp EC, Pieper CF, Snyder DC, Sloane R, et al. Leading the way in exercise and diet (Project LEAD): intervening to improve function among older breast and prostate cancer survivors. Control Clin Trials. 2003;24(2):206–23.
77. Demark-Wahnefried W, Aziz NM, Rowland JH, Pinto BM. Riding the crest of the teachable moment: promoting long-term health after the diagnosis of cancer. J Clin Oncol. 2005;23(24):5814–30.
78. Ganz PA. A teachable moment for oncologists: cancer survivors, 10 million strong and growing! J Clin Oncol. 2005;23(24):5458–60.
79. Doyle C, Kushi LH, Byers T, Courneya KS, Demark-Wahnefried W, Grant B, et al. Nutrition and physical activity during and after cancer treatment: an American Cancer Society guide for informed choices. CA Cancer J Clin. 2006;56(6):323–53.
80. Bellizzi KM, Rowland JH, Jeffery DD, McNeel T. Health behaviors of cancer survivors: examining opportunities for cancer control intervention. J Clin Oncol. 2005;23(34):8884–93.
81. Mayer DK, Terrin NC, Menon U, Kreps GL, McCance K, Parsons SK, et al. Screening practices in cancer survivors. J Cancer Surviv. 2007;1(1):17–26.
82. Coups EJ, Ostroff JS. A population-based estimate of the prevalence of behavioral risk factors among adult cancer survivors and noncancer controls. Prev Med. 2005;40(6):702–11.
83. Blanchard CM, Courneya KS, Stein K. Cancer survivors' adherence to lifestyle behavior recommendations and associations with health-related quality of life: results from the American Cancer Society's SCS-II. J Clin Oncol. 2008;26(13):2198–204.
84. Findley PA, Sambamoorthi U. Preventive health services and lifestyle practices in cancer survivors: a population health investigation. J Cancer Surviv. 2009;3(1):43–58.
85. Demark-Wahnefried W, Peterson B, McBride C, Lipkus I, Clipp E. Current health behaviors and readiness to pursue life-style changes among men and women diagnosed with early stage prostate and breast carcinomas. Cancer. 2000;88(3):674–84.
86. Blanchard CM, Denniston MM, Baker F, Ainsworth SR, Courneya KS, Hann DM, et al. Do adults change their lifestyle behaviors after a cancer diagnosis? Am J Health Behav. 2003;27(3):246–56.
87. Pinto BM, Eakin E, Maruyama NC. Health behavior changes after a cancer diagnosis: what do we know and where do we go from here? Ann Behav Med. 2000;22(1):38–52.
88. Lemon SC, Zapka JG, Clemow L. Health behavior change among women with recent familial diagnosis of breast cancer. Prev Med. 2004;39(2):253–62.
89. National Comprehensive Cancer Network. Clinical practice guidelines in oncology: colon cancer. National Comprehensive Cancer Network, 2010.
90. National Comprehensive Cancer Network. Clinical practice guidelines in oncology: rectal cancer. National Comprehensive Cancer Network, 2010.
91. Oncoline. Prostate cancer: nation wide guideline, version 1 [Internet]. 2007 [cited 2010 Apr 4]. Available from: http://www.oncoline.nl/index.php?pagina=/richtlijn/item/pagina.php&richtlijn_id=575.
92. Grunfeld E, Dhesy-Thind S, Levine M. Clinical practice guidelines for the care and treatment of breast cancer: follow-up after treatment for breast cancer (summary of the 2005 update). CMAJ. 2005;172(10):1319–20.
93. Patterson RE, Neuhouser ML, Hedderson MM, Schwartz SM, Standish LJ, Bowen DJ. Changes in diet, physical activity, and supplement use among adults diagnosed with cancer. J Am Diet Assoc. 2003;103(3):323–8.
94. Satia JA, Campbell MK, Galanko JA, James A, Carr C, Sandler RS. Longitudinal changes in lifestyle behaviors and health status in colon cancer survivors. Cancer Epidemiol Biomark Prev. 2004;13(6):1022–31.
95. Demark-Wahnefried W, Clipp EC, Morey MC, Pieper CF, Sloane R, Snyder DC, et al. Physical function and associations with diet and exercise: results of a cross-sectional survey among elders with breast or prostate cancer. Int J Behav Nutr Phys Act. 2004;1(1):16.
96. Courneya KS, Vallance JK, McNeely ML, Karvinen KH, Peddle CJ, Mackey JR. Exercise issues in older cancer survivors. Crit Rev Oncol Hematol. 2004;51(3):249–61.

97. Holmes MD, Chen WY, Feskanich D, Kroenke CH, Colditz GA. Physical activity and survival after breast cancer diagnosis. JAMA. 2005;293(20):2479–86.
98. Pierce JP, Faerber S, Wright FA, Newman V, Flatt SW, Kealey S, et al. Feasibility of a randomized trial of a high-vegetable diet to prevent breast cancer recurrence. Nutr Cancer. 1997;28(3):282–8.
99. Pierce JP, Newman VA, Flatt SW, Faerber S, Rock CL, Natarajan L, et al. Telephone counseling intervention increases intakes of micronutrient- and phytochemical-rich vegetables, fruit and fiber in breast cancer survivors. J Nutr. 2004;134(2):452–8.
100. Chlebowski RT, Blackburn GL, Elashoff RE, Thomson C, Goodman MT, Shapiro A, et al. Dietary fat reduction in postmenopausal women with primary breast cancer: Phase III Women's Intervention Nutrition Study (WINS). J Clin Oncol (Meeting Abstracts). 2005;23(16_suppl):10.
101. McNeely ML, Campbell KL, Rowe BH, Klassen TP, Mackey JR, Courneya KS. Effects of exercise on breast cancer patients and survivors: a systematic review and meta-analysis. CMAJ. 2006;175(1):34–41.
102. Kangas M, Bovbjerg DH, Montgomery GH. Cancer-related fatigue: a systematic and meta-analytic review of non-pharmacological therapies for cancer patients. Psychol Bull. 2008;134(5):700–41.
103. Schmitz KH, Holtzman J, Courneya KS, Masse LC, Duval S, Kane R. Controlled physical activity trials in cancer survivors: a systematic review and meta-analysis. Cancer Epidemiol Biomark Prev. 2005;14:1588–95.
104. Pinto BM, Floyd A. Theories underlying health promotion interventions among cancer survivors. Semin Oncol Nurs. 2008;24(3):153–63.
105. Cramp F, Daniel J. Exercise for the management of cancer-related fatigue in adults. Cochrane Database Syst Rev 2008. Issue 2. Art. No: DC006145. DOI:10.1002/14651858.CD006145.pub2.
106. Rao A, Cohen HJ. Symptom management in the elderly cancer patient: fatigue, pain, and depression. J Natl Cancer Inst Monogr. 2004;32:150–7.
107. Deimling GT, Bowman KF, Sterns S, Wagner LJ, Kahana B. Cancer-related health worries and psychological distress among older adult, long-term cancer survivors. Psychooncology. 2006;15(4):306–20.
108. Gritz ER, Nisenbaum R, Elashoff RE, Holmes EC. Smoking behavior following diagnosis in patients with stage I non-small cell lung cancer. Cancer Causes Control. 1991;2(2):105–12.
109. Hudson SV, Chubak J, Coups EJ, Blake-Gumbs L, Jacobsen PB, Neugut AI, et al. Identifying key questions to advance research and practice in cancer survivorship follow-up care: a report from the ASPO Survivorship Interest Group. Cancer Epidemiol Biomark Prev. 2009;18(7):2152–4.
110. Rabin C, Pinto B. Cancer-related beliefs and health behavior change among breast cancer survivors and their first-degree relatives. Psychooncology. 2006;15(8):701–12.
111. Pinto BM, Frierson GM, Rabin C, Trunzo JJ, Marcus BH. Home-based physical activity intervention for breast cancer patients. J Clin Oncol. 2005;23(15):3577–87.
112. von Gruenigen VE, Gibbons HE, Kavanagh MB, Janata JW, Lerner E, Courneya KS. A randomized trial of a lifestyle intervention in obese endometrial cancer survivors: quality of life outcomes and mediators of behavior change. Health Qual Life Outcomes. 2009;7:17.
113. Bandura A. Self-efficacy: toward a unifying theory of behavioral change. Psychol Rev. 1977;84(2):191–215.
114. Bandura A. Self-efficacy: the exercise of control. New York: Freeman; 1997.
115. Vallance JK, Courneya KS, Plotnikoff RC, Yasui Y, Mackey JR. Randomized controlled trial of the effects of print materials and step pedometers on physical activity and quality of life in breast cancer survivors. J Clin Oncol. 2007;25(17):2352–9.
116. Bennett JA, Lyons KS, Winters-Stone K, Nail LM, Scherer J. Motivational interviewing to increase physical activity in long-term cancer survivors: a randomized controlled trial. Nurs Res. 2007;56(1):18–27.

117. Boesen EH, Ross L, Frederiksen K, Thomsen BL, Dahlstrom K, Schmidt G, et al. Psychoeducational intervention for patients with cutaneous malignant melanoma: a replication study. J Clin Oncol. 2005;23(6):1270–7.
118. Lane LG, Viney LL. The effects of personal construct group therapy on breast cancer survivors. J Consult Clin Psychol. 2005;73(2):284–92.
119. Mishel MH, Germino BB, Gil KM, Belyea M, Laney IC, Stewart J, et al. Benefits from an uncertainty management intervention for African-American and Caucasian older long-term breast cancer survivors. Psychooncology. 2005;14(11):962–78.
120. Bloom JR, Stewart SL, D'Onofrio CN, Luce J, Banks PJ. Addressing the needs of young breast cancer survivors at the 5 year milestone: can a short-term, low intensity intervention produce change? J Cancer Surviv. 2008;2(3):190–204.
121. Gilbert SM, Miller DC, Hollenbeck BK, Montie JE, Wei JT. Cancer survivorship: challenges and changing paradigms. J Urol. 2008;179(2):431–8.
122. Earle CC. Cancer survivorship research and guidelines: maybe the cart should be beside the horse. J Clin Oncol. 2007;25(25):3800–1.
123. Ayanian JZ, Jacobsen PB. Enhancing research on cancer survivors. J Clin Oncol. 2006;24(32):5149–53.
124. OpenClinical. Clinical practice guidelines [Internet]. 2008 [cited 2010 Apr 10]. Available from: http://www.openclinical.org.guidelines.html [accessed April 10, 2010].
125. Children's Oncology Group. Long-term follow-up guidelines for survivors of childhood, adolescent, and young adult cancers, version 2.0 [Internet]. 2008 [cited 2010 Apr 9]. Available from: http://www.survivorshipguidelines.org.
126. Smith TJ, Hillner BE. Ensuring quality cancer care by the use of clinical practice guidelines and critical pathways. J Clin Oncol. 2001;19(11):2886–97.
127. Khatcheressian JL, Wolff AC, Smith TJ, Grunfeld E, Muss HB, Vogel VG, et al. American Society of Clinical Oncology 2006 update of the breast cancer follow-up and management guidelines in the adjuvant setting. J Clin Oncol. 2006;24(31):5091–7.
128. Association of Community Cancer Centers (ACCC). Cancer Program Guidelines [Internet]. 2008 [2010 Apr 8]. Available from: http://accc-cancer.org/publications/publications-cpguidelines4.asp#Section%2017.
129. Brown J, Byers T, Thompson K, Eldridge B, Doyle C, Williams AM. Nutrition during and after cancer treatment: a guide for informed choices by cancer survivors. CA Cancer J Clin. 2001;51(3):153–87.
130. Smith TJ, Davidson NE, Schapira DV, Grunfeld E, Muss HB, Vogel III VG, et al. American Society of Clinical Oncology 1998 update of recommended breast cancer surveillance guidelines. J Clin Oncol. 1999;17(3):1080–2.
131. Bast Jr RC, Ravdin P, Hayes DF, Bates S, Fritsche Jr H, Jessup JM, et al. 2000 update of recommendations for the use of tumor markers in breast and colorectal cancer: Clinical Practice Guidelines of the American Society of Clinical Oncology. J Clin Oncol. 2001;19(6): 1865–78.
132. Desch CE, Benson III AB, Somerfield MR, Flynn PJ, Krause C, Loprinzi CL, et al. Colorectal cancer surveillance: 2005 update of an American Society of Clinical Oncology Practice Guideline. J Clin Oncol. 2005;23(33):8512–9.
133. American Society of Clinical Oncology. Oncologist-approved cancer information from the American Society of Clinical Oncology [Internet]. 2010 [cited 2010 Apr 9]. Available from: http://www.cancer.net/.
134. National Comprehensive Cancer Network. Clinical Practice Guidelines in Oncology [Internet]. 2010 [cited 2010 Apr 10]. Available from: http://www.nccn.org/professionals/physician_gls/f_guidelines.asp.
135. Grunfeld E, Earle CC. The interface between primary and oncology specialty care: treatment through survivorship. J Natl Cancer Inst Monogr. 2010;2010(40):25–30.
136. Cooper GS, Johnson CC, Lamerato L, Poisson LM, Schultz L, Simpkins J, et al. Use of guideline recommended follow-up care in cancer survivors: routine or diagnostic indications? Med Care. 2006;44(6):590–4.

137. Earle CC. Failing to plan is planning to fail: improving the quality of care with survivorship care plans. J Clin Oncol. 2006;24(32):5112–6.
138. Elston LJ, Simpkins J, Schultz L, Chase GA, Johnson CC, Yood MU, et al. Routine surveillance care after cancer treatment with curative intent. Med Care. 2005;43(6):592–9.
139. Grunfeld E. Primary care physicians and oncologists are players on the same team. J Clin Oncol. 2008;26(14):2246–7.
140. Bober SL, Recklitis CJ, Campbell EG, Park ER, Kutner JS, Najita JS, et al. Caring for cancer survivors: a survey of primary care physicians. Cancer. 2009;115(18 Suppl):4409–18.
141. Cheung WY, Le LW, Zimmermann C. Symptom clusters in patients with advanced cancers. Support Care Cancer. 2009;17(9):1223–30.
142. Miedema B, MacDonald I, Tatemichi S. Cancer follow-up care. Patients' perspectives. Can Fam Physician. 2003;49:890–5.
143. Howell D, Hack T, Chulak T, Oliver TK, Mayo S, Aubin M, et al. A Pan-Canadian guidance on adult cancer survivorship services and psychosocial-supportive care clinical practice. Toronto: Canadian Partnership Against Cancer (Cancer Journey Action Group) and the Canadian Association of Psychosocial Oncology; 2010.
144. Erikson C, Saisber E, Forte G, Bruinooge S, Goldstein M, et al. Future supply and demand for oncologists: challenges to assuring access to oncology services. J Oncol Pract. 2007;3:79–86.
145. Grunfeld E, Gray A, Mant D, Yudkin P, Adewuyi-Dalton R, Coyle D, et al. Follow-up of breast cancer in primary care vs specialist care: results of an economic evaluation. Br J Cancer. 1999;79(7–8):1227–33.
146. Grunfeld E, Whelan TJ, Zitzelsberger L, Willan AR, Montesanto B, Evans WK. Cancer care workers in Ontario: prevalence of burnout, job stress and job satisfaction. CMAJ. 2000;163(2):166–9.
147. Del Giudice ME, Grunfeld E, Harvey BJ, Piliotis E, Verma S. Primary care physicians' views of routine follow-up care of cancer survivors. J Clin Oncol. 2009;27(20):3338–45.
148. Grunfeld E, Mant D, Vessey MP, Fitzpatrick R. Specialist and general practice views on routine follow-up of breast cancer patients in general practice. Fam Pract. 1995;12(1):60–5.
149. Mao JJ, Bowman MA, Stricker CT, DeMichele A, Jacobs L, Chan D, et al. Delivery of survivorship care by primary care physicians: the perspective of breast cancer patients. J Clin Oncol. 2009;27(6):933–8.
150. Grunfeld E. Looking beyond survival: how are we looking at survivorship? J Clin Oncol. 2006;24(32):5166–9.
151. Horning SJ. Follow-up of adult cancer survivors: new paradigms for survivorship care planning. Hematol Oncol Clin North Am. 2008;22(2):201–10. v.
152. Snyder CF, Earle CC, Herbert RJ, Neville BA, Blackford AL, Frick KD. Trends in follow-up and preventive care for colorectal cancer survivors. J Gen Intern Med. 2008;23(3):254–9.
153. Snyder CF, Earle CC, Herbert RJ, Neville BA, Blackford AL, Frick KD. Preventive care for colorectal cancer survivors: a 5-year longitudinal study. J Clin Oncol. 2008;26(7): 1073–9.
154. Earle CC, Burstein HJ, Winer EP, Weeks JC. Quality of non-breast cancer health maintenance among elderly breast cancer survivors. J Clin Oncol. 2003;21(8):1447–51.
155. Earle CC, Neville BA. Under use of necessary care among cancer survivors. Cancer. 2004;101(8):1712–9.
156. Grunfeld E, Fitzpatrick R, Mant D, Yudkin P, Adewuyi-Dalton R, Stewart J, et al. Comparison of breast cancer patient satisfaction with follow-up in primary care versus specialist care: results from a randomized controlled trial. Br J Gen Pract. 1999;49(446):705–10.
157. Grunfeld E, Mant D, Yudkin P, Adewuyi-Dalton R, Cole D, Stewart J, et al. Routine follow up of breast cancer in primary care: randomised trial. BMJ. 1996;313(7058):665–9.
158. Nissen MJ, Beran MS, Lee MW, Mehta SR, Pine DA, Swenson KK. Views of primary care providers on follow-up care of cancer patients. Fam Med. 2007;39(7):477–82.

159. Starfield B, Fryer Jr GE. The primary care physician workforce: ethical and policy implications. Ann Fam Med. 2007;5(6):486–91.
160. Salsberg E, Grover A. Physician workforce shortages: implications and issues for academic health centers and policymakers. Acad Med. 2006;81(9):782–7.
161. Salsberg ES, Forte GJ. Trends in the physician workforce, 1980–2000. Health Aff Millwood. 2002;21(5):165–73.
162. Kindig DA. Strategic issues for managing the future physician workforce. Baxter Health Policy Rev. 1996;2:149–82.
163. Goodman DC, Fisher ES. Physician workforce crisis? Wrong diagnosis, wrong prescription. N Engl J Med. 2008;358(16):1658–61.
164. Potter J, Johnston K. Keeping up with survivors: education across the spectrum of cancer. J Gen Intern Med. 2009;24 Suppl 2:S501–2.
165. McCabe MS, Jacobs L. Survivorship care: models and programs. Sem Oncol Nurs. 2008;24(3):202–7.
166. Nekhlyudov L. "Doc, should I see you or my oncologist?": a primary care perspective on opportunities and challenges in providing comprehensive care for cancer survivors. J Clin Oncol. 2009;27(15):2424–6.
167. Institute of Medicine. Implementing cancer survivorship care planning. Washington, DC: National Academics Press; 2007.
168. Ganz PA, Hahn EE. Implementing a survivorship care plan for patients with breast cancer. J Clin Oncol. 2008;26(5):759–67.
169. CJAP. A brief review of survivorship programs in the United States and Canada. In: Keal S, editor. Cancer Journey Action Group; 2009, pp. 1–23.
170. Canadian Partnership Against Cancer. Cancer journey: boosting integrated person-centred care [Internet]. 2009 [cited 2010 Apr 6]. Available from: http://www.partnershipagainstcancer.ca/person.
171. Rowland JH. What are cancer survivors telling us? Cancer J. 2008;14(6):361–8.
172. Geiger AM, Strom SS, Demark-Wahnefried W, Buist DS. Strategies to maximize the competitiveness of cancer survivorship grant applications: a report from the American Society of Preventive Oncology's Survivorship Interest Group. Cancer Epidemiol Biomark Prev. 2008;17(10):2899–900.
173. Aziz NM. Cancer survivorship research: state of knowledge, challenges and opportunities. Acta Oncol. 2007;46(4):417–32.
174. Buchanan DR, O'Mara AM, Kelaghan JW, Minasian LM. Quality-of-life assessment in the symptom management trials of the National Cancer Institute-supported Community Clinical Oncology Program. J Clin Oncol. 2005;23(3):591–8.
175. Newell SA, Sanson-Fisher RW, Savolainen NJ. Systematic review of psychological therapies for cancer patients: overview and recommendations for future research. J Natl Cancer Inst. 2002;94(8):558–84.

# Chapter 2
# What Is Quality Health Care for Cancer Survivors?

Jennifer Malin, Emma-Jane Sayers, and Michael Jefford

## Introduction

### *Defining Cancer Survivorship*

The term "cancer survivor" has been used to identify different populations affected by cancer [1, 2]. The National Coalition for Cancer Survivorship (NCCS) suggests "an individual is considered a cancer survivor from the time of diagnosis, through the balance of his or her life [3]." This definition, which has been adopted by the National Cancer Institute Office of Cancer Survivorship, covers family members, friends, and caregivers, who are also affected by the survivorship experience. It also acknowledges that cancer affects people for the rest of their lives. Traditionally, to "survive cancer" has meant to be cured of or to appear to be free from cancer. Measures such as 5-year disease-free (or overall) survival [2] have been deployed to mark out the survivor period. More recently, the meaning of "cancer survivorship" has been broadened to signify the period following potentially curative treatments; notably, the influential Institute of Medicine (IOM) report, *From Cancer Patient to Cancer Survivor: Lost in Transition*, focuses on this period [4]. This definition does not explicitly include family and caregivers, so we must remember that cancer also affects those close to the person with cancer. We must also remember that the survivor experience is a continuum, which includes diagnosis and treatment, and may also include recurrence, living with advanced cancer, and death.

J. Malin (✉)
Jonsson Comprehensive Cancer Center, University of California,
Los Angeles and Greater Los Angeles Veterans Administration, Los Angeles, CA, USA
e-mail: drjmalin@gmail.com

M. Feuerstein and P.A. Ganz (eds.), *Health Services for Cancer Survivors*,
DOI 10.1007/978-1-4419-1348-7_2, © Springer Science+Business Media, LLC 2011

## *Importance of Continued Care for Cancer Survivors*

There is increasing awareness of challenges that survivors may experience following completion of primary treatment. They may experience physical, psychological, and social consequences of cancer and its treatments [5–11]. Survivors may feel abandoned by their cancer treatment team and experience fear of cancer recurrence, uncertainty about the future, difficulties returning to work and social situations, financial problems, and issues managing long-term and late effects of treatment [5–11]. The risk of second or recurrent cancers is increased for survivors, who also face illnesses such as heart disease and arthritis that affect older populations [12]. Care beyond the period of acute treatment needs to include appropriate management of such problems to improve survivor outcomes [13, 14]. In its recommendations regarding the transition from cancer patient to cancer survivor, the IOM recommended that "health care providers, patient advocates, and other stakeholders should work to raise awareness of the needs of cancer survivors, establish cancer survivorship as a distinct phase of cancer care, and act to ensure the delivery of appropriate survivorship care" [4]. This chapter provides a discussion of just what "the delivery of appropriate survivorship care" is.

### Current Survivorship Care

Care of cancer survivors appears to be suboptimal [4]. Follow-up care between the oncology specialist (surgical, medical, and radiation oncologists) and primary care provider may be poorly coordinated, meaning that the survivor risks either duplication of effort or gaps in care. A too-narrow medical focus on surveillance for recurrence, metastases, or new primary cancers may overlook late physical and psychosocial effects, including the impact of cancer on the survivor's life. Advice and strategies that promote healthy living and psychosocial well-being are rarely discussed; when they are, this is usually ad hoc, inconsistent, and without a sound evidence base [4, 15, 16].

Patients often lack necessary information and continuing support [7]. In Hewitt's research on posttreatment cancer care, most survivors reported satisfaction with current medical care, but not with how their psychosocial needs were met. At the end of treatment they felt overwhelmed, but were rarely given written information [17].

> I think it's just one of those things that during the treatment period you've got a, like, a schedule that you're running to, and everyone runs to that. There's a plan.
> And everyone knows, "Right, well, I can help this way by I'll drive you to that chemo session. I'll do this on it." And everyone can say "Now, alright, you cook the meals this week; I'll do it that week." All that wonderful support that's around you from your family and friends, you come out of treatment, when you get the sort of "OK, it's all over," no one knew quite what to do. And now, is it all just going to be magically better? And I was all prepared for the amount of time it was going to take for me to feel better after the chemo and that, because it took forever before I felt human again, and no one quite knew what to ask me to do at work, how much more to put back on me, all that sort of thing [6].

> After my good news, a year after treatment, I spat up blood, and I went "Oh dear, it's back." I was taken in; they looked down and couldn't find anything. Patted me on the head and sent me home. For the next five years I was waiting to be spitting up blood again, until I finally did. So I came back here, and they said, "Don't worry about it. It happens." Now, if somebody had told me that five years before, I wouldn't have been worried about it coming back so much [6].

In a large Internet-based study conducted by the Lance Armstrong Foundation, 33% of survivors reported there were few or no resources available to deal with their emotional needs; 70% felt that their physician was unable to assist with identified nonmedical issues [18].

Importantly, optimal survivorship care does not begin as treatment ends. Optimal posttreatment outcomes are strongly influenced by experiences and interventions that take place much earlier, including at diagnosis and during treatment. Identifying and addressing supportive care needs early may result in improved outcomes [15, 16, 19]. For example, meeting informational needs and providing necessary practical and emotional support is likely to reduce distress following treatment completion and into the survivorship phase. Similarly, medical interventions during the treatment phase may prevent later consequences. For example, with appropriate intervention, it may be possible to reduce the risk of premature menopause, infertility, sexual dysfunction, and cognitive problems.

Over the past 15 years, there has been increasing pressure for better services for survivors:

- In 1996, the National Coalition for Cancer Survivorship established 12 principles for delivering quality cancer care [20].
- There has been extensive investigation into the types of changes needed to improve the quality of care, including the 2001 IOM report *Crossing the Quality Chasm: A New Health System for the 21st Century* [21].
- In 2005 the IOM released *From Cancer Patient to Cancer Survivor: Lost in Transition*, which comprehensively examines the need for improved care for survivors [4].

## A Framework for Considering Quality Survivorship Care

The IOM Committee on Health Care Quality in America has defined essential features to guide the redesign of health-care processes [21]. These are shown in Table 2.1.

These general considerations provide a valuable framework for considering ideal care for cancer patients and survivors. Importantly, the above points do not impose a restricted consideration of patient needs. As noted, survivors may encounter a broad range of consequences as a result of cancer and its treatments. Some might clearly be considered within the scope of medical care (treatment of side effects, risk of late effects) and some within the broader scope of supportive care (dealing with fear of recurrence, adjustment issues); however, other issues, for

**Table 2.1** Essential features to guide the redesign of health-care processes [21] (Reprinted with permission from the National Academies Press, Copyright [2001], National Academy of Sciences)

- Care based on continuous healing relationships. The system should be responsive and accessible.
- Customization based on patient needs and values. The system should have the capability to respond to individual patient choices and preferences.
- The patient as the source of control. Patients should be given the necessary information and the opportunity to exercise the degree of control they choose over decisions that affect them.
- Shared knowledge and the free flow of information.
- Evidence-based decision-making.
- Safety as a system property.
- The need for transparency.
- Anticipation of needs. The system should not just react to events.
- Continuous decrease in waste.
- Cooperation among clinicians.

example, returning to school or work or coping with financial consequences, may not be considered the focus of posttreatment care. Perspectives of the survivor, health-care provider, and payer may indeed be quite different regarding what constitutes quality survivorship care. It will be important to continue to debate the scope of "quality health care for cancer survivors."

Considering the range of potential issues affecting survivors and the need for a broad focus, it is worthwhile to highlight the World Health Organization definition of health, that being "a state of complete physical, mental and social well-being and not merely the absence of disease or infirmity [22]." The emphasis on well-being accords with a notion of cancer as a chronic disease and the need for rehabilitation following active cancer treatments.

In addition to advocating for planned and coordinated care to manage the medical and psychosocial difficulties experienced by cancer survivors after completing treatment, the IOM report *From Cancer Patient to Cancer Survivor: Lost in Transition* attempted to further describe and "operationalize" the content of what survivorship care should involve. Four essential components of survivorship care were identified and are presented in Table 2.2 [4].

While these four components may have broad applicability, it should be remembered that every survivor will have a unique experience. Even patients with the same type of cancer may receive quite different treatments, be affected in very different ways, encounter individual difficulties, and be at risk of different consequences. This underscores the need to tailor follow-up to each individual survivor.

## *Prevention of Recurrent and New Cancers, and of Other Late Effects*

Although survivors remain at a heightened risk of developing new cancers, this risk may be reduced through health promotion strategies [14]. There is increasing evidence to support the use of adjuvant medical treatments to reduce the risk of cancer recurrence. In addition, the period after treatment can be seen as a

**Table 2.2** Four essential components of survivorship care

| | |
|---|---|
| 1. | *Prevention* of recurrent and new cancers, and of other late effects |
| 2. | *Surveillance* for cancer spread, recurrence, or second cancers; assessment of medical and psychosocial late effects |
| 3. | *Intervention* for consequences of cancer and its treatment |
| 4. | *Coordination* between specialists and primary care providers to ensure that all of the survivor's health needs are met |

"teachable moment," where changes to health and lifestyle may be more readily adopted in an attempt to prevent disease and ill health [4]. Improved diet, maintaining a healthy weight, ceasing smoking, and increasing physical activity may prevent secondary and recurrent cancers, and may reduce many of the physical and psychosocial consequences of cancer treatment [23, 24]. Information on recommended health and lifestyle strategies should be provided to all cancer survivors [4, 24]. Indeed, the second recommendation of the IOM report (and relevant to each of the four essential components of survivorship care) concerns provision of information: "patients completing primary treatment should be provided with a comprehensive care summary and follow-up plan that is clearly and effectively explained. This 'survivorship care plan' should be written by the principal provider(s) who coordinated oncology treatment. It is recommended that this service/procedure be reimbursed by third-party payors of health care [4]." It is possible that this coordinated effort would provide for a more systematic and even preventive service, reducing the need for mismanaged care.

## *Surveillance for Cancer Spread, Recurrence, or Second Cancers; Assessment of Medical and Psychosocial Late Effects*

Ongoing surveillance is an essential component of follow-up care to ensure that new or recurrent cancers are detected at a time when treatment may be most effective [25]. Guidelines are not available for all cancer types and vary considerably in terms of their comprehensiveness. Many emphasize detection of cancer recurrence, but place little emphasis on the prevention, detection, and amelioration of the consequences of cancer treatments. Many of these guidelines provide inconsistent recommendations about the frequency, duration, and type of follow-up that is required for different survivor groups [25]. The third recommendation from the IOM report was that "Health care providers should use systematically developed evidence-based clinical practice guidelines, assessment tools, and screening instruments to help identify and manage late effects of cancer and its treatment. Existing guidelines should be refined and new evidence-based guidelines should be developed through public- and private-sector efforts [4]."

Surveillance is an ideal opportunity to monitor treatment efficacy and any ongoing physical or psychosocial consequences. It is also a time to provide continuing information and support. Surveillance may also help survivors to feel less anxious about the possibility of cancer returning and more confident about what will happen to them in the future. Surveillance should be tailored, with individuals at high risk of treatment sequelae requiring a higher degree of surveillance [25]. Surveillance also provides an added opportunity to screen for general health issues, as many patients neglect other areas of health due to a heavy focus on cancer and recurrence [26]. Furthermore, it has been suggested that a full review of psychosocial and adjustment issues be incorporated into an optimal model of survivorship care [12].

### Intervention for Consequences of Cancer and Its Treatment

Cancer survivors may require further assistance managing the physical and psychosocial effects of cancer diagnosis and treatment. Patients may have persisting, even long-term effects and be at risk of developing problems at a later time – late effects. Physical issues such as fatigue, pain, urinary and bowel issues, and hot flashes may be successfully managed with medical interventions or self-care strategies [6, 27]. A growing number of psychosocial interventions may improve symptom management and psychological issues as they arise and should be discussed as part of a tailored survivor consultation [28].

## *Coordination Among Specialists and Primary Care Providers*

Follow-up care is often provided by a group of oncology specialists and primary care providers. This system has a number of strengths, if used effectively. Cancer screening services are received more reliably when specialists are involved; however, preventive services for other medical illnesses tend to be neglected [12]. This may be greatly improved when a primary care provider is also involved [12]. Coordinated care between oncologists and primary care providers is essential to ensure that all health needs are met [4, 29]. Regular, effective communication strategies are crucial to the success of such an arrangement. Care plans may assist. Clear delineation of roles is essential. Comprehensive care means that each of the above principles (detection, surveillance, and intervention) should be undertaken, but it is less clear how to optimally allocate these responsibilities in a shared care model.

Elsewhere we have suggested other elements of ideal survivorship care [30]. High-quality care would:

- Be comprehensive and accessible
- Include specialized services
- Be patient-centered
- Be tailored to meet individual needs
- Empower survivors to take a role in their own health management to the extent that they wished
- Be multidisciplinary and collaborative and include oncologists; primary care providers; nurses; rehabilitation specialists such as physiatrists, physical therapists, social workers and psychologists; and survivors and their families

- Recognize the transition from acute care to the community and be designed to facilitate this transition
- Use effective communication strategies to promote planned and coordinated follow-up
- Be holistic and address psychosocial as well as physical needs
- Encompass preventive as well as reactive health management
- Be evidence-based and supported by appropriate guidelines, policies, and research, to ensure that care is outcomes-focused, cost-effective, and sustainable

## Defining and Measuring Quality Survivorship Care

The ultimate objective of good quality cancer care is to achieve desired outcomes for survivors. This includes not only surviving the cancer but also living well. Functional status, quality of life, and the personal cancer care experience emerge as critical and perhaps overlooked outcomes [31, 32]. Thus, important outcomes for cancer survivors include not only overall and disease-free survival but also functional status and quality of life, as well as their experience of care (satisfaction).

The IOM has defined *quality* as "the degree to which health services for individuals and populations increase the likelihood of desired health outcomes and are consistent with current professional knowledge [33]." Of note, this definition refers to health services and health outcomes. Health systems overall tend to be oriented around the acute treatment of ill people, with lesser emphasis on prevention and rehabilitation. Cancer is a leading cause of death. Thus, research and clinical services have developed with the primary focus being effective treatment with the goal of cure. Quality frameworks have emphasized the treatment phase of the cancer journey and focused on safe, effective, well-coordinated medical care. Only quite recently has there been recognition of the posttreatment phase. Survivors may be affected by cancer and its treatments for many decades. As noted previously, survivors' well-being may be strongly influenced by a broad set of consequences, including impact of the illness on work, education, finances, and relationships. Therefore, quality metrics may need to be expanded to recognize the breadth and duration of the survivorship experience. Clarifying definitions is important, as this may strongly affect the orientation of care and services. The fourth recommendation from the IOM report is that "quality of survivorship care measures should be developed through public/private partnerships and quality assurance programs implemented by health systems to monitor and improve the care that all survivors receive [4]."

Moving beyond survival, functional status, quality of life, and the personal cancer care experience emerge as critical and perhaps overlooked outcomes [31, 32]. Cancer survivors have more functional limitations due to their health than age-, gender-, and educational-attainment-matched controls, with 18% unable to work due to health problems (vs 10% for controls), 27% limited in the amount or kind of work that they can do because of health problems (vs 18%), 5% needing help in activities of daily living (vs 3%), and 11% needing help in independent activities of daily living (vs 7%) [34]. Survivors may have other long-term functional limitations.

A high proportion of cancer survivors have limitations in lower-body function, with 56% reporting difficulty in performing at least one of the following activities compared with only 27% of controls: walking one-quarter of a mile; walking up and down ten steps; standing for 2 h; stooping, crouching, or kneeling; and lifting 10 lb [35]. There are opportunities to provide the type of care needed to mitigate the impact of these functional limitations to enhance overall health.

Research is urgently needed to develop evidence-based approaches to improve outcomes for cancer survivors. In addition, however, we must determine what processes and structures of care will produce the highest quality outcomes given *current* scientific knowledge.

## *What Is Known About the Quality of Survivorship Care?*

The ultimate objective of good quality cancer care is to achieve desired outcomes for survivors. This includes not only surviving the cancer but also living well. Thus, important outcomes for cancer survivors include not only overall and disease-free survival, but also functional status and quality of life, as well as their experience of care (satisfaction). Both structure and process of care, along with individual patient characteristics, contribute to outcomes (Fig. 2.1). The only way to improve the quality of outcomes is to improve the quality of the process and structure of care. Process is the set of activities that go on between patients and practitioners and includes both the technical and interpersonal quality of care. The structural dimension of health-care quality includes resources needed to provide medical care, such as the availability of imaging services or the professional education and competence of the providers.

## *Quality Indicators for the Processes of Survivorship Care*

Quality of care can be measured across three dimensions: outcomes, process, and structure of care [36]. Measures of the process of care are referred to as "quality indicators." Quality indicators take the form of an "if-then" statement, which is then represented as a ratio where the "if" is the denominator and the "then" is the numerator:

$$\text{Quality indicator} = \frac{\#\text{ patients who received the specified intervention}}{\#\text{ patients for whom the intervention is indicated} \\ -\#\text{ patients reasonable to exempt from intervention}}$$

The numerator describes the care that should be provided. The denominator identifies the group of patients to whom the care should be provided. For example, when specifying a quality indicator for tamoxifen for breast cancer, it is necessary to determine which patients would be eligible, and in addition to identifying the cohort for whom tamoxifen is indicated, it may be desirable to exclude patients who

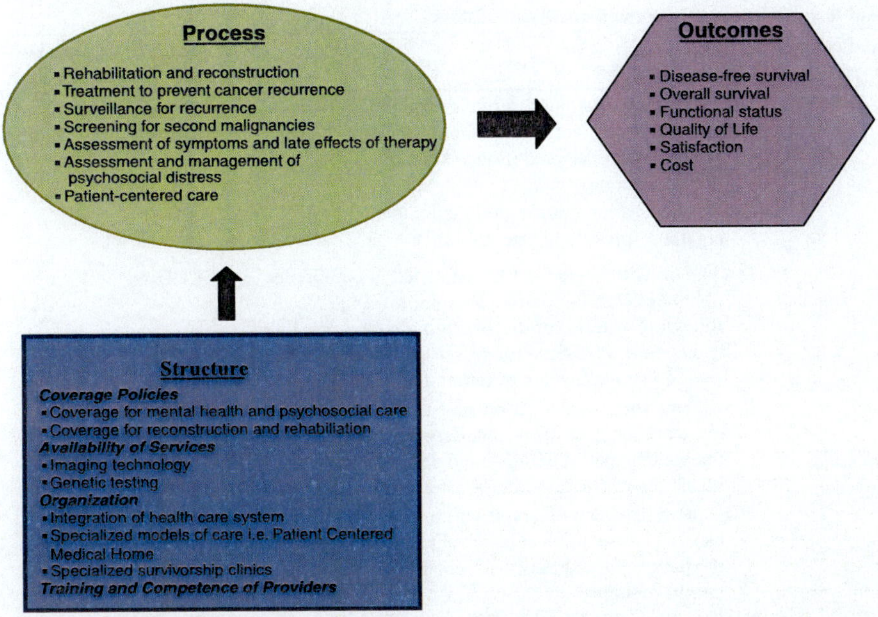


**Fig. 2.1** Structure and processes of care that lead to desired outcomes for cancer survivors

refused. If a patient newly diagnosed with invasive breast cancer meets all of the criteria – is premenauposal, has estrogen receptor–positive or progesterone receptor–positive breast cancer, tumor size greater than 1 cm or involved axillary lymph nodes, and did not refuse tamoxifen – THEN the patient should receive tamoxifen. To operationalize this measure, the THEN statement becomes the numerator and all of the criteria in the IF statement need to be specified in the denominator.

$$\text{Quality indicator} = \frac{\text{\# eligible patients who received tamoxifen}}{\begin{array}{l}\text{\# premenopausal women with ER or PR positive breast}\\ \text{cancer} > 1 \text{ cm or involved axillary lymph nodes}\\ -\text{\# patients who refused tamoxifen}\end{array}}$$

Since the IOM called attention to the quality of cancer care in its 1999 report "Ensuring the Quality of Cancer Care [37]," a number of quality indicator sets have been developed to evaluate the quality of cancer care [38–43]. However, few of these quality indicators address posttreatment survivorship care and most focus on follow-up of people with a history of breast, colorectal, or prostate cancer, or melanoma. Of the four essential components of survivorship care described by the IOM (and discussed above), almost all of the indicators are focused on the second element (surveillance for cancer spread, recurrence, or second cancers; assessment of medical and psychosocial late effects) and most focus on detection of recurrence.

Of the quality indicators that address aspects of survivorship care (see Table 2.3), nine address surveillance (essential component 2) and the domains of prevention (essential component 1), consequences of cancer treatment (essential component 3), and

**Table 2.3** Cancer survivorship quality indicators

| Cancer type | Quality indicator | Indicator set | Level of evidence |
|---|---|---|---|
| All | Chemotherapy treatment summary completed; provided to patient; and communicated or provided to other practitioner(s) within 3 months of chemotherapy end. | QOPI | III |
| | Smoking cessation counseling recommended to cigarette smokers by second office visit. | QOPI | II |
| Breast cancer | If a patient with stage I–III breast cancer who initiates treatment with tamoxifen does not meet the following criteria for discontinuing tamoxifen: there is evidence of disease progression, then the patient should receive 5 years of tamoxifen 20 mg/day. | NICCQ | I |
| | If a patient with stage I–III breast cancer undergoes mastectomy, then prior to undergoing mastectomy the patient should be informed about the option of breast reconstruction after mastectomy. | NICCQ | III |
| | If a patient has been diagnosed with stage I–III breast cancer and has not had bilateral mastectomies, then the patient should have had a mammogram in the last 12 months. | NICCQ | I |
| | Women with a history of breast cancer should have yearly mammography. | QATOOL (RAND) | I |
| | Women diagnosed with breast cancer in the past 5 years should have a clinical breast exam in the past 6 months. | QATOOL (RAND) | III |
| | Women diagnosed with breast cancer more than 5 years ago should have a clinical breast exam in the past year. | QATOOL (RAND) | III |
| Colorectal cancer | If the patient has resection of a stage II or stage III colon rectal cancer, then the patient should be counseled about the need to have first degree relatives undergo colorectal cancer screening. | NICCQ | II |
| | Patients with stage I–III colorectal cancer, then he/she should receive colonoscopy or double contrast barium enema within 1 year of curative surgery if it did not occur within 12 months preoperatively. | QATOOL (RAND) | II |
| | Patients with stage I–III colorectal cancer should receive colonoscopy or double contrast barium enema within 3 years of curative surgery and every 5 years thereafter. | QATOOL (RAND) | I |
| Prostate cancer | Documentation/evidence of communication with patient's primary care physician or provision of continuing care. | RAND prostate | III |
| | At least two visits for follow-up by treating physician during the first posttreatment year. | RAND prostate | III |
| Melanoma | Patients with a personal history of cutaneous melanoma should receive a referral to a dermatologist for surveillance screening. | QATOOL (RAND) | III |

*QOPI* Quality Oncology Practice Initiative, *NICCQ* National Initiative on Cancer Care Quality, *QATOOL* Quality Assessment Tool, *RAND* the RAND Corporation (Research And Development) coordination between specialists and primary care providers (essential component 4) each have just one quality indicator. Additionally, only three are based on Level I evidence (adjuvant therapy with tamoxifen and screening for second cancers with mammography and colonoscopy).

## Are Patients Receiving the Essential Components of Quality Survivorship Care?

Given the paucity of validated quality indicators, our knowledge of the quality of the process of care for cancer survivors is limited. Nevertheless, in recent years, a number of studies provide valuable insights on the quality of survivorship care.

Poor quality of care can result from too little care (underuse), too much care (overuse), or the wrong care (misuse). Most quality measurement has focused on underuse or misuse. Overuse of an intervention is an important indicator of poor quality when the potential for harm exceeds the potential benefit to patients. Overuse that does not have an adverse risk–benefit ratio may not be an indicator of poor quality care for the individual patient but may be undesirable because it results in inefficient resource allocation. Given the paucity of evidence-based quality indicators for survivorship care, our knowledge of the quality of survivorship care is somewhat limited. Nevertheless, the available data suggest that we are falling short on delivering the essential components of survivorship care proposed by the IOM.

## Prevention of Recurrent and New Cancers, and of Other Late Effects

Unfortunately, few strategies currently exist for preventing recurrent or new primary cancers (beyond adjuvant therapy) and little is known about preventing late effects of treatment, although lifestyle factors, such as ceasing cigarette smoking, maintaining a healthy weight range, and regular exercise, may assist [23]. Nevertheless, the available data suggest that prevention efforts are lacking for those cancers where the evidence does demonstrate a benefit. Smoking cessation has been shown specifically to improve the outcomes of patients with lung cancer and head and neck cancer [44]. Additionally, smokers with a non-tobacco-related malignancy may be more receptive to counseling as their experience with cancer providing a "teachable moment [45]." Of course, stopping smoking has many other health benefits. In 2006 American Society of Clinical Oncology (ASCO) began integrating smoking-related measures into the ASCO Quality Oncology Practice Initiative (QOPI), a quality improvement program that enables oncology practices to assess their performance relative to their peers on a menu of quality measures. Among QOPI practices, smoking cessation counseling is offered to smokers only approximately 25% of the time [46]. Given that these are a self-selected group of practices interested in quality improvement, this rate likely overestimates the rate of patients counseled about smoking prevention overall.

Most women with hormone receptor–positive breast cancer are prescribed hormonal therapy with tamoxifen or an aromatase inhibitor at the completion of the initial treatment not only to decrease their risk of distant recurrence but also to prevent local recurrence and second breast cancers. Although the rates of appropriate prescribing of adjuvant hormonal therapy are very high, the available data suggest that the quality of care to ensure that patients continue to receive this important therapy needs to be improved. In the NICCQ study, while 92% of women with hormone receptor breast cancers larger than 1 cm or positive lymph nodes received tamoxifen, only 74% of those who initiated therapy were still taking the medication when surveyed 4 years after diagnosis [47]. Other studies have reported even higher rates of discontinuation of tamoxifen ranging from 31% to 49% in women over 65 [48, 49]. Factors predicting non-adherence include older age and greater comorbidity but also having side effects from the medication [49], not being informed about side effects in advance of starting the medication, and having less support than needed [50], suggesting that adherence may improve with greater attention to the quality of survivorship care.

## *Surveillance for Cancer Spread, Recurrence, or Second Cancers; Assessment of Medical and Psychosocial Late Effects*

There is strong evidence supporting the benefit of surveillance for new primaries for a number of cancers, including breast cancer, colorectal cancer, and consensus regarding the practice for others such as melanoma. While the data concerning the benefits of surveillance for local recurrence are less certain, the same modalities used to screen for a new primary would generally identify a local recurrence (e.g., mammogram and breast exam). Rates of adherence to mammography screening quality indicators are generally very high. In NICCQ, 94% of breast cancer survivors reported having received a mammogram in the prior year [47]. Rates of mammography are lower in older breast cancer survivors but still far exceed the mammography screening rates of women without a cancer history or who have other comorbid conditions (73% vs 59% vs 38%, respectively, for women enrolled in Medicare) [51]. Similarly, among colorectal cancer survivors, most appear to receive recommended colonoscopy screening with overall 74% having at least one colonoscopy within 3 years of diagnosis, with the proportion appropriately declining with age (83% of survivors 66–69 vs 47% of survivors 85 and older) and comorbidity (75% with no comorbid conditions and 69% with three or more comorbid conditions) [52]. Since patients with melanoma are at high risk for a second skin cancer, routine physical examination of the skin is recommended. In one study, more than 90% of Medicare patients diagnosed with melanoma in the US Surveillance, Epidemiology, and End Results (SEER) registry had a visit with a clinician for a skin examination within 2 years of their diagnosis [53]. Thus, while there may still be room for improvement, especially to address areas of health disparities, overall, at least for common cancers where consensus exists on appropriate surveillance, the quality of care for detection of second cancers appears quite good.

Unfortunately, for only a handful of cancers does early identification of distant recurrence appear to result in improved outcomes. Randomized trials have found that for a number of cancers, including breast cancer and ovarian cancer, intensive monitoring for disease recurrence not only does not prolong survival but may worsen quality of life by adding to the number of months of palliative chemotherapy received [54, 55]. Because of this, clinical guidelines recommend against routine surveillance for cancer recurrence using tumor markers or imaging, except in those situations where early treatment has been shown to improve patient outcomes, such as resection of liver metastases in colorectal cancer or high-dose chemotherapy for lymphoma.

Given that until recently, the primary focus of care for cancer survivors has been on identifying relapses, it is perhaps not surprising that there appears to be extensive overuse of testing to detect cancer recurrences. Use of medical imaging in general has been increasing dramatically in recent years, with PET scanning becoming the most widely used imaging for patients with cancer in the USA [56–58]. Much of this increase reflects the overuse of these tests to detect cancer recurrences. In the US National Oncology PET Registry, 65% of PET scans were obtained for detection of recurrences despite the fact that guidelines do not recommend imaging surveillance for any of the nine malignancies that are included [58]. A recent study estimated that while cancer patients represented only 1% of the patients receiving imaging studies in Germany in 2000–2005, they received more than 10% of the effective dose of radiation delivered during that time [59]. The unfortunate irony is that this inappropriate surveillance for a cancer recurrence may place cancer survivors at increased risk for second primaries and other malignancies [60, 61].

Assessment of medical and psychosocial late effects has not been systematically studied, though appears suboptimal. As an illustration, Beaker and Luker studied the nature and content of hospital follow-up for women with early breast cancer [62]. Consultations were generally quite short (mean duration of 6 min) and focused on the detection of cancer recurrence. Unsurprisingly, few opportunities were available to meet supportive care needs. However, patients gained reassurance from these visits, as they were generally very optimistic.

## Intervention for Consequences of Cancer and Its Treatment

Cancer and its treatments are associated with numerous physical and emotional consequences. While effective approaches to mitigate the effects of cancer treatment are sorely lacking, interventions do exist for a growing number. The consequences of often disfiguring cancer surgeries have long been recognized and several quality indicators speak to the need to address these issues. Although only 20–40% of women undergo breast reconstruction following mastectomy [63], over 80% report discussing reconstruction with their physicians [63, 64]. The NICCQ study included a quality indicator for breast reconstruction for women who have a mastectomy which recommends that prior to undergoing mastectomy the patient should be informed about the option of breast reconstruction after mastectomy. In the NICCQ cohort there was widespread variation in adherence to this quality indicator with just over half of the patients receiving the specified care, but across cities this ranged from 39% to 65% [47]. Similarly, for patients with colorectal cancer who receive an ostomy during their primary surgery, reversal of the ostomy is critical for quality of life during survivorship when feasible and while data are limited, they suggest that this is often not performed after the patient completes their initial treatment. In the NICCQ study, 40% of patients with stage II rectal cancer and just 3% of patients with stage III rectal cancer had their ostomy reversed, although this included both patients who had abdominoperineal resections as well as low anterior resections, so some may not have been candidates for ostomy closure [65]. In contrast, a recent study of an intervention to increase the timeliness of ostomy closure by "setting a date" at the time of discharge from their primary surgery reported that 72% of patients undergoing low anterior resections had their ostomies closed [66]. These data suggest that there are widespread problems with the quality of survivorship care in the area of interventions to improve the consequences of cancer and its treatment, even when a well-accepted procedure is available and supported by guidelines.

The prevalence and time course of psychological distress in cancer survivors is not well described. Depression in survivors has been estimated to range from 10% to 58%, anxiety disorders reverse from 23% to 65%, and posttraumatic stress disorder from 0% to 32% [31]. A recent study found that while most patients did not report unmet supportive care needs following completion of their cancer treatment, 30% reported at least one unmet psychological need and for most the need persisted 6 months later [67]. While little is known about how or when to screen for distress [68] nor how best to intervene – currently available guidelines for the psychosocial care of patients with cancer do not address the posttreatment period [69] – this clearly is an area where attention to improving the process of care is needed in parallel to research to improve the tools and services to optimize psychological support for cancer survivors. Additionally, a variety of barriers to access psychosocial service exist, including the availability of providers, health-care coverage for services, as well as patient reluctance to discuss these issues. In the USA, even among patients who are insured, coverage of mental health services may be at lower reimbursement levels or included in behavioral health contracts, separate from medical coverage, posing additional barriers to access [70].

Cancer survivors have more functional limitations due to their health than age-, gender-, and educational-attainment matched controls, with 18% unable to work due to health problems (vs 10% for controls), 27% limited in the amount or kind of work that they can do because of health problems (vs 18%), 5% needing help in activities of daily living (vs 3%), and 11% needing help in independent activities of daily living (vs 7%) [34]. A high proportion of cancer survivors have limitations in lower-body function with 56% reporting difficulty in performing at least one of the following activities compared with only 27% of controls: walking one-quarter of a mile; walking up and down ten steps; standing for 2 h; stooping, crouching or kneeling; and lifting 10 lb [35]. There are opportunities to provide the type of care needed to mitigate the impact of these functional limitations to enhance overall health.

### Coordination Between Specialists and Primary Care Providers

Although data are limited, anecdotal reports and several small studies suggest significant problems in communication between cancer specialists and primary care providers providing ongoing care [29, 71, 72]. A recent study of 300 breast cancer survivors followed at an outpatient clinic of a university hospital found that only 28% thought that their oncologists and primary care providers communicated well [72].

While a majority of cancer survivors continue to follow-up with their oncologist for many years, the proportion of patients receiving their follow-up care solely from primary care physicians increases over time [73, 74]. Despite having to assume primary responsibility for survivorship care for a large proportion of cancer survivors, primary care physicians report uncertainty in their role in caring for survivors as well as lack of knowledge regarding late effects of cancer and its treatment [75, 76]. In a recent survey of primary care physicians, half of them reported feeling unprepared to evaluate and manage late effects of cancer treatment [7].

In 2005, in its seminal report, *From Cancer Patient to Cancer Survivor: Lost in Transition*, the IOM recommended that patients completing primary cancer treatment "be provided with a comprehensive summary of their treatment together with a survivorship follow-up care plan written by the treating health care provider(s)." Although ASCO (available at http://www.asco.org) has developed templates and the Journey Forward, a collaborative effort of the UCLA Cancer Survivorship Center, NCCS, WellPoint, Inc, and Genentech (http://www.JourneyForward.org), has created tools for developing customized survivorship care plans, few oncologists have yet to make the survivorship care plans part of their routine practice. Among patients treated at oncology practices participating in ASCO's Quality Oncology Practice Initiative (QOPI), in chart abstractions only 27% had received a treatment summary and had it communicated to the clinician providing continuing care within 3 months of completing chemotherapy in 2010. This is despite of it being a QOPI quality indicator since 2008. Given the importance placed upon this kind of communication by primary care physicians caring for survivors, it will be critical to develop strategies to overcome the barriers that are inhibiting the acceptance of treatment summaries and survivorship plans by oncologists. Expectations for survivorship care differ between patients and their physicians. A lack of clarity surrounding their respective roles may contribute to suboptimal levels of care [34].

## Opportunities for Improvement

While available information on the quality of the process of care for cancer survivors must be considered very preliminary, it underscores the need to shift the focus of survivorship care from surveillance of disease recurrence, especially distant recurrence, to the other areas of survivorship care identified by the IOM including prevention of recurrence and new cancers; intervention for consequences of cancer and its treatment, including functional impairment, symptom burden, psychological distress; and coordination among specialists of several disciplines and primary care providers. While the quality of care for surveillance for second cancers appears very good (although variation and potential disparities persist), there is substantial overuse of imaging and other tests for surveillance of distant recurrence that have not been shown to improve outcomes and may contribute to the risk of secondary malignancies. Gaps between existing care and ideal care are substantial for survivorship care, highlighting the urgent need of validated quality indicators both to monitor the quality of care and guide quality improvement interventions. Additionally, new models of care need to be explored and systematically studied as ways to deliver higher quality survivorship care more efficiently. Survivorship clinics run by nurse practitioners or physicians assistants and the Patient-Centered Medical Home are two different approaches discussed further in Chaps. 10 and 11.

## *Identifying Barriers to Optimal Care*

There are several reasons why survivorship care may be inadequate. Firstly, there are insufficient means for identifying and addressing issues that are crucial for cancer survivors. Follow-up appointments, often occurring in busy clinics, are often too brief to adequately address the broad range of survivorship issues [62]. There is an urgent need for alternative models of posttreatment care [14, 29, 77]. Clinicians lack comprehensive assessment tools that could be administered in such an environment.

Secondly, responsibilities for follow-up are not clearly delineated between oncologists and primary care providers. Without an established system that includes accountability for each component of care, patients' needs are unmet, and there is a risk they will be lost to follow-up [4]. Even when these roles are delineated, primary care providers may lack training in survivorship issues and may not be able to rely on communication and advice from specialists [4].

Thirdly, although the ASCO is developing guidelines [78], there is currently insufficient evidence about the optimal frequency and content of follow-up appointments. Existing guidelines generally focus on detecting recurrence and second cancers and are not always easy for clinicians to access. Furthermore, evidence is lacking for self-care strategies that might improve management of treatment side effects [27]. To date, interventions have focused on limited health promotional strategies, particularly exercise programs and the reduction of physical side effects [24, 78]. More evidence-based support for psychosocial treatments would greatly improve their promotion and uptake. The IOM report recommended developing strategies to improve both physical and psychosocial outcomes [4].

## Recommended Strategies to Promote Quality Survivorship Care

Much work is needed to improve survivorship care. Several priority areas and strategies have been identified to implement the above principles. Although discussed in greater detail elsewhere in this text, a few key points are described below.

### Clinical Guidelines for Follow-up

There is a clear need for long-term continuous follow-up for cancer survivors. The IOM report revealed limited progress had been made to develop evidence-based guidance for providers of survivorship care. The IOM report recommended the development of "evidence-based clinical practice guidelines, assessment tools and screening instruments to help identify and manage late effects of cancer and its treatment [4]." Guidelines should cover ongoing, repeat assessments and assist clinicians to manage the complex range of survivor issues; this will ensure that health changes related or unrelated to cancer can be detected when treatment or intervention is most likely to be effective [25].

### Screening and Management of Psychosocial Issues

All cancer survivors require screening for distress and unmet needs. Mechanisms are also required that match these needs to interventions and other treatments. Psychosocial outcomes and efficient use of health resources may be enhanced by interventions tailored to the level of distress experienced [79]. Those involved in survivorship care should be encouraged to broaden discussions with survivors to include work, finances, and other social difficulties, and to develop appropriate referral pathways.

### Education and Training

Survivorship issues should be part of the training of all health professionals, and be included in skills development for the current workforce. The IOM report recommended: "The National Cancer Institute, professional associations, and voluntary organizations should expand and coordinate their efforts to provide educational opportunities to health care providers to equip them to address the health care and quality of life issues facing cancer survivors [4]." Improved awareness of the medical and psychosocial difficulties that can occur after cancer treatment will prompt appropriate assessment and intervention. This, combined with a system of increased accountability for follow-up, may give clinicians greater confidence to identify and manage survivor issues directly, rather than allowing patients to be lost in a system of referrals.

### Survivorship Care Plans

Communication between health-care professionals is a serious concern in survivorship care. The IOM report recommended that all patients completing primary treatment be given a comprehensive care summary and follow-up plan. This should be written by those who coordinated oncology treatment [4]. The summary should include all diagnosis and treatment information, plus details about any toxicities and complications experienced [12]. The care plan should recommend the frequency and duration of follow-up and a schedule for appointments, particularly if the survivor was being treated according to a shared care model. It should also provide strategies for dealing with current consequences of cancer and its treatments, health promotion strategies, and a list of support services.

A survivorship care plan is meant for the cancer survivor as well as their health-care providers. Structured care plans potentially will greatly improve communication between specialists and primary care providers; in the absence of such plans, health-care providers often rely on patient recall and understanding. There is widespread support for tailored care plans from survivors, nurses, and physicians, although more investigation is needed to determine the best ways to prepare and implement the plans [17, 80]. Ideally, care plans should be "living" documents that reflect current and projected circumstances.

## *Exploration and Assessment of Alternate Models of Care*

It is critical that various models of follow-up be explored and rigorously evaluated. These models may include shared care models (specialist/primary care provider), specialist survivorship clinics (including long-term follow-up clinics) and nurse-led clinics [14, 29, 77]. Follow-up need not be face-to-face, but may be conducted by telephone or using the Internet. Self-management strategies should also be developed. These models should be studied to determine feasibility, acceptability, and effectiveness (including cost-effectiveness). Ideally, models should be broadly applicable to ensure that the greatest number of survivors is included. The IOM report has recommended that "The Centers for Medicare and Medicaid Services, National Cancer Institute, Agency for Healthcare Research and Quality, the Department of Veterans Affairs, and other qualified organizations should support demonstration programs to test models of coordinated, interdisciplinary survivorship care in diverse communities and across systems of care [4]."

## Conclusion

There is growing recognition of the need to improve the structure and process of care in order to optimize the outcomes of the expanding numbers of cancer survivors. Since much of the care of cancer survivors has heretofore focused on surveillance for recurrence, the development of evidence-based strategies for prevention, consequences of cancer treatment, and coordination of care has lagged, limiting the development of quality indicators in these areas. However, even as research is being conducted to develop evidence-based approaches to improve outcomes for cancer

**Table 2.4** Priority areas to improve quality survivorship care that need immediate attention

| |
|---|
| Evidence-based strategies for detection and management of late-effects of cancer therapy |
| Evidence-based guidelines for comprehensive survivorship care across all cancer types |
| Evidence-based quality indicators for comprehensive survivorship care across all cancer types |
| Development of a comprehensive screening tool to tailor survivorship care to individual patient needs |
| Systematic review to identify best practices for delivering high quality survivorship care |
| Assessment of impact of imaging practices for surveillance on rates of second malignancies |
| Comparative effectiveness research to evaluate models for delivering survivorship care |
| Development of mechanisms to respond to identified gaps in high quality survivorship care |
| Development of quality improvement tools for survivorship care |
| Evaluation of coverage policies that may limit access to critical components of survivorship care (i.e. psychosocial services) |

survivors, we must determine what processes and structures of care will produce the highest quality outcomes given *current* scientific knowledge. Key priority areas to improve quality survivorship care that need immediate attention include (Table 2.4):

- Evidence-based strategies for detection and management of late-effects of cancer therapy
- Evidence-based guidelines for comprehensive survivorship care across all cancer types
- Evidence-based quality indicators for comprehensive survivorship care across all cancer types
- Development of a comprehensive screening tool to tailor survivorship care to individual patient needs
- Systematic review to identify best practices for delivering high-quality survivorship care
- Assessment of impact of imaging practices for surveillance on rates of second malignancies
- Comparative effectiveness research to evaluate models for delivering survivorship care
- Development of mechanisms to respond to identified gaps in high-quality survivorship care
- Development of quality improvement tools for survivorship care
- Evaluation of coverage policies that may limit access to critical components of survivorship care (i.e., psychosocial services).

## References

1. Twombly R. What's in a name: who is a cancer survivor? J Natl Cancer Inst. 2004;96(19):1414–5.
2. Jefford M. Improving outcomes for cancer survivors in Australia. Cancer Forum. 2009;33(3):159–63.

3. National Coalition for Cancer Survivorship (NCCS). Official website of the National Coalition for Cancer Survivorship. [cited 2010 July 31]; Available from: http://www.canceradvocacy.org/about/org/.
4. Hewitt ME, Greenfield S, Stovall E, editors. From cancer patient to cancer survivor: lost in transition. Washington, DC: The National Academies Press; 2006.
5. Boyes A, Hodgkinson K, Aldridge T, Turner J. Issues for cancer survivors in Australia. Cancer Forum. 2009;33(3):164–7.
6. Jefford M, Karahalios E, Pollard A, Baravelli C, Carey M, Franklin J, et al. Survivorship issues following treatment completion–results from focus groups with Australian cancer survivors and health professionals. J Cancer Surviv. 2008;2(1):20–32.
7. Hodgkinson K, Butow P, Hobbs KM, Wain G. After cancer: the unmet supportive care needs of survivors and their partners. J Psychosoc Oncol. 2007;25(4):89–104.
8. Sanson-Fisher R, Girgis A, Boyes A, Bonevski B, Burton L, Cook P. The unmet supportive care needs of patients with cancer. Supportive Care Review Group. Cancer. 2000;88(1):226–37.
9. Foster C, Wright D, Hill H, Hopkinson J, Roffe L. Psychosocial implications of living 5 years or more following a cancer diagnosis: a systematic review of the research evidence. Eur J Cancer Care (England). 2009;18(3):223–47.
10. Gotay CC, Muraoka MY. Quality of life in long-term survivors of adult-onset cancers. J Natl Cancer Inst. 1998;90(9):656–67.
11. Foley KL, Farmer DF, Petronis VM, Smith RG, McGraw S, Smith K, et al. A qualitative exploration of the cancer experience among long-term survivors: comparisons by cancer type, ethnicity, gender, and age. Psychooncology. 2006;15(3):248–58.
12. Ganz PA. Monitoring the physical health of cancer survivors: a survivorship-focused medical history. J Clin Oncol. 2006;24(32):5105–11.
13. Rowland JH, Hewitt M, Ganz PA. Cancer survivorship: a new challenge in delivering quality cancer care. J Clin Oncol. 2006;24(32):5101–4.
14. Oeffinger KC, McCabe MS. Models for delivering survivorship care. J Clin Oncol. 2006;24(32):5117–24.
15. Institute of Medicine, Adler NE, Page AEK, editors. Cancer care for the whole patient: meeting psychosocial health needs. Washington, DC: The National Academies Press; 2008.
16. National Breast Cancer Centre and National Cancer Control Initiative. Clinical practice guidelines for the psychosocial care of adults with cancer. Camperdown, NSW, Australia: National Breast Cancer Centre; 2003.
17. Hewitt ME, Bamundo A, Day R, Harvey C. Perspectives on post-treatment cancer care: qualitative research with survivors, nurses, and physicians. J Clin Oncol. 2007;25(16):2270–3.
18. Wolff SN. The burden of cancer survivorship. A pandemic of treatment success. In: Feuerstein M, editor. Handbook of cancer survivorship. New York: Springer; 2007.
19. Pigott C, Pollard A, Thomson K, Aranda S. Unmet needs in cancer patients: development of a supportive needs screening tool (SNST). Support Care Cancer. 2009;17(1):33–45.
20. Clark EJ, Stovall EL, Leigh S, Siu AL, Austin DK, Rowland JH. Imperatives for quality cancer care: access, advocacy, action, and accountability care: access advocacy, action and accountability. Silver Spring: National Coalition for Cancer Survivorship; 1996.
21. Institute of Medicine. Crossing the quality chasm: a new health system for the 21st century. Washington, DC: The National Academies Press; 2001.
22. World Health Organization. Preamble to the Constitution of the World Health Organization as adopted by the International Health Conference, New York, 19–22 June, 1946; signed on 22 July 1946 by the representatives of 61 States (Official Records of the World Health Organization, no. 2, p. 100) and entered into force on 7 April 1948.
23. Pollard A, Eakin E, Vardy J, Hawkes A. Health behaviour interventions for cancer survivors: an overview of the evidence and contemporary Australian trials. Cancer Forum. 2009;33(3):182–6.
24. Stull VB, Snyder DC, Demark-Wahnefried W. Lifestyle interventions in cancer survivors: designing programs that meet the needs of this vulnerable and growing population. J Nutr. 2007;137(1 Suppl):243S–8.

25. Earle CC. Surveillance after primary therapy. In: Ganz PA, editor. Cancer survivorship: today and tomorrow. New York: Springer; 2007. p. 43–53.
26. Ganz PA. Quality of care and cancer survivorship: the challenge of implementing the institute of medicine recommendations. J Oncol Pract. 2009;5:101–5.
27. Lotfi-Jam K, Carey M, Jefford M, Schofield P, Charleson C, Aranda S. Nonpharmacologic strategies for managing common chemotherapy adverse effects: a systematic review. J Clin Oncol. 2008;26(34):5618–29.
28. Newell SA, Sanson-Fisher RW, Savolainen NJ. Systematic review of psychological therapies for cancer patients: overview and recommendations for future research. J Natl Cancer Inst. 2002;94(8):558–84.
29. Brennan M, Jefford M. General practitioner-based models of post-treatment follow up. Cancer Forum. 2009;33(3):179–82.
30. Lotfi-Jam K, Schofield P, Jefford M. What constitutes ideal survivorship care? Cancer Forum. 2009;33(3):171–4.
31. Stein KD, Syrjala KL, Andrykowski MA. Physical and psychological long-term and late effects of cancer. Cancer. 2008;112(11 Suppl):2577–92.
32. Arora NK. Importance of patient-centered care in enhancing patient well-being: a cancer survivor's perspective. Qual Life Res. 2009;18(1):1–4.
33. Lohr KN, Schroeder SA. A strategy for quality assurance in Medicare. N Engl J Med. 1990;322(10):707–12.
34. Yabroff KR, Lawrence WF, Clauser S, Davis WW, Brown ML. Burden of illness in cancer survivors: findings from a population-based national sample. J Natl Cancer Inst. 2004;96(17):1322–30.
35. Schootman M, Aft R, Jeffe DB. An evaluation of lower-body functional limitations among long-term survivors of 11 different types of cancers. Cancer. 2009;115(22):5329–38.
36. Donabedian A. The quality of medical care: a concept in search of a definition. J Fam Pract. 1979;9(2):277–84.
37. National Cancer Policy Board, Institute of Medicine and Commission on Life Sciences, National Research Council. In: Hewitt M, Simone JV, editors. Ensuring quality cancer care. Washington, DC: The National Academies Press; 1999.
38. Jacobson JO, Neuss MN, McNiff KK, Kadlubek P, Thacker 2nd LR, Song F, et al. Improvement in oncology practice performance through voluntary participation in the Quality Oncology Practice Initiative. J Clin Oncol. 2008;26(11):1893–8.
39. Desch CE, McNiff KK, Schneider EC, Schrag D, McClure J, Lepisto E, et al. American Society of Clinical Oncology/National Comprehensive Cancer Network Quality Measures. J Clin Oncol. 2008;26(21):3631–7.
40. National Quality Forum: Quality of Cancer Care Performance Measures [Internet]. [cited 2008 Nov 20]. Available from: http://www.qualityforum.org/Projects/c-d/Cancer_Care_Phase_II/Cancer_Care_Phase_II.aspx.
41. Spencer BA, Steinberg M, Malin J, Adams J, Litwin MS. Quality-of-care indicators for early-stage prostate cancer. J Clin Oncol. 2003;21(10):1928–36.
42. Gagliardi AR, Fleshner N, Langer B, Stern H, Brown AD. Development of prostate cancer quality indicators: a modified Delphi approach. Can J Urol. 2005;12(5):2808–15.
43. Malin JL, Asch SM, Kerr EA, McGlynn EA. Evaluating the quality of cancer care: development of cancer quality indicators for a global quality assessment tool. Cancer. 2000;88(3):701–7.
44. Rubins J, Unger M, Colice GL. Follow-up and surveillance of the lung cancer patient following curative intent therapy: ACCP evidence-based clinical practice guideline (2nd edition). Chest. 2007;132(3 Suppl):355S–67.
45. Smoking Cessation and Continued Risk in Cancer Patients (PDQ®) [Internet]. National Cancer Institute; [updated 2010 April 14; cited 2010 Mar 23]. Available from: http://www.cancer.gov/cancertopics/pdq/supportivecare/smokingcessation/HealthProfessional/allpages.
46. American Society of Clinical Oncology. Tobacco Cessation and Quality Cancer Care. J Oncol Pract. 2009;5:2–5.

47. Malin JL, Schneider EC, Epstein AM, Adams J, Emanuel EJ, Kahn KL. Results of the National Initiative for Cancer Care Quality: how can we improve the quality of cancer care in the United States? J Clin Oncol. 2006;24(4):626–34.
48. Owusu C, Buist DS, Field TS, Lash TL, Thwin SS, Geiger AM, et al. Predictors of tamoxifen discontinuation among older women with estrogen receptor-positive breast cancer. J Clin Oncol. 2008;26(4):549–55.
49. Lash TL, Fox MP, Westrup JL, Fink AK, Silliman RA. Adherence to tamoxifen over the five-year course. Breast Cancer Res Treat. 2006;99(2):215–20.
50. Kahn KL, Schneider EC, Malin JL, Adams JL, Epstein AM. Patient centered experiences in breast cancer: predicting long-term adherence to tamoxifen use. Med Care. 2007;45(5):431–9.
51. Snyder CF, Frick KD, Kantsiper ME, Peairs KS, Herbert RJ, Blackford AL, et al. Prevention, screening, and surveillance care for breast cancer survivors compared with controls: changes from 1998 to 2002. J Clin Oncol. 2009;27(7):1054–61.
52. Cooper GS, Kou TD, Reynolds Jr HL. Receipt of guideline-recommended follow-up in older colorectal cancer survivors: a population-based analysis. Cancer. 2008;113(8):2029–37.
53. Barzilai DA, Cooper KD, Neuhauser D, Rimm AA, Cooper GS. Geographic and patient variation in receipt of surveillance procedures after local excision of cutaneous melanoma. J Investig Dermatol. 2004;122(2):246–55.
54. Rosselli Del Turco M, Palli D, Cariddi A, Ciatto S, Pacini P, Distante V. Intensive diagnostic follow-up after treatment of primary breast cancer. A randomized trial. National Research Council Project on Breast Cancer follow-up. JAMA. 1994;271(20):1593–7.
55. Weiss M, Loprinzi CL, Creagan ET, Dalton RJ, Novotny P, O'Fallon JR. Utility of follow-up tests for detecting recurrent disease in patients with malignant melanomas. JAMA. 1995;274(21):1703–5.
56. A Data Book: Health Care Spending and the Medicare Program [Internet]. Washington DC: Medicare Payment Advisory Commission [cited 23 Mar 2010]. 2009. http://www.medpac.gov/documents/Jun09DataBookEntireReport.pdf.
57. Miles KA. Cancer imaging: is it cost-effective? Cancer Imaging. 2004;4(2):97–103.
58. Hillner BE, Siegel BA, Shields AF, Liu D, Gareen IF, Hunt E, et al. Relationship between cancer type and impact of PET and PET/CT on intended management: findings of the national oncologic PET registry. J Nucl Med. 2008;49(12):1928–35.
59. Brix G, Nissen-Meyer S, Lechel U, Nissen-Meyer J, Griebel J, Nekolla EA, et al. Radiation exposures of cancer patients from medical X-rays: how relevant are they for individual patients and population exposure? Eur J Radiol. 2009;72(2):342–7.
60. Berrington de Gonzalez A, Mahesh M, Kim KP, Bhargavan M, Lewis R, Mettler F, et al. Projected cancer risks from computed tomographic scans performed in the United States in 2007. Arch Intern Med. 2009;169(22):2071–7.
61. Smith-Bindman R, Lipson J, Marcus R, Kim KP, Mahesh M, Gould R, et al. Radiation dose associated with common computed tomography examinations and the associated lifetime attributable risk of cancer. Arch Intern Med. 2009;169(22):2078–86.
62. Beaver K, Luker KA. Follow-up in breast cancer clinics: reassuring for patients rather than detecting recurrence. Psychooncology. 2005;14(2):94–101.
63. Greenberg CC, Schneider EC, Lipsitz SR, Ko CY, Malin JL, Epstein AM, et al. Do variations in provider discussions explain socioeconomic disparities in postmastectomy breast reconstruction? J Am Coll Surg. 2008;206(4):605–15.
64. Chen JY, Malin J, Ganz PA, Ko C, Tisnado D, Tao ML, et al. Variation in physician-patient discussion of breast reconstruction. J Gen Intern Med. 2009;24(1):99–104.
65. Schneider EC, Malin JL, Kahn KL, Ko CY, Adams J, Epstein AM. Surviving colorectal cancer: patient-reported symptoms 4 years after diagnosis. Cancer. 2007;110(9):2075–82.
66. Chand M, Nash GF, Talbot RW. Timely closure of loop ileostomy following anterior resection for rectal cancer. Eur J Cancer Care (England). 2008;17(6):611–5.
67. Armes J, Crowe M, Colbourne L, Morgan H, Murrells T, Oakley C, et al. Patients' supportive care needs beyond the end of cancer treatment: a prospective, longitudinal survey. J Clin Oncol. 2009;27(36):6172–9.

68. Vodermaier A, Linden W, Siu C. Screening for emotional distress in cancer patients: a systematic review of assessment instruments. J Natl Cancer Inst. 2009;101(21):1464–88.
69. Jacobsen PB. Clinical practice guidelines for the psychosocial care of cancer survivors: current status and future prospects. Cancer. 2009;115(18 Suppl):4419–29.
70. Hewitt M, Herdman R, Holland J, editors. National Research Council. Meeting psychosocial needs of women with breast cancer. Washington, DC: National Academy Press, 2004. http://www.nap.edu/catalog/10909.html. Accessed 2010 Aug 11.
71. Cheung WY, Neville BA, Cameron DB, Cook EF, Earle CC. Comparisons of patient and physician expectations for cancer survivorship care. J Clin Oncol. 2009;27(15):2489–95.
72. Mao JJ, Bowman MA, Stricker CT, DeMichele A, Jacobs L, Chan D, et al. Delivery of survivorship care by primary care physicians: the perspective of breast cancer patients. J Clin Oncol. 2009;27(6):933–8.
73. Haggstrom DA, Arora NK, Helft P, Clayman ML, Oakley-Girvan I. Follow-up care delivery among colorectal cancer survivors most often seen by primary and subspecialty care physicians. J Gen Intern Med. 2009;24 Suppl 2:S472–9.
74. Snyder CF, Earle CC, Herbert RJ, Neville BA, Blackford AL, Frick KD. Preventive care for colorectal cancer survivors: a 5-year longitudinal study. J Clin Oncol. 2008;26(7):1073–9.
75. Bober SL, Recklitis CJ, Campbell EG, Park ER, Kutner JS, Najita JS, et al. Caring for cancer survivors: a survey of primary care physicians. Cancer. 2009;115(18 Suppl):4409–18.
76. Lynch T, Goldberg W, Carey J, Varga J. A preliminary examination of primary care providers' self-reported ability and comfort with coordinating care for cancer survivors. American Psychosocial Oncology Society Annual Conference in New Orleans, Louisiana; February 19, 2010.
77. Gates P, Krishnasamy M. Nurse-led survivorship care. Cancer Forum. 2009;33(3):175–8.
78. American Society of Clinical Oncology 2009. Clinical Practice Guidelines. 2009. http://www.asco.org/ASCOv2/Practice+%26+Guidelines/Guidelines/Clinical+Practice+Guidelines. Accessed 2009 Sept 17.
79. Hutchison SD, Steginga SK, Dunn J. The tiered model of psychosocial intervention in cancer: a community based approach. Psychooncology. 2006;15(6):541–6.
80. Baravelli C, Krishnasamy M, Pezaro C, Schofield P, Lotfi-Jam K, Rogers M, et al. The views of bowel cancer survivors and health care professionals regarding survivorship care plans and post treatment follow up. J Cancer Surviv. 2009;3(2):99–108.

# Part II
# Targets for Improved Health Care

# Chapter 3
# Managing Symptoms over Time

**Elena M. Kouri and Nancy L. Keating**

## Description of the Problem

### *Overview*

The importance of quality of life (QOL) among cancer survivors is second only to survival [1]. A cancer survivor's general well-being significantly impacts his or her ability to successfully engage in everyday activities and to adapt to living with cancer [2], and it has been shown to be a powerful predictor of survival and treatment-related toxicity among cancer survivors [3–7]. How well a cancer survivor copes with the changes resulting from the cancer and its treatment depends on a variety of physical and psychosocial factors that determine the cancer survivor's overall QOL.

Cancer survivors generally report lower QOL than individuals without a history of cancer. Studies using population-based data from the National Health Interview Survey have found that cancer survivors, compared with individuals without a history of cancer, report more functional disabilities and limitations in activities of daily living [8] and serious psychological distress [9], and they are more likely to report fair or poor health, days lost from work, and inability to work [10]. Similarly, analysis of population-based data from the Behavioral Risk Factor Surveillance System questionnaire has shown that among all individuals who reported any activity limitations, those with limitations due to cancer had worse health status than those whose limitations were due to cardiovascular disease or emotional problems [11]. The findings from these and other studies [12–17] suggest that cancer survivors can experience significant long-term psychological and physical effects of their cancer, and highlight the importance of effective symptom monitoring after cancer treatment to prevent and manage late effects and ultimately improve QOL in cancer survivors.

E.M. Kouri (✉)
Department of Health Care Policy, Harvard Medical School, Boston, MA, USA
e-mail: kouri@hcp.med.harvard.edu

M. Feuerstein and P.A. Ganz (eds.), *Health Services for Cancer Survivors*,
DOI 10.1007/978-1-4419-1348-7_3, © Springer Science+Business Media, LLC 2011

## *General Symptoms*

Even though the concept of QOL has no universal definition, most conceptual QOL models incorporate multiple domains that include the individual's physical, psychological, social, and spiritual well-being [18–21]. One example of a conceptual model of QOL for cancer survivors, developed by Dr. Betty Ferrell, is shown in Fig. 3.1 [21].

### Physical Symptoms

As depicted in Ferrell's QOL model, cancer survivors can experience a variety of physical symptoms, including fatigue, pain, new health conditions, and fertility problems. Symptoms in cancer survivors rarely occur in isolation; most symptoms occur in clusters with interrelated symptoms that can vary in frequency, intensity, and level of perceived distress within a cluster [22–25]. The interaction of symptoms in a cluster can influence functional status, QOL, disease progression, and survival [26].

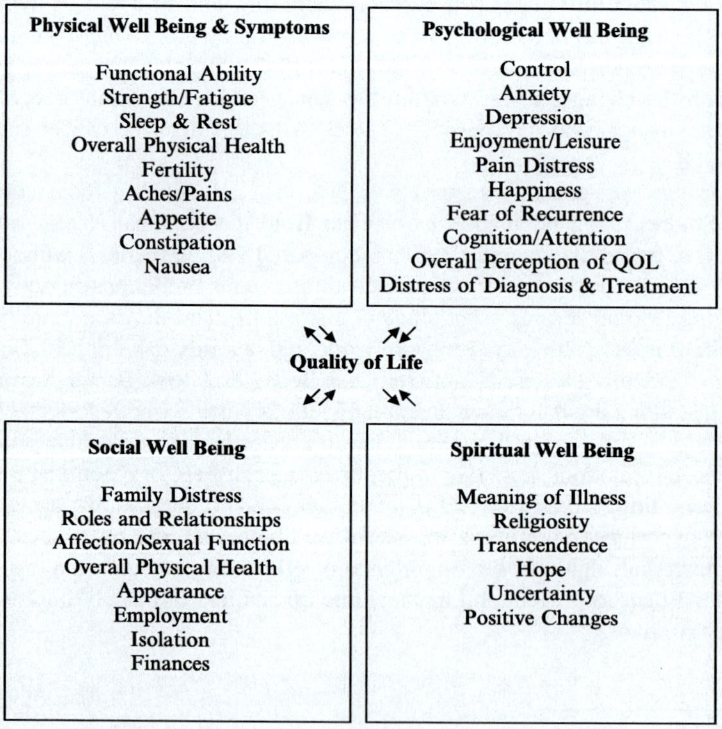


**Fig. 3.1** QOL in cancer survivors (Reprinted with permission from Ferrel et al. [21]. Available at http://prc.coh.org/pdf/cancer_survivor_QOL.pdf)

It is estimated that up to one-third of cancer survivors experience elevated levels of fatigue [27–30] that can persist for months or years after successful completion of cancer treatment [30–34]. Fatigue is identified by many cancer survivors as the most distressing cancer-related symptom [13, 16, 35–38] as it can significantly interfere with daily functioning [39, 40], ability to return to work [41, 42], and QOL [43–46]. There are different definitions of cancer-related fatigue, but most include significant tiredness [47, 48], exhaustion, weakness, and lack of energy in spite of adequate amounts of rest and sleep [49, 50]. Fatigue in cancer survivors has been shown to be associated with depression [38, 40], anxiety [40], and pain [51].

Effective management of fatigue among cancer survivors begins with an assessment of the underlying causes of the fatigue. For example, if fatigue is related to conditions such as anemia or hypoxia, targeted treatments that include blood transfusion, supplemental oxygen, or medications that increase production of red blood cells may be prescribed. In addition, changes in nutrition and exercise regimens can help maintain muscle strength, increase energy, and play an important role in decreasing fatigue among cancer survivors.

Another physical symptom commonly experienced by cancer survivors is chronic pain. Pain in cancer survivors is often caused by residual tissue damage from the cancer or the cancer treatment. The most common type of cancer-treatment-related pain is neuropathy secondary to surgery, radiation therapy, or chemotherapy. Radiation-related pain syndromes are caused by neural damage or tissue fibrosis and may persist for many years after the initial treatment [52, 53]. Surgery-related chronic pain syndromes vary in severity and prevalence depending on the type of surgery. For example, it is estimated that during the initial 12 months after surgery, 50% of breast cancer patients who receive a mastectomy experience chronic pain [54], compared to 39% of patients who receive breast conserving surgery [55–57]. Estimates of pain during the first 3 years after breast cancer surgery range between 10% and 47% [58, 59] and have been shown to remain significantly higher than those from the general population for up to 5 years after surgery [57].

In addition to being largely dependent on treatment-related factors, chronic pain among cancer survivors is also influenced by the type of cancer, the cancer stage at the time of diagnosis, the patient's age and comorbid medical conditions (e.g., diabetes, obesity, and chronic obstructive pulmonary disease) [60–63]. For example, patients with more advanced stage, comorbid conditions (particularly diabetes), and lung vs. breast, colon, or prostate cancers, experience more pain than others [60, 62].

Effective management of chronic pain among cancer survivors should involve a comprehensive assessment of the nature and magnitude of the pain, an evaluation of conditions such as comorbid illnesses that may exacerbate the pain and the development of pharmacologic and non-pharmacologic interventions to treat the pain.

Cancer survivors are also at increased risk for cancer, either through recurrence of the primary cancer or development of a secondary cancer. The increased risk for developing a second cancer can be a result of the treatment received for the primary cancer, genetic susceptibilities, lifestyle factors, environmental exposures, or an interaction among these. For example, compared to the general population, breast cancer survivors have an 18% increased risk of developing a second cancer [64]. Both chemotherapy and radiation therapy are associated with an increased risk of developing leukemia [65]. One of the most comprehensively studied treatment-related malignancies is leukemia, following chemotherapy for Hodgkin's lymphoma. Estimates of the overall relative risk of leukemia for Hodgkin's lymphoma patients treated with chemotherapy range from 3.5 to 24 (95% cl, 0.8 to 225) compared to patients treated with radiation therapy alone [66–69]. Hormonal cancer therapies have also been associated with an increased risk for developing other cancers. For example, breast cancer survivors treated with tamoxifen have a two- to threefold increase in the risk of developing endometrial cancer [70, 71].

These and other estimates of risk for developing second cancers vary depending on the type and cumulative dose of the agents used during treatment. Research will continue to identify the treatment regimens associated with increased risk of secondary malignancies and to characterize patient characteristics that may increase these risks.

Management plans for cancer among cancer survivors should include regular screening, education, and prevention strategies. Other physical symptoms experienced by cancer survivors are system-specific symptoms, such as organ damage, endocrine damage, or compromised immune systems. Specific treatment-related effects are described in more detail below.

As mentioned earlier in this chapter, one important factor affecting the pattern and extent of physical symptoms experienced by cancer survivors is the age when the cancer was diagnosed. Older survivors may experience different late effects than younger survivors because of the higher prevalence of comorbid illnesses such as diabetes, heart disease, obstructive pulmonary disease, arthritis, or hypertension [72, 73]. Any of these comorbid illnesses can potentially affect treatment choices [74], increase the risk of treatment-related complications [75], and affect prognosis and survival. Therefore, a comprehensive assessment of patients' type and severity of preexisting conditions should be performed and taken into account when treatment decisions are made.

## Psychological Symptoms

Psychological symptoms experienced by cancer survivors include fear of recurrence, anxiety, depression, cognitive difficulties, distress, and loneliness. The pattern of psychological symptoms experienced by cancer survivors is similar regardless of the cancer site, the age when cancer was diagnosed, and the number of years since the diagnosis [76–79].

Depression is commonly experienced after cancer diagnosis, and approximately 25% of older adult long-term cancer survivors experience clinical levels of depression 5 or more years after their initial cancer diagnosis [79]. The strongest predictor of depression in this population is current cancer-related symptoms, such as pain and fatigue. Cancer survivors who continue to experience cancer-related symptoms are significantly more likely to experience depression than those who do not have symptoms [79].

Cancer survivors can experience cognitive deficits related to a variety of cancer treatments including cranial radiation, standard chemotherapy, and high-dose chemotherapy. The majority of studies examining cognitive function following cancer treatment have focused on patients treated with chemotherapy for breast cancer. However, cognitive impairments have also been documented following chemotherapy treatment for other cancers including lung cancer [80] and lymphoma [81]. The reported cognitive deficits associated with chemotherapy treatment are positively correlated with duration of chemotherapy treatment [82], most pronounced following high doses of chemotherapy [83], and during the first 2 years after chemotherapy treatment [83–85]. However, some reports indicate that memory and concentration impairments can persist for many years after treatment [86–88] and can contribute to functional disability in older cancer survivors [89].

Fear of recurrence and associated anxiety has been reported in up to 97% of cancer survivors [90, 91] and can result in persistent anxiety and difficulties in planning for the future [92]. Other factors influencing the extent and severity of psychological symptoms experienced by cancer survivors include poor coping strategies, lack of social support systems, and the number and severity of other comorbidities [93–95].

### Social Well-Being

The effect of a cancer diagnosis and its related treatment is not isolated to the individual with cancer; it impacts the needs and lives of the entire family and other members of an individual's social network. Some of the social symptoms experienced by cancer survivors include changes in the family structure, interpersonal relations, and social supports. Some of these changes are related to the stressors associated with a cancer diagnosis and its treatment while others are related to physical symptoms. For example, changes in physical appearance and sexual function related to cancer treatment can affect interpersonal relationships, self-esteem, and social adjustment among cancer survivors [96, 97]. A cancer diagnosis and its treatment can also result in changes in employment status or ability to work, which can affect the individual's financial condition and increase concern about treatment costs, contributing to feelings of distress among survivors [98–100]. Factors that have been shown to facilitate psychological and social adaptation to living with cancer include optimism, perceived control over the illness, generalized self-esteem, availability and utilization of social support [101–104]. The perception of the availability of social support appears to be more important in predicting social well-being among cancer survivors than the actual support received [105, 106].

### Spiritual Well-Being

Cancer survivorship may also influence an individual's spirituality and spiritual well-being. Following a cancer diagnosis, many individuals focus on their faith [107] and rely on their trust in God as an important coping strategy [108].

Although some patients may experience some spiritual uncertainty, many cancer survivors experience positive spiritual effects from coping with their cancer. Some of the positive effects of surviving cancer include changes in religiosity, outlook on life purpose, and existential concerns of surviving a life-threatening illness [21, 109, 110]. Surviving cancer can lead to a reevaluation of life priorities such that relationships with others and giving back to society become more important priorities [111].

## *Treatment-Related Symptoms*

As mentioned earlier, many of the symptoms experienced by cancer survivors are late effects of the cancer treatment itself. Treatment-related symptoms in cancer survivors can occur immediately after treatment or sometime after treatment has been completed.

### Surgery-Related Late Effects

Advances in surgical techniques have contributed to the successful treatment of many cancers. However, many of the diagnostic and curative cancer surgeries result in short- and long-term effects that can impact the cancer survivor's QOL. For example, breast cancer survivors who had lymph nodes removed are at risk for lymphedema, a chronic, progressive, and incurable condition that results in limb swelling, discomfort, and arm function impairments [112, 113]. Lymphedema incidence rates following surgery for breast cancer vary between 6% and 70% depending on the criteria used to define lymphedema and the post-surgery window of time used in the assessment [114, 115]. Also, different types of breast cancer surgery are associated with different risks of developing lymphedema. For example, sentinel-node biopsy is associated with a lower risk of lymphedema than axillary dissection surgery [116].

Many prostate cancer survivors treated with a prostatectomy experience urinary incontinence and erectile dysfunction as long-term complications of surgery. Estimated rates of erectile dysfunction after prostatectomy range from 40% to 85% [117, 118], and these rates are influenced by the patient's age and preoperative potency status [119]. Rectal cancer survivors who undergo surgery may have chronic colostomy bags, which can require adjustment and can be associated with bowel irregularities.

### Chemotherapy-Related Late Effects

Receipt of chemotherapy for cancer treatment has been associated with adverse cardiac events and cardiovascular toxicity. Adverse cardiac events associated with chemotherapy vary in incidence and can occur during treatment, within days or weeks after treatment or months after completion of treatment. Cardiovascular toxicity can also occur as a late effect of chemotherapy that manifests many years after treatment, although this is less common. Individuals who experience reduced cardiac function within 6 months of completing chemotherapy are at increased risk for the development of late adverse cardiovascular events [120], including changes in blood pressure, thrombosis, arrhythmias, cardiac failure, and congestive heart failure [121]. For example, it is estimated that between 0.5% and 1% of breast cancer patients treated with standard anthracycline-based chemotherapy regimens will develop congestive heart failure [71]. These anthracycline-related cardiac effects are potentially irreversible and may appear years or decades after the completion of the chemotherapy treatment [122]. The risk of developing chemotherapy-related cardiovascular toxicity depends on the type of chemotherapy agents used, the dose used during each course of treatment and the cumulative dose, as well as patient characteristics including age, history of cardiovascular disease, and other comorbid illnesses [123]. Patients treated with cardio-toxic chemotherapy should undergo baseline cardiac assessments to identify those at increased risk of cardiovascular complications, and measures should be taken to prevent, monitor, and treat adverse events.

Chemotherapy treatment can also result in a series of cognitive impairments that include inability to concentrate and pay attention, memory loss, and difficulty in thinking. This condition has been referred to as "chemobrain" and it can have a significant impact on a cancer survivor's QOL and daily functioning [124]. The chemotherapy-related cognitive impairments are most pronounced after higher doses [83], longer duration of treatment [82], and during the initial 2 years after treatment [125–127]. These posttreatment cognitive impairments have been well documented in the literature but their nature and etiology are not well understood [128–132].

Changes in sexual function and fertility are also associated with chemotherapy treatment. The risk for infertility after chemotherapy is strongly dependent on the types of agents used and the cumulative dose. For example, chemotherapy regimens that include alkylating agents and procarbazine carry a significantly higher risk of sterility for both men and women compared with chemotherapy regimens that do not [133].

## Radiation-Related Late Effects

Radiation therapy can result in short- and long-term pulmonary, cardiac, ischemic, skeletal, and functional effects that vary depending on the type, targeted organ, dose, and duration of the radiation therapy, as well as patient characteristics. Radiation therapy can also increase the risk of developing second cancers, particularly after higher doses and longer duration of radiation treatment [134, 135]. For example, in a population-based study of breast cancer patients, women treated with surgery and radiation therapy had a 1.45 relative risk for developing a second cancer compared with women treated with surgery alone. Risks of developing second cancers were higher among women receiving high-radiation doses (1+ Gy) compared with those receiving medium (0.5–0.99 Gy) or low (<0.5 Gy) doses [135]. As with chemotherapy, some of the patient characteristics that can modify the risk of radiation-related effects are the type of cancer, age, smoking status, and comorbid illnesses [136–138]. For example, young breast cancer survivors have a higher risk of developing other cancers after radiation therapy than older survivors and this risk decreases with increasing age, becoming particularly low among postmenopausal women [134, 139].

Radiation-related effects on the skeletal system include bone fractures and alterations in bone growth. Estimates of radiation-related bone fractures range between 4% and 29% among adults [140, 141] and between 10% and 23% among children [142, 143]. Alterations in bone growth are particularly important in children receiving radiation therapy as they can result in facial asymmetry, extremity and clavicular shortening, long bone asymmetry, and growth of flat bones [144–146]. Radiation therapy can also increase the risk of developing other cancers. For example, breast and lung cancer risks are increased following radiation treatment for Hodgkin's lymphoma [147, 148].

Effects of radiation on the cardiovascular system include myocardial infarction, pericardial thickening, congestive heart failure, and valvular disorders [149–151] that can persist for decades after completion of radiation therapy even in the absence of symptoms [152]. The risk of radiation-induced cardiotoxicity is proportional to the volume of the heart irradiated and the dose received [153, 154]. However, other risk factors of radiation-induced cardiac toxicity are the relative field weighting, type of radiation source, younger age at exposure, other cardiac risk factors such as smoking and diabetes, and the radiation technique used [155]. Many of the radiation-induced cardiovascular complications reported in the literature are the result of older radiotherapy equipment and techniques [155–157]; the incidence of cardiovascular complications is likely to decrease as newer radiation therapies are used.

Fatigue is commonly experienced by individuals receiving radiation therapy. It is estimated that 70% of cancer patients receiving radiation therapy and chemotherapy experience fatigue during the treatment [158] and more than 65% report problems with fatigue 1 year after the initial cancer diagnosis [13].

## *Cancer-Specific Symptoms*

Much of the literature on long-term cancer survival has focused on breast cancer [159–163], prostate cancer [15, 164, 165], colorectal cancer [166–170], and Hodgkin's lymphoma [171]. We will review what is understood about symptoms in cancer survivors with these conditions.

### Breast Cancer

**Case Study** Mrs. S. is a 50-year-old woman who was diagnosed with a stage II breast cancer 4 years ago. She underwent mastectomy with sentinel lymph node biopsy and was then treated with chemotherapy. Following chemotherapy, she started on tamoxifen, which she will take for 5 years. She returned to work as an accountant following her chemotherapy and has continued to work about 40 h per week. She is married and has two children who are in high school. She reports that overall she is doing okay, but has persistent fatigue. She is always tired, even though she thinks she is sleeping enough. Working full-time and coordinating schedules of her children, she finds herself falling asleep on the sofa by 8:30 p.m. She also reports some difficulty with concentration, which she says has been the case ever since getting the chemotherapy. She also reports low libido and inability to enjoy sex, which was never a problem before her cancer diagnosis. She says her mood is okay, but that she does worry a lot about what she would do if her cancer recurred.

## Symptoms

**Physical Symptoms.** Fatigue is frequently reported among breast cancer survivors [172], ranging in prevalence from 41% to 76% [35, 173–175] and sometimes lasting for up to 10 years after the initial cancer diagnosis [12, 31, 176]. For example, in a study of disease-free breast cancer survivors who had finished treatment for an average of 29 months, 38% of cancer survivors reported severe fatigue compared to 11% of women without a history of cancer. The severely fatigued breast cancer survivors in this study also scored higher on measures of depression and sleep problems and lower on levels of physical activity [33].

The severity of fatigue in cancer survivors is associated with the type of cancer treatment received. Breast cancer patients who received both chemotherapy and radiation appear to experience greater fatigue than those treated with chemotherapy alone [36] or radiation therapy alone [31, 177, 178], although these differences appear to dissipate over time [31]. Also, survivors treated with radiation therapy alone or chemotherapy alone report higher levels of fatigue following completion of treatment than those treated with surgery alone [31].

Many breast cancer survivors experience chronic pain. In a recent study of breast cancer survivors treated with mastectomy or lumpectomy, 47% reported experiencing regular pain 2–3 years after their surgery, 13% of the women reported severe pain, 39% had moderate pain, and 48% had light pain [59]. Post-surgery chronic pain among breast cancer survivors appears to be more prevalent among younger patients [179, 180], patients treated with radiation therapy compared to chemotherapy [57, 180], and those receiving axillary node dissection compared to sentinel node biopsy [181, 182].

Post-surgery pain is estimated to occur in 20–43% of breast cancer patients who receive a mastectomy [183–185]. Post-mastectomy pain is usually related to nerve injury or dysfunction and can involve lancinating pain, paresthesia, dysesthesia, hyperalgesia or allodynia, edema, muscle weakness, and skin irritations [55].

As described earlier in this chapter, lymphedema and related long-term inflammatory changes are relatively common among breast cancer survivors. Lymphedema is a chronic condition that often results in arm swelling, impaired arm function, pain, and discomfort [186–188], and it can occur as a result of the removal of lymph nodes for biopsy [189]. It is estimated that approximately 25% of breast cancer survivors develop lymphedema within 1 year of cancer treatment [189] and up to 42% within 5 years of treatment [190, 191]. Breast cancer patients who undergo axillary dissections (with mastectomy or breast-conserving surgery) have a threefold increase in the risk of developing lymphedema compared with patients with no dissection, and as many as 60% of patients who undergo axillary lymph node resection and radiation eventually develop lymphedema [192]. The risk of lymphedema and other associated impairments in arm mobility appear much lower with use of sentinel node biopsy compared with axillary dissection [193]. For instance, in a study of motion restriction among breast cancer patients, limitations in shoulder range of motion was limited in 45% of patients who received sentinel node biopsy compared to 86% of patients who received axillary dissections [194].

Even though there is no cure for lymphedema, treatments that effectively decrease the discomfort and functional impairments include early detection, regular use of a compression arm sleeve, elevation of the arm, pneumatic compression, and lymph drainage [195]. Moreover, data from a recent study suggest that a slowly progressive weight-lifting program decreases the incidence of exacerbations of lymphedema, reduces symptoms, and increases arm strength without affecting limb swelling among breast cancer survivors suffering from lymphedema [196].

Breast cancer patients are at increased risk of treatment-induced menstrual dysfunction that can be prolonged or permanent. The probability of premature menopause in breast cancer patients depends on the age of the patient and the treatments used. For example, the estimated probability of a 45-year-old breast cancer survivor experiencing menopause during the first year after the initial cancer diagnosis is 10% if treated with chemotherapy, 80% if treated with hormonal therapy, and 90% if treated with chemotherapy and hormonal therapy combined [197]. Menopausal symptoms in breast cancer survivors are usually more severe than during the normal transition into menopause because treatment-induced menopause happens relatively fast. These symptoms include hot flashes, sweats, vaginal dryness, pain during intercourse, mood changes, and sleep disturbances [198].

Breast cancer survivors also can experience changes in sexual function and problems with body image. Changes in sexual functioning among breast cancer survivors have been shown to occur shortly after initiation of cancer treatment and to decline during the first year after cancer treatment completion [199, 200]. Patients treated with chemotherapy appear to experience greater impairments in sexual functioning than those not treated with chemotherapy, regardless of the type of breast cancer surgery received [201]. Some of the factors that contribute to sexual dysfunction among breast cancer survivors include lack of sexual interest, difficulty becoming sexually aroused, problems with body image, and vaginal dryness [202]. Women who received a mastectomy are more likely to report dissatisfaction with body image than those treated with breast-conserving surgery [200, 203, 204].

Treatment with aromatase inhibitors to reduce estrogen levels in postmenopausal women with breast cancer has been shown to induce bone loss and increase the risk of fractures [205, 206]. Fractures and bone loss among older women can significantly affect morbidity and mortality, as approximately 25% of older patients with hip fractures die within 1 year after the fracture [207]. Successful management of aromatase inhibitor-induced bone loss in breast cancer survivors can be achieved with good nutrition and age-appropriate intake of calcium and vitamin D as well as addition of a bisphosphonate [208]. Aromatase inhibitors are also associated with arthralgias, or severe joint pain, which can lead to discontinuation of therapy in up to 20% of women taking them [209].

Studies suggest that breast cancer survivors also experience cognitive deficits, including impaired concentration and memory [83, 210]. These deficits appear to be dose-related, with patients who received high-dose chemotherapy experiencing more significant deficits than those who received a standard dose of chemotherapy [83], and to typically improve over time [84], although they can still be present a decade after completion of treatment in a subset of women [81]. The incidence of cognitive impairments among breast cancer survivors previously treated with chemotherapy has been reported between 28% and 75% [81, 84, 85]. The etiology of the treatment-related cognitive impairments among breast cancer survivors is not well understood. It has been suggested that the impairments may not be the direct result of chemotherapy treatment but instead the result of the combination of surgery and anesthesia, menopause, anxiety, depression, fatigue, genetic predisposition, and comorbid medical conditions [211].

Chemotherapy for breast cancer can also cause cardiac disease. As described above, anthracycline chemotherapy, as well as trastuzumab, a newer monoclonal antibody directed at Human Epidermal Growth Factor Receptor 2 (HER2) – receptor for women with HER2-positive breast cancer, can have significant cardiac toxicity, including congestive heart failure, an infrequent but serious complication.

**Psychosocial Symptoms**. Some level of psychological distress among breast cancer survivors is common [163, 198]. One study on a large cohort of cancer patients reported that the prevalence of depression among breast cancer survivors was about 33% [77]. Anxiety and depression usually improve during the first 24 months after diagnosis [212] and breast cancer survivors ultimately experience good QOL [213]. Younger women, those with a history of depression or anxiety and those with inadequate social supports are more likely to experience psychological distress [214–217].

Up to 30% of breast cancer survivors experience poor body image, decreased sexuality and fear of disease recurrence years after the completion of treatment [86, 161, 212, 218–220].

Despite the high prevalence of psychological morbidity and major depressive symptoms in breast cancer survivors, these are frequently misdiagnosed or undertreated, leading to diminished QOL and affecting compliance with medical therapies, which could potentially reduce survival [221].

## Prostate Cancer

**Case Study** Mr. H is a 70-year-old man with a history of prostate cancer diagnosed 4 years ago. He was treated with radical prostatectomy. He has done well since then, although he reports persistent difficultly with sexual function since his surgery. He had some urinary incontinence for about 6 months after his surgery requiring him to wear a pad, but this has resolved. Last year he was started on Lupron by his urologist for a small increase in his Prostate Specific Antigen (PSA) score.

## Symptoms

**Physical Symptoms**. The available treatments for localized prostate cancer can affect patients' urinary, sexual and bowel function [222]. Nearly all men with prostate cancer experience urinary dysfunction in the period immediately following treatment but these symptoms usually improve during the first 2 years after therapy [223]. Older age and a high PSA score are associated with worse urinary incontinence after prostate cancer treatment [224]. In addition, the severity, nature, and duration of urinary dysfunction in prostate cancer survivors vary by treatment. Men treated with external beam radiation or brachytherapy often experience urgency and pain with urination, while men treated with radical prostatectomies are more likely to experience urinary leakage while coughing [222, 225]. Even though urinary incontinence among prostate cancer survivors is usually associated with the treatment received, it can also be the result of the cancer itself, as prostate cancer patients who did not receive aggressive treatments for their cancer and instead chose watchful waiting have also been shown to experience urinary incontinence [223].

Another physical symptom experienced by many prostate cancer survivors is erectile dysfunction. Its severity and prevalence vary depending on the treatment used. For example, rates of erectile dysfunction among prostate cancer survivors 1 year after treatment have been reported as 75% after non-nerve-sparing prostatectomy, 24% after brachytherapy, 40% after brachytherapy with external beam radiation, and 40% after external beam radiation alone [226]. Receipt of androgen-supression therapy in addition to external beam radiotherapy is associated with worse recovery of sexual function after treatment compared to radiotherapy alone [224]. Other factors associated with worse sexual function after treatment are older age, larger prostate size, and high pretreatment PSA score [224].

Prostate cancer patients treated with external beam radiation therapy or brachytherapy sometimes experience significant bowel dysfunction if the radiation damages normal bowel tissue. The symptoms can include rectal urgency, abdominal cramping, diarrhea, and bowel necrosis [223]. Up to 10% of prostate cancer survivors treated with radiation may have severe bowel symptoms [227]. Treatment with anti-inflammatory drugs, such as corticosteroids, can reduce acute inflammatory symptoms and aid in the management of symptoms.

The urinary, sexual, and bowel dysfunction symptoms in prostate cancer survivors are exacerbated by obesity, large prostate size, a high pretreatment PSA score, and older age [224].

Chronic fatigue is also experienced by many prostate cancer survivors following treatment [225, 228, 229]. Up to 40% of prostate cancer patients treated with radiation therapy report severe fatigue even 16 months after initiation of radiation therapy [230]. Posttreatment chronic fatigue is higher among prostate cancer survivors treated with radiation therapy compared with those treated with radical prostatectomy [231]

Androgen deprivation therapy is increasingly used as a treatment for prostate cancer. The goal of the treatment is to induce a hypogonadal state to decrease any hormonal stimulation of prostate cancer. This hypogonadal state results in several systemic side effects of androgen deprivation therapy that can significantly impact survivorship and QOL [37, 232–234]. Vasomotor flushing, loss of libido, gynecomastia, and erectile dysfunction are common side effects experienced secondary to the induced hypogonadism. The decrease in serum androgens has also been linked to significant clinical manifestations including osteopenia and osteoporosis [235], fractures [236], anemia [237], and increased body mass index [238]. More recent data have identified an increased risk of central obesity and decreased lean body mass, insulin resistance, and lipid abnormalities [239], and recent data suggest that androgen deprivation therapy may be associated with increased risk of diabetes, coronary heart disease, myocardial infarction, and stroke [240–242].

**Psychosocial Symptoms**. Prostate cancer survivors experience increased levels of anxiety, depression, and fear of recurrence [243] that can persist for up to 2 years after completion of treatment [244]. Because of the adverse effects of prostate cancer treatment on sexual function, prostate cancer survivors often experience changes in body image, self-esteem, and loss of self-image [245, 246]. Similarly, treatment-related physical effects can significantly impact psychosocial well-being among prostate cancer survivors. Prostate cancer patients who experience urinary incontinence following radical prostatectomy report higher levels of depression, anger, and a reduced sense of well-being 1 year after surgery compared with presurgery levels [247]. The negative psychological effects of prostate cancer appear to be most pronounced during the first 3 months following surgery [246] and gradually subside over time [248].

Addressing the psychological needs of prostate cancer survivors through support groups and educational interventions aimed at increasing prostate cancer knowledge have been shown to successfully improve general physical functioning and improved QOL related to sexual dysfunction among prostate cancer survivors [249]. In addition, because prostate cancer can significantly affect the relationship between the patient and his partner or spouse [250, 251], interventions targeting the spouse have been shown to have a positive impact on the psychological well-being of prostate cancer survivors and their families [243].

## Colorectal Cancer

**Case Study** Mr. P is a 68-year-old man with a history of stage III rectal cancer diagnosed in 2003. He underwent surgical resection requiring permanent colostomy. Although this troubled him for some time, he has become quite adept at managing the colostomy. He also underwent adjuvant chemotherapy and radiation therapy. He is divorced and not in a relationship, so is not too troubled by his sexual dysfunction. But he remains worried about recurrence because he knows his cancer was somewhat advanced when it was diagnosed.

## Symptoms

**Physical Symptoms**. Treatment of colorectal cancer can involve the temporary or permanent exteriorization of the small or large bowel through an intestinal stoma. Patients receiving a stoma can experience profound changes in their daily functioning and well-being that result in lower QOL [252–254] related to problems with sexuality [255, 256], psychological well-being [257, 258], satisfaction with appearance [259, 260], and spirituality [261]. For patients with permanent colostomies, higher levels of distress related to having to adjust to living with a colostomy have been reported [262].

Colorectal cancer survivors sometimes experience frequent bowel movements, diarrhea, and digestive problems that can interfere with everyday activities [166, 168]. These may be more notable in patients who undergo radiation, as they are at risk for radiation proctitis [263, 264]. Radiation for rectal cancer is also associated with erectile dysfunction [265]. Recent evidence also suggests that individuals with rectal cancer who undergo radiation therapy are at increased risk of hip fracture [266] and small bowel obstruction [267].

**Psychosocial Symptoms**. Most colorectal cancer survivors experience good QOL following their treatment [166]. Nevertheless, it is estimated that approximately 25% of colorectal cancer survivors with a stoma experience significant, clinically meaningful psychological symptoms [268]. These symptoms include depression, fear of recurrence, anxiety, and decreased intimacy; they can be present even 5 years after the initial cancer diagnosis and are more pronounced among women survivors compared with men [168, 269].

## Hodgkin's Disease

**Case Study** Ms. R. is a 41-year-old woman with a history of stage IA Hodgkin's disease (HD) diagnosed at age 22. She was treated with mantle radiation and has remained disease-free since then. She is married and has two young children. She takes levoxyl for hypothyroidism, which she was told was a result of her radiation therapy. She has been told that she is at increased risk for breast cancer, and has been undergoing regular mammograms since her early 30s. She is taking pravastatin because she has a history of high cholesterol and her doctor told her that she is at increased risk of heart disease.

### Symptoms

**Physical Symptoms**. Survival rates for HD are quite high, with 5-year survival of 90% for patients with stage I/II, 80% for patients with stage III, and 65% for patients with stage IV disease [270]. Late effects of HD are primarily associated with its treatment, and include decreased fertility, hormonal disturbances, cardiac and pulmonary toxicity, thyroid disease, arthritis, and secondary malignancies [271, 272]. However, longer-term complications are becoming less severe in light of continuing success in finding effective but less toxic chemotherapy regimens and with use of lower doses of radiation.

Survivors of HD who were treated with mediastinal radiation therapy are at increased risk of adverse cardiovascular events including congestive heart failure, pericardial fibrosis, myocardial infarction, coronary artery disease, and valvular disorders [149, 273] that can persist for up to 20 years or more [152]. The prevalence of these cardiovascular disorders is estimated between 25% and 72% depending on the volume, dose, and technique of the radiation therapy used and whether chemotherapy was also received [150, 152, 274]. Newer techniques that involve radiation intensity modulation, decreased fraction size, and total dose have resulted in significantly less cardiac complications associated with radiation therapy. For example, a study comparing cardiovascular disease among HD patients treated between 1940 and 1966 and HD patients treated between 1967 and 1985 showed a decrease in the relative risk of fatal myocardial infarction from 6.3 to 2.0 [156].

Survivors of HD are also at increased risk of developing other cancers and secondary malignancies are the primary cause of mortality among HD survivors [275, 276]. One of the most important prognostic risk factors for developing secondary malignancies among HD survivors is the patient's age at HD treatment. Younger patients, especially those treated before the age of 20, have a significantly higher risk of developing a second cancer after HD than patients treated at older ages [277–280]. Other factors that influence the risk for developing second cancers among HD survivors are treatment with radiation therapy [281–283], treatment with certain chemotherapy agents [284, 285], hormonal factors [286, 287], and genetic influences [288]. The most common secondary malignancy among female HD survivors is breast cancer. Female HD survivors have a two- to fivefold increased risk for breast cancer [277, 289, 290], with higher risks observed among women diagnosed with HD at age 30 or younger who have had chest radition [284, 286, 291, 292]. HD survivors who received mantle and upper abdominal radiation are also at higher risk for lung, stomach, and thyroid cancer [289, 290] even 25 years after the initial cancer diagnosis [276]. These increased risks for secondary solid tumors appear after 10 years of the initial HD diagnosis and remain elevated for decades [276, 290].

HD survivors treated with radiation therapy or chemotherapy can also experience endocrine effects related to sexual function and fertility. The risk of infertility and premature menopause among HD survivors depends on the chemotherapy agents used, the cumulative chemotherapy and/or radiation dose, and the age of the patient when treatment was received [133, 293].

Radiation therapy can also result in thyroid function abnormalities among HD survivors. Hypothyroidism and hyperthyroidism has been reported in up to 50% of HD survivors 10–15 years after radiation treatment [294, 295].

Changes in radiation therapy techniques and chemotherapy regimens for the treatment of HD in recent decades should result in a decrease in the treatment-related late effects among HD survivors. However, because many individuals were treated with regimens known today to be associated with significant late effects, all HD survivors should undergo regular, comprehensive screening for cardiovascular toxicity and secondary cancers even in the absence of any symptoms.

**Psychosocial Symptoms.** Survivors of HD can experience psychological symptoms associated with their diagnosis and treatment which can persist for decades after successful treatment. For example, a study of HD survivors and their siblings found that HD survivors were 1.6–1.7 times more likely to report symptomatic levels of depression and somatic distress more than a decade after their diagnosis, than their siblings without a history of cancer [296]. Similarly, levels of posttraumatic stress disorder among long-term survivors of HD are estimated between 7.4% and 7.9% [297], more than three times higher than the estimated prevalence rates of 2.4% in the general population [298].

## *Effective Management of Cancer-Related Symptoms: Potential Solutions*

Because of the emotional, social, and physical symptoms often associated with cancer and its treatment, cancer survivors have unique health care needs. The importance of comprehensive assessment and management of symptoms among cancer survivors is evident in the Institute of Medicine Report *From Cancer Patient to Cancer Survivor: Lost in Transition* [299] where it is stated that "knowledge of the medical, functional and psychological consequences of cancer and its treatment is essential if the best possible outcomes are to be achieved."

As the numbers of cancer survivors continue to increase, health care providers must work closely with patients to develop a survivorship care plan that includes non-cancer-related medical care (disease prevention and vaccination, chronic care, unrelated cancer screening), cancer-related medical care (surveillance for recurrence, complications of treatment, related cancer screening), and monitoring of psychosocial issues (QOL, financial burden, family/genetic counseling). Particular attention should be paid to the potentially confounding effects of the normal aging process or other health problems related to advancing age among cancer survivors. Interventions that focus on the patient's lifestyle and concentrate on healthy choices such as improved nutrition, increased physical activity, and smoking cessation can further impact QOL among cancer survivors. New strategies for delivering care should be considered and studied. For example, team-based approaches to survivorship care that include nutritionists, physical therapists, and social workers working in conjunction with physicians, nurse practitioners, and physicians' assistants may be best suited to improving QOL and managing symptoms that arise from cancer or its treatment.

Potential barriers to successful management of symptoms for cancer survivors include lack of education, training, and expertise among health care professionals, cost of medications, patient beliefs that the symptoms cannot be controlled, and patient's fear of addiction to medications such as opiates for pain management [300]. Oncologists, primary care physicians, nurses, and mental health workers must work closely with cancer survivors and their families to implement a comprehensive survivorship plan that focuses not only on the length of survival but also on the quality of survival.

Some organizations that provide resources for cancer survivors and their families include:

National Cancer Institute: Office of Cancer Survivorship http://dccps.nci.nih.gov/ocs
National Coalition for Cancer Survivorship http://www.canceradvocacy.org
National Cancer Survivors Day Foundation http://www.ncsdf.org
Lance Armstrong Foundation: Livestrong http://www.livestrong.org
CancerCare http://www.cancercare.org

## *Future Research*

Additional research is needed to better characterize the long-term effects of cancer and its treatment. Current data primarily focus on patients with a few select cancers. Moreover, even conditions that have been relatively well studied, such as cognitive function associated with chemotherapy, remain poorly understood. Finally, little research focuses on interventions to address the physical and psychosocial symptoms experienced by cancer survivors.

Population-based studies that allow for long-term follow-up should be supported by the National Cancer Institute (NCI) and other funders. The Cancer Care Outcomes and Research Surveillance (CanCORS) Consortium [301] is an example of a population-based study that will provide information on symptom and QOL of lung and colorectal cancer survivors up to 7 years after their diagnosis. Long-term follow-up of patients enrolled in clinical trials would also help to better characterize the time course of symptoms and adverse events associated with treatments.

Also needed are more studies designed to identify behaviors to improve the QOL of cancer survivors and treatments for patients with existing symptoms. In addition, studies of the best models to follow, manage, and treat patients are essential. As early diagnosis and treatment of cancer improves and as the population continues to age, the numbers of cancer survivors will continue to grow. Maximizing the health of this growing population will be crucial to improving the health of society.

## References

1. Oncology, ASoC. Outcomes of cancer treatment for technology assessment and cancer treatment guidelines. J Clin Oncol. 1996;14:671–9.
2. Loescher LJ, Clark L, Atwood JR, Leigh S, Lamb G. The impact of the cancer experience on long-term survivors. Oncol Nurs Forum. 1990;17(2):223–9.
3. Herndon 2nd JE, Fleishman S, Kornblith AB, Kosty M, Green MR, Holland J. Is quality of life predictive of the survival of patients with advanced nonsmall cell lung carcinoma? Cancer. 1999;85(2):333–40.
4. Gotay CC, Kawamoto CT, Bottomley A, Efficace F. The prognostic significance of patient-reported outcomes in cancer clinical trials. J Clin Oncol. 2008;26(8):1355–63.

5. Efficace F, Bottomley A, Smit EF, Lianes P, Legrand C, Debruyne C, et al. Is a patient's self-reported health-related quality of life a prognostic factor for survival in non-small-cell lung cancer patients? A multivariate analysis of prognostic factors of EORTC study 08975. Ann Oncol. 2006;17(11):1698–704.
6. Efficace F, Innominato PF, Bjarnason G, Coens C, Humblet Y, Tumolo S, et al. Validation of patient's self-reported social functioning as an independent prognostic factor for survival in metastatic colorectal cancer patients: results of an international study by the Chronotherapy Group of the European Organisation for Research and Treatment of Cancer. J Clin Oncol. 2008;26(12):2020–6.
7. Montazeri A, Milroy R, Hole D, McEwen J, Gillis CR. Quality of life in lung cancer patients: as an important prognostic factor. Lung Cancer. 2001;31(2–3):233–40.
8. Hewitt M, Rowland JH, Yancik R. Cancer survivors in the United States: age, health, and disability. J Gerontol A Biol Sci Med Sci. 2003;58(1):82–91.
9. Hoffman KE, McCarthy EP, Recklitis CJ, Ng AK. Psychological distress in long-term survivors of adult-onset cancer: results from a national survey. Arch Intern Med. 2009;169(14):1274–81.
10. Yabroff KR, Lawrence WF, Clauser S, Davis WW, Brown ML. Burden of illness in cancer survivors: findings from a population-based national sample. J Natl Cancer Inst. 2004;96(17):1322–30.
11. Richardson LC, Wingo PA, Zack MM, Zahran HS, King JB. Health-related quality of life in cancer survivors between ages 20 and 64 years: population-based estimates from the Behavioral Risk Factor Surveillance System. Cancer. 2008;112(6):1380–9.
12. Bower JE, Ganz PA, Desmond KA, Bernaards C, Rowland JH, Meyerowitz BE, et al. Fatigue in long-term breast carcinoma survivors: a longitudinal investigation. Cancer. 2006;106(4):751–8.
13. Baker F, Denniston M, Smith T, West MM. Adult cancer survivors: how are they faring? Cancer. 2005;104(11 Suppl):2565–76.
14. Cella D, Davis K, Breitbart W, Curt G. Cancer-related fatigue: prevalence of proposed diagnostic criteria in a United States sample of cancer survivors. J Clin Oncol. 2001;19(14):3385–91.
15. Mols F, van de Poll-Franse LV, Vingerhoets AJ, Hendrikx A, Aaronson NK, Houterman S, et al. Long-term quality of life among Dutch prostate cancer survivors: results of a population-based study. Cancer. 2006;107(9):2186–96.
16. Denlinger CS, Barsevick AM. The challenges of colorectal cancer survivorship. J Natl Compr Cancer Netw. 2009;7(8):883–93.
17. Ganz PA. Psychological and social aspects of breast cancer. Oncology (Williston Park). 2008;22(6):642–46.
18. Ferrans CE. Development of a quality of life index for patients with cancer. Oncol Nurs Forum. 1990;17(3 Suppl):15–19.
19. Padilla GV, Ferrell B, Grant MM, Rhiner M. Defining the content domain of quality of life for cancer patients with pain. Cancer Nurs. 1990;13(2):108–15.
20. Spiker B. Quality of life assessments in clinical trials. New York: Raven; 1990.
21. Ferrell BR, Dow KH, Grant M. Measurement of the quality of life in cancer survivors. Qual Life Res. 1995;4(6):523–31.
22. Armstrong TS. Symptoms experience: a concept analysis. Oncol Nurs Forum. 2003;30(4):601–6.
23. Barsevick AM. The concept of symptom cluster. Semin Oncol Nurs. 2007;23(2):89–98.
24. Barsevick AM. The elusive concept of the symptom cluster. Oncol Nurs Forum. 2007;34(5):971–80.
25. Dodd MJ, Miaskowski C, Paul SM. Symptom clusters and their effect on the functional status of patients with cancer. Oncol Nurs Forum. 2001;28(3):465–70.
26. Cleeland CS, Reyes-Gibby CC. When is it justified to treat symptoms? Measuring symptom burden. Oncology (Williston Park). 2002;16(9 Suppl 10):64–70.
27. Kuhnt S, Ernst J, Singer S, Ruffer JU, Kortmann RD, Stolzenburg JU, et al. Fatigue in cancer survivors – prevalence and correlates. Onkologie. 2009;32(6):312–7.

28. Hjermstad MJ, Oldervoll L, Fossa SD, Holte H, Jacobsen AB, Loge JH. Quality of life in long-term Hodgkin's disease survivors with chronic fatigue. Eur J Cancer. 2006;42(3):327–33.
29. Hjermstad MJ, Fossa SD, Oldervoll L, Holte H, Jacobsen AB, Loge JH. Fatigue in long-term Hodgkin's Disease survivors: a follow-up study. J Clin Oncol. 2005;23(27):6587–95.
30. Orre IJ, Fossa SD, Bremnes R, Dahl O, Klepp O, et al. Chronic cancer-related fatigue in long-term survivors of testicular cancer. J Psychosom Res. 2008;64(4):363–71.
31. Bower JE, Ganz PA, Desmond KA, Rowland JH, Meyerowitz BE, Belin TR. Fatigue in breast cancer survivors: occurrence, correlates, and impact on quality of life. J Clin Oncol. 2000;18(4):743–53.
32. Ganz PA, Moinpour CM, Pauler DK, Kornblith AB, Gaynor ER, Balcerzak SP, et al. Health status and quality of life in patients with early-stage Hodgkin's disease treated on Southwest Oncology Group Study 9133. J Clin Oncol. 2003;21(18):3512–9.
33. Servaes P, van der Werf S, Prins J, Verhagen S, Bleijenberg G. Fatigue in disease-free cancer patients compared with fatigue in patients with chronic fatigue syndrome. Support Care Cancer. 2001;9(1):11–7.
34. Ruffer JU, Flechtner H, Tralls P, Josting A, Sieber M, Lathan B, et al. Fatigue in long-term survivors of Hodgkin's lymphoma; a report from the German Hodgkin Lymphoma Study Group (GHSG). Eur J Cancer. 2003;39(15):2179–86.
35. Curt GA, Breitbart W, Cella D, Groopman JE, Horning SJ, Itri LM, et al. Impact of cancer-related fatigue on the lives of patients: new findings from the Fatigue Coalition. Oncologist. 2000;5(5):353–60.
36. Schwartz AL. Fatigue in long-term cancer survivors. Oncology (Williston Park). 2009;23(8 Suppl):27. 33–4.
37. Saylor PJ, Keating NL, Smith MR. Prostate cancer survivorship: prevention and treatment of the adverse effects of androgen deprivation therapy. J Gen Intern Med. 2009;24 Suppl 2:S389–94.
38. Andrykowski MA, Curran SL, Lightner R. Off-treatment fatigue in breast cancer survivors: a controlled comparison. J Behav Med. 1998;21(1):1–18.
39. Richardson A. Fatigue in cancer patients: a review of the literature. Eur J Cancer Care (Engl). 1995;4(1):20–32.
40. Hann DM, Jacobsen PB, Azzarello LM, Martin SC, Curran SL, Fields KK, et al. Measurement of fatigue in cancer patients: development and validation of the Fatigue Symptom Inventory. Qual Life Res. 1998;7(4):301–10.
41. Verbeek J, Spelten E, Kammeijer M, Sprangers M. Return to work of cancer survivors: a prospective cohort study into the quality of rehabilitation by occupational physicians. Occup Environ Med. 2003;60(5):352–7.
42. Spelten ER, Verbeek JH, Uitterhoeve AL, Ansink AC AC, Van der Lelie J, de Reijke TM, et al. Cancer, fatigue and the return of patients to work-a prospective cohort study. Eur J Cancer. 2003;39(11):1562–7.
43. Bjordal K, Kaasa S, Mastekaasa A. Quality of life in patients treated for head and neck cancer: a follow-up study 7 to 11 years after radiotherapy. Int J Radiat Oncol Biol Phys. 1994;28(4):847–56.
44. Norum J, Wist EA. Quality of life in survivors of Hodgkin's disease. Qual Life Res. 1996;5(3):367–74.
45. Hann DM, Jacobsen PB, Martin SC, Kronish LE, Azzarello LM, Fields KK. Fatigue in women treated with bone marrow transplantation for breast cancer: a comparison with women with no history of cancer. Support Care Cancer. 1997;5(1):44–52.
46. Broeckel JA, Jacobsen PB, Horton J, Balducci L, Lyman GH. Characteristics and correlates of fatigue after adjuvant chemotherapy for breast cancer. J Clin Oncol. 1998;16(5):1689–96.
47. Piper BF, Dibble SL, Dodd MJ, Weiss MC, Slaughter RE, Paul SM. The revised Piper Fatigue Scale: psychometric evaluation in women with breast cancer. Oncol Nurs Forum. 1998;25(4):677–84.
48. Piper BF, Lindsey AM, Dodd MJ. Fatigue mechanisms in cancer patients: developing nursing theory. Oncol Nurs Forum. 1987;14(6):17–23.

49. Aistars J. Fatigue in the cancer patient: a conceptual approach to a clinical problem. Oncol Nurs Forum. 1987;14(6):25–30.
50. Winningham ML, Nail LM, Burke MB, Brophy L, Cimprich B, Jones LS, et al. Fatigue and the cancer experience: the state of the knowledge. Oncol Nurs Forum. 1994;21(1):23–36.
51. Karabulu N, Erci B, Ozer N, Ozdemir S. Symptom clusters and experiences of patients with cancer. J Adv Nurs. 2010;66(5):1011–21.
52. Evensen JF, Bjordal K, Knutsen BH, Olsen DR, Store G, Tausjo JE. Side effects and quality of life after inadvertent radiation overdosage in brachytherapy of head-and-neck cancer. Int J Radiat Oncol Biol Phys. 2002;52(4):944–52.
53. Small Jr W, Kachnic L. Postradiotherapy pelvic fractures: cause for concern or opportunity for future research? JAMA. 2005;294(20):2635–7.
54. Jung BF, Ahrendt GM, Oaklander AL, Dworkin RH. Neuropathic pain following breast cancer surgery: proposed classification and research update. Pain. 2003;104(1–2):1–13.
55. Tasmuth T, von Smitten K, Hietanen P, Kataja M, Kalso E. Pain and other symptoms after different treatment modalities of breast cancer. Ann Oncol. 1995;6(5):453–9.
56. Tasmuth T, von Smitten K, Kalso E. Pain and other symptoms during the first year after radical and conservative surgery for breast cancer. Br J Cancer. 1996;74(12):2024–31.
57. Peuckmann V, Ekholm O, Rasmussen NK, Groenvold M, Christiansen P, Moller S, et al. Chronic pain and other sequelae in long-term breast cancer survivors: nationwide survey in Denmark. Eur J Pain. 2009;13(5):478–85.
58. Perkins FM, Kehlet H. Chronic pain as an outcome of surgery. A review of predictive factors. Anesthesiology. 2000;93(4):1123–33.
59. Gartner R, Jensen MB, Nielsen J, Ewertz M, Kroman N, Kehlet H. Prevalence of and factors associated with persistent pain following breast cancer surgery. JAMA. 2009;302(18):1985–92.
60. Given CW, Given B, Azzouz F, Kozachik S, Stommel M. Predictors of pain and fatigue in the year following diagnosis among elderly cancer patients. J Pain Symptom Manage. 2001;21(6):456–66.
61. Visovsky C. Chemotherapy-induced peripheral neuropathy. Cancer Investig. 2003;21(3): 439–51.
62. Visovsky C, Meyer RR, Roller J, Poppas M. Evaluation and management of peripheral neuropathy in diabetic patients with cancer. Clin J Oncol Nurs. 2008;12(2):243–7.
63. Visovsky C, Daly BJ. Clinical evaluation and patterns of chemotherapy-induced peripheral neuropathy. J Am Acad Nurse Pract. 2004;16(8):353–9.
64. Curtis RE, Ron E, Hankey BF, Hoover RN. New malignancies following breast cancer. In: Institute NC, editor. New malignancies among cancer survivors: SEER Cancer Registries 1973–2000. Bethesda: National Cancer Institute; 2006. p. 181–205.
65. Jaffe ES, Harris NL, Stein H, Vardiman JW. World Health Organization classification of tumours: pathology and genetics of haematopoietic and lymphoid tissues. Lyon: IARC Press; 2001.
66. Delwail V, Jais JP, Colonna P, Andrieu JM. Fifteen-year secondary leukaemia risk observed in 761 patients with Hodgkin's disease prospectively treated by MOPP or ABVD chemotherapy plus high-dose irradiation. Br J Haematol. 2002;118(1):189–94.
67. van Leeuwen FE, Chorus AM, van den Belt-Dusebout AW, Hagenbeek A, Noyon R, van Kerkhoff EH, et al. Leukemia risk following Hodgkin's disease: relation to cumulative dose of alkylating agents, treatment with teniposide combinations, number of episodes of chemotherapy, and bone marrow damage. J Clin Oncol. 1994;12(5):1063–73.
68. Henry-Amar M. Second cancers after treatment of Hodgkin's disease: experience at the International Database on Hodgkin's disease (IDHD). Bull Cancer. 1992;79(4):389–91.
69. Kaldor JM, Day NE, Clarke EA, Van Leeuwen FE, Henry-Amar M, Fiorentino MV, et al. Leukemia following Hodgkin's disease. N Engl J Med. 1990;322(1):7–13.
70. Matesich SM, Shapiro CL. Second cancers after breast cancer treatment. Semin Oncol. 2003;30(6):740–8.
71. Burstein HJ, Winer EP. Primary care for survivors of breast cancer. N Engl J Med. 2000;343(15):1086–94.

72. Janssen-Heijnen ML, Houterman S, Lemmens VE, Louwman MW, Maas HA, Coebergh JW. Prognostic impact of increasing age and co-morbidity in cancer patients: a population-based approach. Crit Rev Oncol Hematol. 2005;55(3):231–40.
73. van Spronsen DJ, Janssen-Heijnen ML, Lemmens VE, Peters WG, Coebergh JW. Independent prognostic effect of co-morbidity in lymphoma patients: results of the population-based Eindhoven Cancer Registry. Eur J Cancer. 2005;41(7):1051–7.
74. Vulto AJ, Lemmens VE, Louwman MW, Janssen-Heijnen ML, Poortmans PH, Lybeert ML, et al. The influence of age and comorbidity on receiving radiotherapy as part of primary treatment for cancer in South Netherlands, 1995 to 2002. Cancer. 2006;106(12):2734–42.
75. Shahir MA, Lemmens VE, van de Poll-Franse LV, Voogd AC, Martijn H, Janssen-Heijnen ML. Elderly patients with rectal cancer have a higher risk of treatment-related complications and a poorer prognosis than younger patients: a population-based study. Eur J Cancer. 2006;42(17):3015–21.
76. Le Corroller-Soroano AG, Bouhnik AD, Preau M, Malavolti L, Julian-Reynier C, Auquier P, et al. Does cancer survivors' health-related quality of life depend on cancer type? Findings from a large French national sample 2 years after cancer diagnosis. Eur J Cancer Care (Engl). 2011;20(1):132–40.
77. Zabora J, BrintzenhofeSzoc K, Curbow B, Hooker C, Piantadosi S. The prevalence of psychological distress by cancer site. Psychooncology. 2001;10(1):19–28.
78. Ciaramella A, Poli P. Assessment of depression among cancer patients: the role of pain, cancer type and treatment. Psychooncology. 2001;10(2):156–65.
79. Deimling GT, Kahana B, Bowman KF, Schaefer ML. Cancer survivorship and psychological distress in later life. Psychooncology. 2002;11(6):479–94.
80. Komaki R, Meyers CA, Shin DM, Garden AS, Byrne K, Nickens JA, et al. Evaluation of cognitive function in patients with limited small cell lung cancer prior to and shortly following prophylactic cranial irradiation. Int J Radiat Oncol Biol Phys. 1995;33(1):179–82.
81. Ahles TA, Saykin AJ, Furstenberg CT, Cole B, Mott LA, Skalla K, et al. Neuropsychologic impact of standard-dose systemic chemotherapy in long-term survivors of breast cancer and lymphoma. J Clin Oncol. 2002;20(2):485–93.
82. Wieneke MH, Dienst ER. Neuropsychological assessment of cognitive functioning following chemotherapy for breast cancer. Psychooncology. 1995;4:61–6.
83. van Dam FS, Schagen SB, Muller MJ, Boogerd W, vd Wall E, Droogleever Fortuyn ME, et al. Impairment of cognitive function in women receiving adjuvant treatment for high-risk breast cancer: high-dose versus standard-dose chemotherapy. J Natl Cancer Inst. 1998;90(3):210–8.
84. Brezden CB, Phillips KA, Abdolell M, Bunston T, Tannock IF. Cognitive function in breast cancer patients receiving adjuvant chemotherapy. J Clin Oncol. 2000;18(14):2695–701.
85. Schagen SB, van Dam FS, Muller MJ, Boogerd W, Lindeboom J, Bruning PF. Cognitive deficits after postoperative adjuvant chemotherapy for breast carcinoma. Cancer. 1999;85(3):640–50.
86. Ferrell BR, Grant MM, Funk B, Otis-Green S, Garcia N. Quality of life in breast cancer survivors as identified by focus groups. Psychooncology. 1997;6(1):13–23.
87. Ferrell BR, Hassey Dow K. Quality of life among long-term cancer survivors. Oncology (Williston Park). 1997;11(4):565–8, 571.
88. Meyers CA. Neurocognitive dysfunction in cancer patients. Oncology (Williston Park). 2000;14(1):75–9.
89. Kvale EA, Clay OJ, Ross-Meadows LA, McGee JS, Edwards JD, Unverzagt FW, et al. Cognitive speed of processing and functional declines in older cancer survivors: an analysis of data from the ACTIVE trial. Eur J Cancer Care (Engl). 2010;19(1):110–7.
90. van den Beuken-van Everdingen MH, Peters ML, de Rijke JM, Schouten HC, van Kleef M, Patijn J. Concerns of former breast cancer patients about disease recurrence: a validation and prevalence study. Psychooncology. 2008;17(11):1137–45.
91. Johnson Vickberg SM. Fears about breast cancer recurrence. Cancer Pract. 2001;9(5):237–43.

92. Lee-Jones C, Humphris G, Dixon R, Hatcher MB. Fear of cancer recurrence – a literature review and proposed cognitive formulation to explain exacerbation of recurrence fears. Psychooncology. 1997;6(2):95–105.
93. Clough-Gorr KM, Ganz PA, Silliman RA. Older breast cancer survivors: factors associated with change in emotional well-being. J Clin Oncol. 2007;25(11):1334–40.
94. Baider L, Andritsch E, Uziely B, Goldzweig G, Ever-Hadani P, Hofman G, et al. Effects of age on coping and psychological distress in women diagnosed with breast cancer: review of literature and analysis of two different geographical settings. Crit Rev Oncol Hematol. 2003;46(1):5–16.
95. Knobf MT. Psychosocial responses in breast cancer survivors. Semin Oncol Nurs. 2007;23(1):71–83.
96. Ganz PA. Late effects of cancer and its treatment. Semin Oncol Nurs. 2001;17(4):241–8.
97. Ferrell BR, Dow KH, Leigh S, Ly J, Gulasekaram P. Quality of life in long-term cancer survivors. Oncol Nurs Forum. 1995;22(6):915–22.
98. McEvoy MD, McCorkle R. Quality of life issues in patients with disseminated breast cancer. Cancer. 1990;66(6 Suppl):1416–21.
99. Kornblith AB. Psychosocial adaptation of cancer survivors. New York: Oxford University Press; 1998.
100. Hoffman B. Cancer survivors at work: job problems and illegal discrimination. Oncol Nurs Forum. 1989;16(1):39–43.
101. Taylor SE. Adjustment to threatening events: a theory of cognitive adaptation. Am Psychol. 1983;38:1161–73.
102. Pinquart M, Frohlich C. Psychosocial resources and subjective well-being of cancer patients. Psychol Health. 2009;24(4):407–21.
103. Carver CS, Smith RG, Antoni MH, Petronis VM, Weiss S, Derhagopian RP. Optimistic personality and psychosocial well-being during treatment predict psychosocial well-being among long-term survivors of breast cancer. Health Psychol. 2005;24(5):508–16.
104. Tedeschi, RG, Park CL, Lawrence LW, eds. Posttraumatic growth: Positive changes in the aftermath of crisis. Mahwah, NJ: Erlbaum; 1998, JA Schaefer and RH Moos. The context for posttraumatic growth: Life crises, individual and social resources and coping.
105. Bloom JR, Stewart SL, Johnston M, Banks P, Fobair P. Sources of support and the physical and mental well-being of young women with breast cancer. Soc Sci Med. 2001;53(11):1513–24.
106. Schroevers MJ, Ranchor AV, Sanderman R. The role of social support and self-esteem in the presence and course of depressive symptoms: a comparison of cancer patients and individuals from the general population. Soc Sci Med. 2003;57(2):375–85.
107. Norum J, Risberg T, Solberg E. Faith among patients with advanced cancer. A pilot study on patients offered "no more than" palliation. Support Care Cancer. 2000;8(2):110–4.
108. Halstead MT, Fernsler JI. Coping strategies of long-term cancer survivors. Cancer Nurs. 1994;17(2):94–100.
109. Bellizzi KM, Miller MF, Arora NK, Rowland JH. Positive and negative life changes experienced by survivors of non-Hodgkin's lymphoma. Ann Behav Med. 2007;34(2):188–99.
110. Bellizzi KM, Blank TO. Cancer-related identity and positive affect in survivors of prostate cancer. J Cancer Surviv. 2007;1(1):44–8.
111. Gall TL, Cornblat MW. Breast cancer survivors give voice: a qualitative analysis of spiritual factors in long-term adjustment. Psychooncology. 2002;11(6):524–35.
112. Hayes SC, Janda M, Cornish B, Battistutta D, Newman B. Lymphedema after breast cancer: incidence, risk factors, and effect on upper body function. J Clin Oncol. 2008;26(21):3536–42.
113. Warren AG, Brorson H, Borud LJ, Slavin SA. Lymphedema: a comprehensive review. Ann Plast Surg. 2007;59(4):464–72.
114. Vignes S, Arrault M, Dupuy A. Factors associated with increased breast cancer-related lymphedema volume. Acta Oncol. 2007;46(8):1138–42.
115. Armer JM, Stewart BR. A comparison of four diagnostic criteria for lymphedema in a post-breast cancer population. Lymphat Res Biol. 2005;3(4):208–17.

116. Golshan M, Martin WJ, Dowlatshahi K. Sentinel lymph node biopsy lowers the rate of lymphedema when compared with standard axillary lymph node dissection. Am Surg. 2003;69(3):209–11.
117. Walsh PC, Marschke P, Ricker D, Burnett AL. Patient-reported urinary continence and sexual function after anatomic radical prostatectomy. Urology. 2000;55(1):58–61.
118. Catalona WJ, Carvalhal GF, Mager DE, Smith DS. Potency, continence and complication rates in 1, 870 consecutive radical retropubic prostatectomies. J Urol. 1999;162(2):433–8.
119. Quinlan DM, Epstein JI, Carter BS, Walsh PC. Sexual function following radical prostatectomy: influence of preservation of neurovascular bundles. J Urol. 1991;145(5):998–1002.
120. Goorin AM, Borow KM, Goldman A, Williams RG, Henderson IC, Sallan SE, et al. Congestive heart failure due to adriamycin cardiotoxicity: its natural history in children. Cancer. 1981;47(12):2810–6.
121. Pai VB, Nahata MC. Cardiotoxicity of chemotherapeutic agents: incidence, treatment and prevention. Drug Saf. 2000;22(4):263–302.
122. Ewer MS, Lippman SM. Type II chemotherapy-related cardiac dysfunction: time to recognize a new entity. J Clin Oncol. 2005;23(13):2900–2.
123. Monsuez JJ, Charniot JC, Vignat N, Artigou JY. Cardiac side-effects of cancer chemotherapy. Int J Cardiol. 2010;144(1):3–15.
124. Grober SE. Resources for treatment of chemotherapy-related cognitive difficulty. Cancer Pract. 2002;10(4):216–8.
125. de Jong N, Candel MJ, Schouten HC, Abu-Saad HH, Courtens AM. Prevalence and course of fatigue in breast cancer patients receiving adjuvant chemotherapy. Ann Oncol. 2004;15(6):896–905.
126. Jansen CE, Miaskowski C, Dodd M, Dowling G, Kramer J. A metaanalysis of studies of the effects of cancer chemotherapy on various domains of cognitive function. Cancer. 2005;104(10):2222–33.
127. Wampler MA, Hamolsky D, Hamel K, Melisko M, Topp KS. Case report: painful peripheral neuropathy following treatment with docetaxel for breast cancer. Clin J Oncol Nurs. 2005;9(2):189–93.
128. Nelson CJ, Nandy N, Roth AJ. Chemotherapy and cognitive deficits: mechanisms, findings, and potential interventions. Palliat Support Care. 2007;5(3):273–80.
129. Kannarkat G, Lasher EE, Schiff D. Neurologic complications of chemotherapy agents. Curr Opin Neurol. 2007;20(6):719–25.
130. Tangpong J, Cole MP, Sultana R, Estus S, Vore M, St Clair W, et al. Adriamycin-mediated nitration of manganese superoxide dismutase in the central nervous system: insight into the mechanism of chemobrain. J Neurochem. 2007;100(1):191–201.
131. Shilling V, Jenkins V, Morris R, Deutsch G, Bloomfield D. The effects of adjuvant chemotherapy on cognition in women with breast cancer – preliminary results of an observational longitudinal study. Breast. 2005;14(2):142–50.
132. Jenkins V, Shilling V, Deutsch G, Bloomfield D, Morris R, Allan S, et al. A 3-year prospective study of the effects of adjuvant treatments on cognition in women with early stage breast cancer. Br J Cancer. 2006;94(6):828–34.
133. Bonadonna G, Bonfante V, Viviani S, Di Russo A, Villani F, Valagussa P. ABVD plus subtotal nodal versus involved-field radiotherapy in early-stage Hodgkin's disease: long-term results. J Clin Oncol. 2004;22(14):2835–41.
134. Stovall M, Smith SA, Langholz BM, Boice JD, Shore RE, Andersson M, et al. Dose to the contralateral breast from radiotherapy and risk of second primary breast cancer in the WECARE study. Int J Radiat Oncol Biol Phys. 2008;72(4):1021–30.
135. de Berrington Gonzalez A, Curtis RE, Gilbert E, Berg CD, Smith SA, Stovall M, et al. Second solid cancers after radiotherapy for breast cancer in SEER cancer registries. Br J Cancer. 2010;102(1):220–6.
136. Moreno M, Aristu J, Ramos LI, Arbea L, Lopez-Picazo JM, Cambeiro M, et al. Predictive factors for radiation-induced pulmonary toxicity after three-dimensional conformal chemoradiation in locally advanced non-small-cell lung cancer. Clin Transl Oncol. 2007;9(9):596–602.

137. Kocak Z, Evans ES, Zhou SM, Miller KL, Folz RJ, Shafman TD, et al. Challenges in defining radiation pneumonitis in patients with lung cancer. Int J Radiat Oncol Biol Phys. 2005;62(3):635–8.
138. Krasin MJ, Constine LS, Friedman DL, Marks LB. Radiation-related treatment effects across the age spectrum: differences and similarities or what the old and young can learn from each other. Semin Radiat Oncol. 2010;20(1):21–9.
139. Preston DL, Mattsson A, Holmberg E, Shore R, Hildreth NG, Boice Jr JD. Radiation effects on breast cancer risk: a pooled analysis of eight cohorts. Radiat Res. 2002;158(2):220–35.
140. Coletti D, Ord RA. Treatment rationale for pathological fractures of the mandible: a series of 44 fractures. Int J Oral Maxillofac Surg. 2008;37(3):215–22.
141. Engleman MA, Woloschak G, Small Jr W. Radiation-induced skeletal injury. Cancer Treat Res. 2006;128:155–69.
142. Paulino AC. Late effects of radiotherapy for pediatric extremity sarcomas. Int J Radiat Oncol Biol Phys. 2004;60(1):265–74.
143. Indelicato DJ, Keole SR, Shahlaee AH, Shi W, Morris CG, Marcus Jr RB. Definitive radiotherapy for ewing tumors of extremities and pelvis: long-term disease control, limb function, and treatment toxicity. Int J Radiat Oncol Biol Phys. 2008;72(3):871–7.
144. Silber JH, Littman PS, Meadows AT. Stature loss following skeletal irradiation for childhood cancer. J Clin Oncol. 1990;8(2):304–12.
145. Eifel PJ, Donaldson SS, Thomas PR. Response of growing bone to irradiation: a proposed late effects scoring system. Int J Radiat Oncol Biol Phys. 1995;31(5):1301–7.
146. Merchant TE, Nguyen L, Nguyen D, Wu S, Hudson MM, Kaste SC. Differential attenuation of clavicle growth after asymmetric mantle radiotherapy. Int J Radiat Oncol Biol Phys. 2004;59(2):556–61.
147. Travis LB, Hill DA, Dores GM, Gospodarowicz M, van Leeuwen FE, Holowaty E, et al. Breast cancer following radiotherapy and chemotherapy among young women with Hodgkin disease. JAMA. 2003;290(4):465–75.
148. Travis LB, Gospodarowicz M, Curtis RE, Clarke EA, Andersson M, Glimelius B, et al. Lung cancer following chemotherapy and radiotherapy for Hodgkin's disease. J Natl Cancer Inst. 2002;94(3):182–92.
149. Aleman BM, van den Belt-Dusebout AW, De Bruin ML, van't Veer MB, Baaijens MH, de Boer JP, et al. Late cardiotoxicity after treatment for Hodgkin lymphoma. Blood. 2007;109(5):1878–86.
150. Glanzmann C, Kaufmann P, Jenni R, Hess OM, Huguenin P. Cardiac risk after mediastinal irradiation for Hodgkin's disease. Radiother Oncol. 1998;46(1):51–62.
151. Heidenreich PA, Hancock SL, Lee BK, Mariscal CS, Schnittger I. Asymptomatic cardiac disease following mediastinal irradiation. J Am Coll Cardiol. 2003;42(4):743–9.
152. Machann, W, Beer M, Breunig M, et al. Cardiac magnetic resonance imaging findings in 20-year survivors of mediastinal radiotherapy for Hodgkin's disease. Int J Radiat Oncol Biol Phys. 2011;79(4):1117–23.
153. Vallis KA, Pintilie M, Chong N, Holowaty E, Douglas PS, Kirkbride P, et al. Assessment of coronary heart disease morbidity and mortality after radiation therapy for early breast cancer. J Clin Oncol. 2002;20(4):1036–42.
154. Rutqvist LE, Liedberg A, Hammar N, Dalberg K. Myocardial infarction among women with early-stage breast cancer treated with conservative surgery and breast irradiation. Int J Radiat Oncol Biol Phys. 1998;40(2):359–63.
155. Gaya AM, Ashford RF. Cardiac complications of radiation therapy. Clin Oncol (R Coll Radiol). 2005;17(3):153–9.
156. Boivin JF, Hutchison GB, Lubin JH, Mauch P. Coronary artery disease mortality in patients treated for Hodgkin's disease. Cancer. 1992;69(5):1241–7.
157. Hancock SL, Tucker MA, Hoppe RT. Factors affecting late mortality from heart disease after treatment of Hodgkin's disease. JAMA. 1993;270(16):1949–55.
158. Vogelzang NJ, Breitbart W, Cella D, Curt GA, Groopman JE, Horning SJ, et al. Patient, caregiver, and oncologist perceptions of cancer-related fatigue: Results of a tripart assessment survey. The fatigue coalition. Semin Hematol. 1997;34(3 Suppl 2):4–12.

159. Ganz PA, Coscarelli A, Fred C, Kahn B, Polinsky ML, Petersen L. Breast cancer survivors: psychosocial concerns and quality of life. Breast Cancer Res Treat. 1996;38(2):183–99.
160. Ahn SH, Park BW, Noh DY, Nam SJ, Lee ES, Lee MK, et al. Health-related quality of life in disease-free survivors of breast cancer with the general population. Ann Oncol. 2007;18(1):173–82.
161. Kornblith AB, Herndon 2nd JE, Weiss RB, Zhang C, Zuckerman EL, Rosenberg S, et al. Long-term adjustment of survivors of early-stage breast carcinoma, 20 years after adjuvant chemotherapy. Cancer. 2003;98(4):679–89.
162. Dorval M, Maunsell E, Deschenes L, Brisson J, Masse B. Long-term quality of life after breast cancer: comparison of 8-year survivors with population controls. J Clin Oncol. 1998;16(2):487–94.
163. Ganz PA, Desmond KA, Leedham B, Rowland JH, Meyerowitz BE, Belin TR. Quality of life in long-term, disease-free survivors of breast cancer: a follow-up study. J Natl Cancer Inst. 2002;94(1):39–49.
164. Blank TO, Bellizzi KM. After prostate cancer: predictors of well-being among long-term prostate cancer survivors. Cancer. 2006;106(10):2128–35.
165. Miller DC, Sanda MG, Dunn RL, Montie JE, Pimentel H, Sandler HM, et al. Long-term outcomes among localized prostate cancer survivors: health-related quality-of-life changes after radical prostatectomy, external radiation, and brachytherapy. J Clin Oncol. 2005;23(12):2772–80.
166. Ramsey SD, Berry K, Moinpour C, Giedzinska A, Andersen MR. Quality of life in long term survivors of colorectal cancer. Am J Gastroenterol. 2002;97(5):1228–34.
167. Ramsey SD, Andersen MR, Etzioni R, Moinpour C, Peacock S, Potosky A, et al. Quality of life in survivors of colorectal carcinoma. Cancer. 2000;88(6):1294–303.
168. Rauch P, Miny J, Conroy T, Neyton L, Guillemin F. Quality of life among disease-free survivors of rectal cancer. J Clin Oncol. 2004;22(2):354–60.
169. Sapp AL, Trentham-Dietz A, Newcomb PA, Hampton JM, Moinpour CM, Remington PL. Social networks and quality of life among female long-term colorectal cancer survivors. Cancer. 2003;98(8):1749–58.
170. Trentham-Dietz A, Remington PL, Moinpour CM, Hampton JM, Sapp AL, Newcomb PA. Health-related quality of life in female long-term colorectal cancer survivors. Oncologist. 2003;8(4):342–9.
171. Heutte N, Flechtner HH, Mounier N, Mellink WA, Meerwaldt JH, Eghbali H, et al. Quality of life after successful treatment of early-stage Hodgkin's lymphoma: 10-year follow-up of the EORTC-GELA H8 randomised controlled trial. Lancet Oncol. 2009;10(12):1160–70.
172. Minton O, Stone P. How common is fatigue in disease-free breast cancer survivors? A systematic review of the literature. Breast Cancer Res Treat. 2008;112(1):5–13.
173. Meeske K, Smith AW, Alfano CM, McGregor BA, McTiernan A, Baumgartner KB, et al. Fatigue in breast cancer survivors two to five years post diagnosis: a HEAL Study report. Qual Life Res. 2007;16(6):947–60.
174. Kim SH, Son BH, Hwang SY, Han W, Yang JH, Lee S, et al. Fatigue and depression in disease-free breast cancer survivors: prevalence, correlates, and association with quality of life. J Pain Symptom Manage. 2008;35(6):644–55.
175. Haghighat S, Akbari ME, Holakouei K, Rahimi A, Montazeri A. Factors predicting fatigue in breast cancer patients. Support Care Cancer. 2003;11(8):533–8.
176. Robb C, Haley WE, Balducci L, Extermann M, Perkins EA, Small BJ, et al. Impact of breast cancer survivorship on quality of life in older women. Crit Rev Oncol Hematol. 2007;62(1):84–91.
177. Mast ME. Correlates of fatigue in survivors of breast cancer. Cancer Nurs. 1998;21(2):136–42.
178. Woo B, Dibble SL, Piper BF, Keating SB, Weiss MC. Differences in fatigue by treatment methods in women with breast cancer. Oncol Nurs Forum. 1998;25(5):915–20.
179. Katz J, Poleshuck EL, Andrus CH, Hogan LA, Jung BF, Kulick DI, et al. Risk factors for acute pain and its persistence following breast cancer surgery. Pain. 2005;119(1–3):16–25.
180. Poleshuck EL, Katz J, Andrus CH, Hogan LA, Jung BF, Kulick DI, et al. Risk factors for chronic pain following breast cancer surgery: a prospective study. J Pain. 2006;7(9):626–34.

181. Sclafani LM, Baron RH. Sentinel lymph node biopsy and axillary dissection: added morbidity of the arm, shoulder and chest wall after mastectomy and reconstruction. Cancer J. 2008;14(4):216–22.
182. Steegers MA, Wolters B, Evers AW, Strobbe L, Wilder-Smith OH. Effect of axillary lymph node dissection on prevalence and intensity of chronic and phantom pain after breast cancer surgery. J Pain. 2008;9(9):813–22.
183. Carpenter JS, Andrykowski MA, Sloan P, Cunningham L, Cordova MJ, Studts JL, et al. Postmastectomy/postlumpectomy pain in breast cancer survivors. J Clin Epidemiol. 1998;51(12):1285–92.
184. Macdonald L, Bruce J, Scott NW, Smith WC, Chambers WA. Long-term follow-up of breast cancer survivors with post-mastectomy pain syndrome. Br J Cancer. 2005;92(2):225–30.
185. Smith WC, Bourne D, Squair J, Phillips DO, Chambers WA. A retrospective cohort study of post mastectomy pain syndrome. Pain. 1999;83(1):91–5.
186. Hayes SC, Janda M, Cornish B, Newman B. Lymphedema following breast cancer. J Clin Oncol. 2009;27(17):2890.
187. Hayes SC, Reul-Hirche H, Turner J. Exercise and secondary lymphedema: safety, potential benefits, and research issues. Med Sci Sports Exerc. 2009;41(3):483–9.
188. Ahmed RL, Prizment A, Lazovich D, Schmitz KH, Folsom AR. Lymphedema and quality of life in breast cancer survivors: the Iowa Women's Health Study. J Clin Oncol. 2008;26(35):5689–96.
189. Smoot B, Wong J, Cooper B, Wanek L, Topp K, Byl N, et al. Upper extremity impairments in women with or without lymphedema following breast cancer treatment. J Cancer Surviv. 2010;4(2):167–78.
190. Norman SA, Localio AR, Potashnik SL, Simoes Torpey HA, Kallan MJ, Weber AL, et al. Lymphedema in breast cancer survivors: incidence, degree, time course, treatment, and symptoms. J Clin Oncol. 2009;27(3):390–7.
191. Engel J, Kerr J, Schlesinger-Raab A, Sauer H, Holzel D. Axilla surgery severely affects quality of life: results of a 5-year prospective study in breast cancer patients. Breast Cancer Res Treat. 2003;79(1):47–57.
192. Armer JM, Stewart BR, Shook RP. 30-month post-breast cancer treatment lymphoedema. J Lymphoedema. 2009;4(1):14–8.
193. Tsai RJ, Dennis LK, Lynch CF, Snetselaar LG, Zamba GK, Scott-Conner C. The risk of developing arm lymphedema among breast cancer survivors: a meta-analysis of treatment factors. Ann Surg Oncol. 2009;16(7):1959–72.
194. Leidenius M, Leppanen E, Krogerus L, von Smitten K. Motion restriction and axillary web syndrome after sentinel node biopsy and axillary clearance in breast cancer. Am J Surg. 2003;185(2):127–30.
195. Johansson K, Branje E. Arm lymphoedema in a cohort of breast cancer survivors 10 years after diagnosis. Acta Oncol. 2010;49(2):166–73.
196. Schmitz KH, Ahmed RL, Troxel A, Cheville A, Smith R, Lewis-Grant L, et al. Weight lifting in women with breast-cancer-related lymphedema. N Engl J Med. 2009;361(7):664–73.
197. Goodwin PJ, Ennis M, Pritchard KI, Trudeau M, Hood N. Risk of menopause during the first year after breast cancer diagnosis. J Clin Oncol. 1999;17(8):2365–70.
198. Ganz PA. Breast cancer, menopause, and long-term survivorship: critical issues for the 21st century. Am J Med. 2005;118(Suppl 12B):136–41.
199. Andrykowski MA, Curran SL, Carpenter JS, Studts JL, Cunningham L, McGrath PC, et al. Rheumatoid symptoms following breast cancer treatment: a controlled comparison. J Pain Symptom Manage. 1999;18(2):85–94.
200. Yurek D, Farrar W, Andersen BL. Breast cancer surgery: comparing surgical groups and determining individual differences in postoperative sexuality and body change stress. J Consult Clin Psychol. 2000;68(4):697–709.
201. Ganz PA, Kwan L, Stanton AL, Krupnick JL, Rowland JH, Meyerowitz BE, et al. Quality of life at the end of primary treatment of breast cancer: first results from the moving beyond cancer randomized trial. J Natl Cancer Inst. 2004;96(5):376–87.

202. Fobair P, Stewart SL, Chang S, D'Onofrio C, Banks PJ, Bloom JR. Body image and sexual problems in young women with breast cancer. Psychooncology. 2006;15(7):579–94.
203. Arora NK, Gustafson DH, Hawkins RP, McTavish F, Cella DF, Pingree S, et al. Impact of surgery and chemotherapy on the quality of life of younger women with breast carcinoma: a prospective study. Cancer. 2001;92(5):1288–98.
204. Avis NE, Crawford S, Manuel J. Psychosocial problems among younger women with breast cancer. Psychooncology. 2004;13(5):295–308.
205. Eastell R, Adams JE, Coleman RE, Howell A, Hannon RA, Cuzick J, et al. Effect of anastrozole on bone mineral density: 5-year results from the anastrozole, tamoxifen, alone or in combination trial 18233230. J Clin Oncol. 2008;26(7):1051–7.
206. Eastell R, Hannon RA, Cuzick J, Dowsett M, Clack G, Adams JE. Effect of an aromatase inhibitor on bmd and bone turnover markers: 2-year results of the Anastrozole, Tamoxifen, Alone or in Combination (ATAC) trial (18233230). J Bone Miner Res. 2006;21(8):1215–23.
207. National Osteoporosis Foundation: Fast Facts. Available at http://www.nof.org/node/40. Last accessed on March 7, 2011.
208. Van Poznak C, Hannon RA, Mackey JR, Campone M, Apffelstaedt JP, Clack G, et al. Prevention of aromatase inhibitor-induced bone loss using risedronate: the SABRE trial. J Clin Oncol. 2010;28(6):967–75.
209. Presant CA, Bosserman L, Young T, Vakil M, Horns R, Upadhyaya G, et al. Aromatase inhibitor-associated arthralgia and/or bone pain: frequency and characterization in non-clinical trial patients. Clin Breast Cancer. 2007;7(10):775–8.
210. Fan HG, Houede-Tchen N, Yi QL, Chemerynsky I, Downie FP, Sabate K, et al. Fatigue, menopausal symptoms, and cognitive function in women after adjuvant chemotherapy for breast cancer: 1- and 2-year follow-up of a prospective controlled study. J Clin Oncol. 2005;23(31):8025–32.
211. Hurria A, Somlo G, Ahles T. Renaming "chemobrain". Cancer Investig. 2007;25(6):373–7.
212. Kornblith AB, Ligibel J. Psychosocial and sexual functioning of survivors of breast cancer. Semin Oncol. 2003;30(6):799–813.
213. Mols F, Vingerhoets AJ, Coebergh JW, van de Poll-Franse LV. Quality of life among long-term breast cancer survivors: a systematic review. Eur J Cancer. 2005;41(17):2613–9.
214. Maunsell E, Brisson J, Deschenes L. Psychological distress after initial treatment of breast cancer. Assessment of potential risk factors. Cancer. 1992;70(1):120–5.
215. Ganz PA, Lee JJ, Sim MS, Polinsky ML, Schag CA. Exploring the influence of multiple variables on the relationship of age to quality of life in women with breast cancer. J Clin Epidemiol. 1992;45(5):473–85.
216. Schag CA, Ganz PA, Polinsky ML, Fred C, Hirji K, Petersen L. Characteristics of women at risk for psychosocial distress in the year after breast cancer. J Clin Oncol. 1993;11(4):783–93.
217. Ganz PA, Hirji K, Sim MS, Schag CA, Fred C, Polinsky ML. Predicting psychosocial risk in patients with breast cancer. Med Care. 1993;31(5):419–31.
218. Hartl K, Janni W, Kastner R, Sommer H, Strobl B, Rack B, et al. Impact of medical and demographic factors on long-term quality of life and body image of breast cancer patients. Ann Oncol. 2003;14(7):1064–71.
219. King CR, Haberman M, Berry DL, Bush N, Butler L, Dow KH, et al. Quality of life and the cancer experience: the state-of-the-knowledge. Oncol Nurs Forum. 1997;24(1):27–41.
220. Ferrell BR, Grant M, Funk B, Otis-Green S, Garcia N. Quality of life in breast cancer. Part I: Physical and social well-being. Cancer Nurs. 1997;20(6):398–408.
221. Somerset W, Stout SC, Miller AH, Musselman D. Breast cancer and depression. Oncology (Williston Park). 2004;18(8):1021–34.
222. Penson DF, Litwin MS. The physical burden of prostate cancer. Urol Clin North Am. 2003;30(2):305–13.
223. Penson DF, Litwin MS. Quality of life after treatment for prostate cancer. Curr Urol Rep. 2003;4(3):185–95.

224. Sanda MG, Dunn RL, Michalski J, Sandler HM, Northouse L, Hembroff L, et al. Quality of life and satisfaction with outcome among prostate-cancer survivors. N Engl J Med. 2008;358(12):1250–61.
225. Penson DF, Litwin MS, Aaronson NK. Health related quality of life in men with prostate cancer. J Urol. 2003;169(5):1653–61.
226. Robinson JW, Moritz S, Fung T. Meta-analysis of rates of erectile function after treatment of localized prostate carcinoma. Int J Radiat Oncol Biol Phys. 2002;54(4):1063–8.
227. Krupski T, Petroni GR, Bissonette EA, Theodorescu D. Quality-of-life comparison of radical prostatectomy and interstitial brachytherapy in the treatment of clinically localized prostate cancer. Urology. 2000;55(5):736–42.
228. Stone P, Hardy J, Huddart R, A'Hern R, Richards M. Fatigue in patients with prostate cancer receiving hormone therapy. Eur J Cancer. 2000;36(9):1134–41.
229. Herr HW, O'Sullivan M. Quality of life of asymptomatic men with nonmetastatic prostate cancer on androgen deprivation therapy. J Urol. 2000;163(6):1743–6.
230. Monga U, Kerrigan AJ, Thornby J, Monga TN, Zimmermann KP. Longitudinal study of quality of life in patients with localized prostate cancer undergoing radiotherapy. J Rehabil Res Dev. 2005;42(3):391–9.
231. Kyrdalen AE, Dahl AA, Hernes E, Cvancarova M, Fossa SD. Fatigue in hormone-naive prostate cancer patients treated with radical prostatectomy or definitive radiotherapy. Prostate Cancer Prostatic Dis. 2010;13(2):144–50.
232. Sharifi N, Gulley JL, Dahut WL. Androgen deprivation therapy for prostate cancer. JAMA. 2005;294(2):238–44.
233. Taylor LG, Canfield SE, Du XL. Review of major adverse effects of androgen-deprivation therapy in men with prostate cancer. Cancer. 2009;115(11):2388–99.
234. Schwandt A, Garcia JA. Complications of androgen deprivation therapy in prostate cancer. Curr Opin Urol. 2009;19(3):322–6.
235. Daniell HW, Dunn SR, Ferguson DW, Lomas G, Niazi Z, Stratte PT. Progressive osteoporosis during androgen deprivation therapy for prostate cancer. J Urol. 2000;163(1):181–6.
236. Shahinian VB, Kuo YF, Freeman JL, Goodwin JS. Risk of fracture after androgen deprivation for prostate cancer. N Engl J Med. 2005;352(2):154–64.
237. Strum SB, McDermed JE, Scholz MC, Johnson H, Tisman G. Anaemia associated with androgen deprivation in patients with prostate cancer receiving combined hormone blockade. Br J Urol. 1997;79(6):933–41.
238. Lee H, McGovern K, Finkelstein JS, Smith MR. Changes in bone mineral density and body composition during initial and long-term gonadotropin-releasing hormone agonist treatment for prostate carcinoma. Cancer. 2005;104(8):1633–7.
239. Smith MR, O'Malley AJ, Keating NL. Gonadotrophin-releasing hormone agonists, diabetes and cardiovascular disease in men with prostate cancer: which metabolic syndrome? BJU Int. 2008;101(11):1335–6.
240. Keating NL, O'Malley AJ, Smith MR. Diabetes and cardiovascular disease during androgen deprivation therapy for prostate cancer. J Clin Oncol. 2006;24(27):4448–56.
241. Lage MJ, Barber BL, Markus RA. Association between androgen-deprivation therapy and incidence of diabetes among males with prostate cancer. Urology. 2007;70(6):1104–8.
242. Alibhai SM, Duong-Hua M, Sutradhar R, Fleshner NE, Warde P, Cheung AM, et al. Impact of androgen deprivation therapy on cardiovascular disease and diabetes. J Clin Oncol. 2009;27(21):3452–8.
243. Manne SL. Prostate cancer support and advocacy groups: their role for patients and family members. Semin Urol Oncol. 2002;20(1):45–54.
244. Mehta SS, Lubeck DP, Pasta DJ, Litwin MS. Fear of cancer recurrence in patients undergoing definitive treatment for prostate cancer: results from CaPSURE. J Urol. 2003;170(5):1931–3.
245. Billington A. Prostate cancer and its effect on sexuality. Community Nurse. 1998;4(10):33–4.
246. Moore KN, Estey A. The early post-operative concerns of men after radical prostatectomy. J Adv Nurs. 1999;29(5):1121–9.

247. Braslis KG, Santa-Cruz C, Brickman AL, Soloway MS. Quality of life 12 months after radical prostatectomy. Br J Urol. 1995;75(1):48–53.
248. Jonler M, Madsen FA, Rhodes PR, Sall M, Messing EM, Bruskewitz RC. A prospective study of quantification of urinary incontinence and quality of life in patients undergoing radical retropubic prostatectomy. Urology. 1996;48(3):433–40.
249. Lepore SJ, Helgeson VS, Eton DT, Schulz R. Improving quality of life in men with prostate cancer: a randomized controlled trial of group education interventions. Health Psychol. 2003;22(5):443–52.
250. Butler L, Downe-Wamboldt B, Marsh S, Bell D, Jarvi K. Behind the scenes: partners' perceptions of quality of life post radical prostatectomy. Urol Nurs. 2000;20(4):254–8.
251. Heyman EN, Rosner TT. Prostate cancer: an intimate view from patients and wives. Urol Nurs. 1996;16(2):37–44.
252. Engel J, Kerr J, Schlesinger-Raab A, Eckel R, Sauer H, Holzel D. Quality of life in rectal cancer patients: a four-year prospective study. Ann Surg. 2003;238(2):203–13.
253. Fucini C, Gattai R, Urena C, Bandettini L, Elbetti C. Quality of life among five-year survivors after treatment for very low rectal cancer with or without a permanent abdominal stoma. Ann Surg Oncol. 2008;15(4):1099–106.
254. Gosselink MP, Busschbach JJ, Dijkhuis CM, Stassen LP, Hop WC, Schouten WR. Quality of life after total mesorectal excision for rectal cancer. Colorectal Dis. 2006;8(1):15–22.
255. Borwell B. The psychosexual needs of stoma patients. Prof Nurse. 1997;12(4):250–5.
256. Hojo K, Vernava 3rd AM, Sugihara K, Katumata K. Preservation of urine voiding and sexual function after rectal cancer surgery. Dis Colon Rectum. 1991;34(7):532–9.
257. Hurny C, Holland J. Psychosocial sequelae of ostomies in cancer patients. CA Cancer J Clin. 1985;35(3):170–83.
258. Thomas C, Madden F, Jehu D. Psychological effects of stomas – I. Psychosocial morbidity one year after surgery. J Psychosom Res. 1987;31(3):311–6.
259. Krouse R, Grant M, Ferrell B, Dean G, Nelson R, Chu D. Quality of life outcomes in 599 cancer and non-cancer patients with colostomies. J Surg Res. 2007;138(1):79–87.
260. Krouse RS, Grant M, Wendel CS, Mohler MJ, Rawl SM, Baldwin CM, et al. A mixed-methods evaluation of health-related quality of life for male veterans with and without intestinal stomas. Dis Colon Rectum. 2007;50(12):2054–66.
261. Baldwin CM, Grant M, Wendel C, Rawl S, Schmidt CM, Ko C, et al. Influence of intestinal stoma on spiritual quality of life of U.S. veterans. J Holist Nurs. 2008;26(3):185–94.
262. Sprangers MA, Taal BG, Aaronson NK, te Velde A. Quality of life in colorectal cancer. Stoma vs. nonstoma patients. Dis Colon Rectum. 1995;38(4):361–9.
263. Pikarsky AJ, Belin B, Efron J, Weiss EG, Nogueras JJ, Wexner SD. Complications following formalin installation in the treatment of radiation induced proctitis. Int J Colorectal Dis. 2000;15(2):96–9.
264. Buchi K. Radiation proctitis: therapy and prognosis. JAMA. 1991;265(9):1180.
265. Bruheim K, Guren MG, Dahl AA, Skovlund E, Balteskard L, Carlsen E, et al. Sexual function in males after radiotherapy for rectal cancer. Int J Radiat Oncol Biol Phys. 2010;76(4):1012–7.
266. Baxter NN, Habermann EB, Tepper JE, Durham SB, Virnig BA. Risk of pelvic fractures in older women following pelvic irradiation. JAMA. 2005;294(20):2587–93.
267. Baxter NN, Hartman LK, Tepper JE, Ricciardi R, Durham SB, Virnig BA. Postoperative irradiation for rectal cancer increases the risk of small bowel obstruction after surgery. Ann Surg. 2007;245(4):553–9.
268. White CA, Hunt JC. Psychological factors in postoperative adjustment to stoma surgery. Ann R Coll Surg Engl. 1997;79(1):3–7.
269. Krouse RS, Herrinton LJ, Grant M, Wendel CS, Green SB, Mohler MJ, et al. Health-related quality of life among long-term rectal cancer survivors with an ostomy: manifestations by sex. J Clin Oncol. 2009;27(28):4664–70.
270. American Cancer Society. Hodgkin Disease. Available at http://www.cancer.org/acs/groups/cid/documents/webcontent/003105-pdf.pdf. Last accessed on March 7, 2011.

271. Schultz PN, Beck ML, Stava C, Vassilopoulou-Sellin R. Health profiles in 5836 long-term cancer survivors. Int J Cancer. 2003;104(4):488–95.
272. Arden-Close E, Pacey A, Eiser C. Health-related quality of life in survivors of lymphoma: a systematic review and methodological critique. Leuk Lymphoma. 2010;51(4):628–40.
273. King V, Constine LS, Clark D, Schwartz RG, Muhs AG, Henzler M, et al. Symptomatic coronary artery disease after mantle irradiation for Hodgkin's disease. Int J Radiat Oncol Biol Phys. 1996;36(4):881–9.
274. Lund MB, Ihlen H, Voss BM, Abrahamsen AF, Nome O, Kongerud J, et al. Increased risk of heart valve regurgitation after mediastinal radiation for Hodgkin's disease: an echocardiographic study. Heart. 1996;75(6):591–5.
275. Mauch PM, Kalish LA, Marcus KC, Shulman LN, Krill E, Tarbell NJ, et al. Long-term survival in Hodgkin's disease relative impact of mortality, second tumors, infection, and cardiovascular disease. Cancer J Sci Am. 1995;1(1):33–42.
276. Dores GM, Metayer C, Curtis RE, Lynch CF, Clarke EA, Glimelius B, et al. Second malignant neoplasms among long-term survivors of Hodgkin's disease: a population-based evaluation over 25 years. J Clin Oncol. 2002;20(16):3484–94.
277. Meattini I, Livi L, Saieva C, Marrazzo L, Rampini A, Iermano C, et al. Breast cancer following Hodgkin's disease: the experience of the university of Florence. Breast J. 2010;16(3):290–6.
278. Aleman BM, van Leeuwen FE. Are we improving the long-term burden of Hodgkin's lymphoma patients with modern treatment? Hematol Oncol Clin North Am. 2007;21(5):961–75.
279. Aleman BM, van den Belt-Dusebout AW, Klokman WJ, Van't Veer MB, Bartelink H, van Leeuwen FE. Long-term cause-specific mortality of patients treated for Hodgkin's disease. J Clin Oncol. 2003;21(18):3431–9.
280. Lee CK, Aeppli D, Nierengarten ME. The need for long-term surveillance for patients treated with curative radiotherapy for Hodgkin's disease: university of Minnesota experience. Int J Radiat Oncol Biol Phys. 2000;48(1):169–79.
281. Foss Abrahamsen A, Andersen A, Nome O, Jacobsen AB, Holte H, Foss Abrahamsen J, et al. Long-term risk of second malignancy after treatment of Hodgkin's disease: the influence of treatment, age and follow-up time. Ann Oncol. 2002;13(11):1786–91.
282. Tinger A, Wasserman TH, Klein EE, Miller EA, Roberts T, Piephoff JV, et al. The incidence of breast cancer following mantle field radiation therapy as a function of dose and technique. Int J Radiat Oncol Biol Phys. 1997;37(4):865–70.
283. Swerdlow AJ, Barber JA, Hudson GV, Cunningham D, Gupta RK, Hancock BW, et al. Risk of second malignancy after Hodgkin's disease in a collaborative British cohort: the relation to age at treatment. J Clin Oncol. 2000;18(3):498–509.
284. Tucker MA, Coleman CN, Cox RS, Varghese A, Rosenberg SA. Risk of second cancers after treatment for Hodgkin's disease. N Engl J Med. 1988;318(2):76–81.
285. Cellai E, Magrini SM, Masala G, Alterini R, Costantini AS, Rigacci L, et al. The risk of second malignant tumors and its consequences for the overall survival of Hodgkin's disease patients and for the choice of their treatment at presentation: analysis of a series of 1524 cases consecutively treated at the Florence University Hospital. Int J Radiat Oncol Biol Phys. 2001;49(5):1327–37.
286. Hill DA, Gilbert E, Dores GM, Gospodarowicz M, van Leeuwen FE, Holowaty E, et al. Breast cancer risk following radiotherapy for Hodgkin lymphoma: modification by other risk factors. Blood. 2005;106(10):3358–65.
287. van Leeuwen FE, Klokman WJ, Stovall M, Dahler EC, van't Veer MB, Noordijk EM, et al. Roles of radiation dose, chemotherapy, and hormonal factors in breast cancer following Hodgkin's disease. J Natl Cancer Inst. 2003;95(13):971–80.
288. M'Kacher R, Girinsky T, Koscielny S, Dossou J, Violot D, Béron-Gaillard N, et al. Baseline and treatment-induced chromosomal abnormalities in peripheral blood lymphocytes of Hodgkin's lymphoma patients. Int J Radiat Oncol Biol Phys. 2003;57(2):321–6.
289. Metayer C, Lynch CF, Clarke EA, Glimelius B, Storm H, Pukkala E, et al. Second cancers among long-term survivors of Hodgkin's disease diagnosed in childhood and adolescence. J Clin Oncol. 2000;18(12):2435–43.

290. Ng AK, Bernardo MP, Weller E, Backstrand KH, Silver B, Marcus KC, et al. Long-term survival and competing causes of death in patients with early-stage Hodgkin's disease treated at age 50 or younger. J Clin Oncol. 2002;20(8):2101–8.
291. Travis LB, Hill D, Dores GM, Gospodarowicz M, van Leeuwen FE, Holowaty E, et al. Cumulative absolute breast cancer risk for young women treated for Hodgkin lymphoma. J Natl Cancer Inst. 2005;97(19):1428–37.
292. Bhatia S, Robison LL, Oberlin O, Greenberg M, Bunin G, Fossati-Bellani F, et al. Breast cancer and other second neoplasms after childhood Hodgkin's disease. N Engl J Med. 1996;334(12):745–51.
293. Sklar C. Maintenance of ovarian function and risk of premature menopause related to cancer treatment. J Natl Cancer Inst Monogr. 2005;34:25–7.
294. Sklar C, Whitton J, Mertens A, Stovall M, Green D, Marina N, et al. Abnormalities of the thyroid in survivors of Hodgkin's disease: data from the Childhood Cancer Survivor Study. J Clin Endocrinol Metab. 2000;85(9):3227–32.
295. Khoo VS, Liew KH, Crennan EC, D'Costa IM, Quong G. Thyroid dysfunction after mantle irradiation of Hodgkin's disease patients. Australas Radiol. 1998;42(1):52–7.
296. Zebrack BJ, Zeltzer LK, Whitton J, Mertens AC, Odom L, Berkow R, et al. Psychological outcomes in long-term survivors of childhood leukemia, Hodgkin's disease, and non-Hodgkin's lymphoma: a report from the Childhood Cancer Survivor Study. Pediatrics. 2002;110 (1 Pt 1):42–52.
297. Smith SK, Zimmerman S, Williams CS, Preisser JS, Clipp EC. Post-traumatic stress outcomes in non-Hodgkin's lymphoma survivors. J Clin Oncol. 2008;26(6):934–41.
298. United States Department of Veterans Affairs, National Center for Posttraumatic Stress Disorder: How Common is PTSD? Available at http://www.ptsd.va.gov/public/pages/how-common-is-ptsd.asp. Last accessed on March 7, 2011.
299. Hewitt M, Greenfield S, Stovall E, editors. From cancer patient to cancer survivor: lost in transition. Washington, DC: National Academy Press; 2005.
300. Lyne ME, Coyne PJ, Watson AC. Pain management issues for cancer survivors. Cancer Pract. 2002;10 Suppl 1:S27–32.
301. National Cancer Institute. Cancer care outcomes research and surveillance consortium. http://healthservices.cancer.gov/cancors/ (2010). Last assessed 4 May 2010.

# Chapter 4
# Health Behaviors and Wellness

**Robyn Osborn, Tricia L. Psota, Jaesin Sa, and Tracy Sbrocco**

## Introduction

Optimizing the health and quality of life for people who have survived cancer requires a continuing focus on health promotion and behavior change to reduce behavioral health risks. A focus on optimizing health behavior is critical for people surviving cancer because they are at increased risk for the development of chronic health conditions. Some of these conditions may develop from previous cancer therapy, called late effects, and include effects on the cardiovascular, respiratory, and endocrine systems [1–8]. Recurrence of primary cancers or the development of secondary cancers, are also of concern. In addition, survivors are vulnerable to preexisting risk factors such as older age, preexisting comorbidities, genetic risks, as well as behavioral and lifestyle factors [9, 10].

Behavior change is difficult for almost all of us. It is important to acknowledge this as we work with patients to assist them and support them in the difficult task of optimizing their health. Aspects of behavior change may be particularly difficult for people surviving cancer. For example, staying physically active may be extra challenging for someone whose is experiencing fatigue or has cardiorespiratory changes as the result of late effects. Compounding these difficulties, behavior change can be even more difficult for certain segments of our population, those from certain racial/ethnic and socioeconomic groups. In this chapter, we describe the key behavioral risk factors; smoking, nutrition, and exercise, that are important to attend to among those who have survived cancer. In addition, we provide specific patient-focused strategies to encourage behavior change with this population.

In addition to risk of recurrence, cancer survivors are at greater risk for developing numerous health complications and chronic diseases, specifically second malignancies, cardiovascular disease, diabetes, and osteoporosis [1–8], many of which are related to lifestyle and behavioral factors.

R. Osborn (✉)
Center for Health Disparities, Department Medical and Clinical Psychology, Uniformed Services University of Health Sciences, 4301 Jones Bridge Road B-1022, Bethesda, MD 20814, USA
e-mail: rosborn@usuhs.mil

M. Feuerstein and P.A. Ganz (eds.), *Health Services for Cancer Survivors*,
DOI 10.1007/978-1-4419-1348-7_4, 

## *Decreasing Modifiable Risk Behavior for Cancer*

While the influence of genetics on cancer risk is well-established, most of the variation in cancer risk across populations and among individuals is due to modifiable factors [11]. In particular, the behavioral factors of cigarette smoking, being physically active, and consuming foods from a certain dietary pattern can substantially affect one's cancer risk. A recent survey of over 32,000 cancer survivors revealed high rates of behavioral risk factors across all types of cancers, including poor diet (e.g., high fat, low fiber, few fruits and vegetables), current body mass index (BMI) $\geq 25$ kg/m$^2$, limited amounts of physical activity, and current smoking behavior [12]. In addition, the prevalence of these health behaviors varies across racial and ethnic groups.

According to the 2008 National Health Interview Survey [13], a multipurpose health survey conducted annually by the Centers for Disease Control and Prevention, the prevalence of adult cigarette smoking was highest for American Indians and Alaska Natives (23%), followed by Whites (21%), African Americans (21%), and Asians (10%) when results are considered by single race without regard to ethnicity. In terms of alcohol drinking status, the prevalence of adult alcohol use was highest for non-Hispanic Whites (56%), followed by Hispanics (42%) and non-Hispanic African Americans (37%) when results are considered by race and ethnicity. Asians were more likely to be lifetime abstainers than other racial/ethnic groups. With regard to the prevalence of leisure-time physical activity among adults, non-Hispanic Whites were more active than Hispanics or non-Hispanic African Americans when all leisure-time physical activity is considered by ethnicity. Accordingly, the prevalence of obesity is highest among non-Hispanic black men (37%) and women (50%) and lowest among non-Hispanic white men (32%) and women (33%) [14]. Body weight differences between ethnic and racial groups also may be attributed to dietary intake and food accessibility which also varies by racial and socioeconomic status [15, 16].

In addition to the sequelae of cancer treatments, high rates of behavioral risk factors among cancer survivors may contribute to higher reports of poor health and disability compared to noncancer survivors [17]. Furthermore, certain subgroups of cancer survivors are at increased risk of problems following diagnosis and treatment which parallels disparities among racial and ethnic groups for these risk factors. For example, African Americans/Blacks suffer the greatest burden in terms of incidence and death from the most common types of cancer [18]. And, as Deimling and colleagues have reported, African-American survivors have poorer functional health/physical functioning following cancer, as well as higher comorbidities [19]. Moreover, minority patients are less likely to express worry and distress following cancer, which may make them less likely to seek medical attention for new symptoms or to stay in touch with their health-care provider [20].

Interventions targeting dietary intake, activity level, maintenance of a healthy body weight, and smoking cessation have been successful in promoting lifestyle modifications which decrease cancer risk and improve health outcomes of cancer survivors.

Although recently diagnosed cancer survivors tend to be highly motivated toward improving their lifestyle behaviors, research indicates that the health behaviors of long-term cancer survivors are more similar to the general population than once thought [12]. Therefore, it is essential that those involved in cancer-survivor health care encourage long-term behavior change and reinforce healthy lifestyle factors over time. In addition, discussions of self-monitoring and behavior change principles may have particular relevance to this population as a means of improving outcomes following treatment.

## Health Behaviors of Cancer Survivors

Nearly two-thirds of cancer deaths that occur in the USA are attributable to tobacco use, unhealthy diet, physical activity habits, and alcohol consumption [21–23].

### *Tobacco Use*

Tobacco is one of the strongest cancer-promoting agents, accounting for at least 30% of all cancer deaths in the USA [21, 24, 25]. Smoking is responsible for about 90% of lung cancer deaths among men and approximately 80% of lung cancer deaths among women [25]. In addition to lung cancer, smokers are at greater risk of other types of cancer including cancers of the mouth, lips, nasal cavity (nose) and sinuses, larynx (voice box), pharynx (throat), esophagus (swallowing tube), stomach, pancreas, kidney, bladder, uterine cervix, and acute myeloid leukemia [21].

According to the National Cancer Institute [26], a significant number of people with a cancer history keep smoking after experiencing cancer. A randomized control trial investigated the impact of a peer-delivered smoking cessation intervention on smoking among childhood cancer survivors and found that the quit rate of a peer-delivered smoking counseling group was significantly higher than that of a self-help group [27]. Given the result of the randomized control trial, consideration needs to be directed toward adoption of interventions for cancer survivors that involve increasing peer support to help cancer survivors quit smoking and increase perceptions of risk for cancer recurrence or new cancers [26–28].

### *Physical Activity*

Various studies have demonstrated that physical activity not only helps cancer survivors improve cardiovascular fitness, muscle strength [29–31], physical functioning [32, 33], body image [34], and quality of life [35], but it also helps them decrease body fat [31, 36] and reduce fatigue [30, 31]. A meta-analysis examined efficacy of physical activity interventions in cancer survivors by calculating effect sizes (i.e., standardized mean differences between an intervention group and a control group) of each intervention [37]. In the review, effect sizes were interpreted using the criteria developed by Cohen [38]. The review showed a moderate effect of physical activity programs on cardiorespiratory fitness after cancer treatment (mean effect size = 0.65, $p < 0.01$).

## *Nutrition*

Currently, the two key nutritional concerns recognized among cancer survivors are diet composition and relative body weight. Although an established evidence base exists describing the relationships between different dietary components and cancer risk, research exploring weight management among cancer patients and survivors is on the rise.

### Diet Composition

Numerous epidemiological studies have investigated the associations of individual nutrients, foods, food groups, or dietary patterns with cancer risk. Overall, high intakes of fiber, folate, vitamin D, fruits and vegetables, legumes, and whole grains tend to be protective against cancer [39–44]; while greater intakes of total energy, saturated fat, *trans* fat, red meat, processed meat, and alcohol increase cancer risk [45–49]. Current research indicates that diets high in a specific nutrient and/or food considered protective against cancer typically are high in other nutrients and foods associated with decreased cancer risk; while the same is true for those associated with increasing cancer risk. For example, a greater intake of fruits and vegetables is associated with higher intakes of fiber, folate, calcium, and vitamin D, and lower intakes of alcohol and red meat [50]. Furthermore, these established dietary patterns are indicative of one's risk for cancer [51, 52]. In particular, a "healthy" dietary pattern, consisting of high intakes of fruits, vegetables, whole grains, low-fat dairy products, fish, poultry, olive oil, and/or legumes, is associated with decreased cancer risk. While a "meat and potatoes" diet, consisting of greater intakes of animal fat and meat, in particular high-fat processed meat, along with preferential consumption of potatoes over other vegetables, high-sugar, and high-fat food items such as fast food, pizza, and desserts, and refined grain products, increases one's risk for cancer.

While there is great interest in the effects of a variety of nutrients, food components, and foods (e.g., antioxidants, phytochemicals, coffee, tea, and soy products) on cancer risk, more research is needed to determine these relationships [22, 53]. One area of oncology nutrition that is of particular interest is vitamin and mineral supplement use among cancer patients and survivors.

Findings indicate that 50-85% of cancer survivors use dietary supplements and that 78% of supplement users take more than one supplement [54, 55]. However, at this time there is no evidence to suggest that supplements can reduce cancer risk. In addition, caution regarding supplement use in cancer patients and survivors is warranted due to their potential effects on existing cancers, effects on factors that may influence carcinogenesis, and their interactions with cancer treatment, specifically chemotherapy and radiation [53].

## Weight Management

Historically, under-nutrition and cancer-related cachexia, due to appetite loss and inadequate food intake, were the primary nutritional concerns in regards to cancer. While these issues remain important for survivors of gastrointestinal, lung, and head and neck cancers, excess body weight is the main nutritional concern facing most cancer patients and survivors today [22]. Being overweight or obese is proposed to increase cancer risk through an array of mechanisms altering nutrient metabolism, immune function, hormone production and action, and cell proliferation and growth [22]. Excess body weight not only increases risk for developing many cancers (e.g., breast, colon, and kidney [56]), obesity significantly increases risk for cancer mortality (relative risks: 1.15–1.61; $p$-values $\leq 0.05$) [57–62]. In addition, being overweight or obese at cancer diagnosis is associated with significantly worse disease-specific outcomes and poorer overall health outcomes [63, 64]. Another issue contributing to the challenge of weight management amongst cancer patients and survivors is weight gain during and after treatment. A substantial portion of cancer patients are overweight or obese at diagnosis and the prevalence of excess body weight during treatment and remission is of particular concern in regards to certain cancers [65]. Weight gain during these times is attributed to some forms of treatment and also to physical inactivity as a result of treatment-related fatigue and weakness [61, 66].

Due to the adverse effects of being overweight or obese on cancer survival, general health outcomes, and quality of life, weight management is a priority for cancer survivors [22, 56, 66–68]. Ongoing behavioral interventions targeting lifestyle factors which affect weight management, specifically nutrition and physical activity, are of great interest. To date the majority of oncology nutrition research studies among cancer survivors have focused on targeting dietary factors associated with decreased cancer risk – caloric and fat restriction and/or primarily plant-based diets [69–77]. The most successful dietary interventions among cancer survivors have utilized intensive, individualized dietary counseling by dietitians, opposed to less rigorous intervention and/or group counseling, to promote dietary change and improvements in biomarkers of chronic disease (e.g., serum lipids) and body weight [73, 77, 78].

The most effective approach to achieving energy balance is through diet and exercise together rather than either component alone [79–82]. Accumulating evidence suggests that exercise is a strong predictor of weight loss among cancer survivors and thus is an important aspect of weight management programs [56, 61]. Furthermore, recent findings demonstrate that physical activity, dietary behaviors, and overall quality of life increased significantly among older, overweight long-term cancer survivors receiving a diet and exercise intervention compared with the control group ($p$-values $\leq 0.001$) [83]. These improvements were associated with a decreased rate of self-reported functional decline. Accordingly, the current American Cancer Society (ACS)'s guidelines to decrease cancer incidence and mortality and to improve the quality of life of cancer survivors focus on dietary and physical activity patterns among Americans [22].

### *Alcohol Consumption*

Alcohol consumption increases the chances of developing cancers of the mouth, pharynx, larynx, esophagus, liver, and breast [21, 24, 84, 85]. The combination of alcohol consumption and smoking is associated with an increased risk of cancers of the mouth, larynx, and esophagus even more than either drinking or smoking alone [21].

## Practical Behavior Change Strategies

Educating survivors about the risk of maintaining unhealthy behaviors is important; however, helping them achieve behavior change can be challenging due to time constraints and uncertainty about the best strategies to assist with these changes [86]. Moreover, such behaviors may be unintentionally overlooked among survivors because they do not carry the same sense of urgency associated with a diagnosis of cancer, or may seem less relevant for individuals with advanced stage cancer or for whom immediate treatment and care remains crucial. However, it has become increasingly clear that changes in behavioral risk factors affect cancer-related and noncancer-related morbidity and mortality, mood, and quality of life of survivors and, therefore, should be targeted by primary care providers, oncologists, nurse practioners, psychologists, and others who work with this ever-growing population.

### *Three Guiding Principles*

When working with cancer survivors on behavior change, providers must be aware that patients may or may not be ready to change [87]. Survivors may prefer and be more responsive to education regarding the benefits of lifestyle change as it fits within his/her individual health profile. Still, others may benefit from their providers encouraging them to make changes. As such, providers may benefit from developing strategies for assisting patients with behavior change if referral to a behavior change expert (i.e., health psychologist) is not possible or unacceptable to the patient.

A few basic premises must be considered in the context of working with survivors on behavior change. First, social support is critical in helping them achieve behavior change [88]. Many patients experience a deluge of support after initial diagnosis, but this high level of support tends to diminish over time [89]. Therefore, providers should encourage survivors to talk directly with family members, friends, and colleagues about his/her concerns not just during the initial stages of diagnosis and treatment but well into the years of survivorship that follow [89].

Second, many cancer survivors continue to experience cancer-related distress and worry long after treatment has ended [90]. Such distress and worry are likely to impact efforts at health behavior change and have been linked to more serious mental health conditions, including clinical depression and anxiety [90]. Screening for distress, however, has become easier with the development of several brief (<5 questions) questionnaires which can be used as initial screening tools. Such tools are a valid means of assessing distress among survivors [91]. Use of such methods, including the Distress Thermometer, which asks patients to indicate his/her level of distress using a visual scale ranging from 0 to 10 along a drawing of a thermometer, may facilitate discussion and offer opportunities for patients to be triaged to other services (e.g., mental health providers, support groups) if needed [92]. Providers can access the National Comprehensive Cancer Network (http://www.nccn.org) for specific information and guidelines on using such tools with cancer survivors.

Finally, making health behavior changes such as healthful eating, exercising more, and smoking cessation are hard for all people, not just cancer survivors. Helping patients prioritize their goals can help reduce anxiety associated with change and can increase the chances of success. Survivors should not be asked to undertake numerous health behavior changes at one time. Providers can empower survivors in their process of change by helping them identify one area they feel most confident in changing [86] (e.g., exercise 3 days/week) rather than bombarding them with a litany of changes they "should" make (e.g., exercise 3 days/week, quit smoking, increase fruit and vegetable consumption, reduce fat consumption).

## *The Five A's*

There are several methods available to assist providers in talking with their patients about behavior change. One method that has been suggested [12, 93] to assist providers in understanding cancer survivors goals and abilities for behavior change is to use the "5 A's," which were initially developed for the purposes of smoking cessation [94].

> The "5 A's" include *Ask*, *Advise*, *Assess*, *Assist*, and *Arrange*.

### Ask

Asking patients about their current health behaviors and about their desire or preferences to make behavior change is a key place to start a discussion. Questions should be targeted, rather than vague, and can begin with an acknowledgment that behavior change is difficult.

"Many of the patients I work with have trouble exercising consistently; do you find this challenging as well?"

"Have you been considering exercising more/quitting smoking/eating more fruits and vegetables to improve your health? Have you already been trying? Which of these changes do you think you would like to start with?"

### Advise

After learning about your patient's current behavior and/or goals for change, provide concrete information and specific recommendations. While simple advice giving is a common, yet often ineffective, communication style among health-care providers [86], there is room for the provision of information in a supportive, nonjudgmental, targeted manner. Vague statements such as "You should increase your exercise" are less helpful than statements that directly relate to the patient's area of need and provide information based on identified sources. Providing information without telling patients what you think they "should" do can reduce resistance because it relies less on persuasion and more on information exchange [86].

"You said you would like to increase your activity. The American College of Sports Medicine currently recommends exercising 30 minutes five days/week or vigorous-intensity aerobic physical activity for a at least 20 minutes three days/week [95]."

### Assess/Agree

Assessing how important behavior change is to your patient, along with how confident he or she feels about making the change can lead to enhanced likelihood of change [86]. If a survivor describes interest in increasing exercise and you have provided information on the current recommendations, yet you discover that he or she has little confidence in his or her ability to make this change, then your intervention will have to change. It will not be very helpful to spend time assisting in change or arranging for follow-up if the patient has low confidence in his or her ability to change or feels that change is unimportant. If a patient does not feel confident in making change, then try to determine why his or her confidence is low. For example, he or she may not have access to a gym or may not know how to use gym equipment. Finding out these types of barriers to change can provide the opportunity to problem solve (e.g., educate patient that a walking program can be an effective exercise routine that does not require a gym membership).

"How confident do you feel that you could make these changes that we have discussed today, on a scale of 1–10 where 10 is very confident?"

"We have discussed many important things today, and I know you are still working on managing some health concerns related to your cancer treatment. I am curious how important it is to you right now to make changes in your exercise routine?"

If, on the other hand, you determine that making a change is not very important to your patient, you can begin to explore importance [86]. At this point, it is important to keep in mind that the goal of an interaction can vary depending on the patient. It may be enough to just get the patient *thinking* about change, rather than starting change immediately [86]. You may explore change by asking questions such as "What would have to happen for it to become more important to you?"

If you have determined both that behavior change is important to the patient and he or she feels confident that he or she could attempt to make a change, then you can agree on some specifics. This is the *Who*, *What*, *Where*, *When* of behavior change. Help the patient identify a specific time, place, and activity they will complete. Being specific about these details is important. For example, as a health-care provider, one would never say "take some of this medication at some point during the day." Rather, providers use specific details, such as "take 1 pill when you wake up in the morning and 1 pill at night before bed." Being specific about behavior change is just as important. Rather than saying "get more exercise," it will likely be more effective for a provider to work with the patient to identify the details of the new exercise routine which might end with a statement like "Great! So your plan is to exercise 3 times per week by walking for 30-minutes during your lunch break at work."

### Assist

Survivors will likely need assistance while making behavior changes. This assistance can be something as simple as helping them problem solve barriers to their behavior change. For example, providers can model brainstorming, trying out solutions and assessing how those solutions worked. In a recent pilot study, nearly 90% of cancer survivors rated a problem-solving intervention as very or somewhat helpful [96].

### Arrange

Arrange for a follow-up visit or for additional services that may help your patient make the changes he or she has identified. Use the follow-up visits to check in on the patient's progress toward goals. Even a phone call or email to check in with the patient in the days following the initial appointment can provide valuable support and the opportunity to problem solve should the patient be in need. In addition to support, the accountability provided by regular follow-up visits can provide additional support as patients attempt to make behavior change.

## *Tackling Common Obstacles to Change*

Below are some common questions/statements that providers may hear when discussing the importance of behavior change their patients. In addition to the difficulties experienced by most individuals in adopting behavior change, people surviving cancer may have a unique psychological "mindset" along with physical or cognitive limitations that serve as obstacles to behavior change. The descriptions that follow could apply to changes in diet, exercise, smoking, or other important health behaviors. We have provided some sample strategies that may facilitate open and honest discussions between patients and providers to assist patients as they work toward change.

### "Why Bother?"

When a survivor responds to a provider's advice to change behavior with a sentiment like "why bother?" they may be experiencing some level of hopelessness toward the future. They may be thinking, "I have already had cancer, so what difference would it make if I quit smoking/started exercising/changed my diet, etc.?" Understanding the beliefs underlying this thought is critical. For example, they may have a belief and a fear that their cancer will recur (or was not fully treated) and that they will soon become ill again. As such, they may think that any health improvements gained from these difficult behavior changes are not worth the effort. They also could be communicating a belief that changing their behavior is unimportant or too difficult to try. Using the five A's to address this question may look like this:

*Ask*: "There are so many things to think about during this phase of your cancer treatment. I am wondering if there is a particular area you have been thinking you would like to change? Many survivors worry that efforts to exercise/improve nutrition may be not be worthwhile, perhaps because they worry it won't make much of a difference. I am wondering if you are having any of these thoughts or concerns?"

*Advise*: "It definitely takes a lot of work to make these changes and I know how hard it can be. The current guidelines for increasing your exercise suggest exercising 30 minutes a day five days a week."

*Assess/Agree*: "Those recommended guidelines I just gave you may sound like quite a bit of work! Given those recommendations, I wonder how confident you feel that you could start taking some steps towards reaching those guidelines, on a scale from 1–10, where 1 is not confident at all and 10 is very confident?" "Do you think you could start walking a few times a week for 15–20 minutes, until you feel stronger and ready to increase the intensity and frequency of your activity?" "Would it seem possible to walk for 15 minutes around your neighborhood in the morning on Mondays, Wednesdays, and Fridays?"

*Assist*: "We just came up with a plan to increase your level of activity, but I am wondering if you can see anything that might get in the way of you being able to follow through with our plan, such as not feeling safe walking alone in your neighborhood?" "I am thinking of a few ideas to get around that issue, like walking inside your local mall, or asking a friend to join you. Do those sound possible? Let's try one or two of those options this week."

*Arrange*: "Myself or someone from my office will give you a call in a few days to check in on your progress. And before you leave, how about scheduling a follow-up appointment in two or three weeks so we can check in and see how it is going?"

## "It Is in God's Hands. There Is Nothing I Can Do"

Spirituality can affect health behaviors in many ways [97]. Spiritual beliefs regarding health and health behaviors have been described as either an active approach to health care where God (or a higher power) is considered to empower an individual to take healthy actions or a more passive approach, where an individual relies on God to protect or maintain his/her health [98]. When God is seen from this passive perspective, such when patients consider caring for their health by "turning it over to the Lord [99] providers face particularly difficult challenges."

At such times, it is important to consider spirituality or religiosity can provide patients with strength to deal with daily challenges and stressors, including those associated with cancer or health behavior change. Thus, reliance on spirituality can be seen as a positive source of emotional support. Importantly, many places of worship (e.g., churches, temples, mosques) have identified health ministries which can be a source of additional support and follow-up for patients who regularly attend such for prayer or worship [100]. Such places also may provide instrumental social support, such as child care and transportation which can come in handy during doctors' appointments or follow-up care [100]. Some churches have even begun incorporating exercise programs into their weekly services [101]. And, data show that weight loss programs delivered in church settings have been met with success [102]. With certain patients, like those who may have a strong religious belief and/or find comfort in their church or religious community, providers can view places of worship as a partner in health care. Use of the 5 A's to address this issue may look like this:

*Ask*: "Some of my patients turn to religion or spirituality in times of stress. Cancer diagnosis and survivorship can be very stressful and may seem overwhelming at times. I wonder if religion/spirituality is important to you during your treatment and recovery?"

*Advise*: "I am aware that many churches or places of worship have health ministries and may provide emotional and physical or instrumental support to individuals in need. Contacting your church or place of worship to learn about what options may be available to you might be helpful."

*Assess/Agree*: "There are many ways to view religion or spirituality in regards to making health changes. Sometimes when people feel overwhelmed, they may be tempted to leave their health in God's (or higher power) hands, as you have said. I can tell your faith is important to you and I wonder if you think it would be possible to view religion as providing support to you as you make health behavior changes?"

*Assist*: "It seems you regularly attend church on the weekends, and you feel that your connection to the church is quite valuable. Could you contact your church to find out if there is a walking group or exercise class being offered that you might be able to join? Or, perhaps you could speak to your pastor or spiritual leader, other congregants or members, or health ministry to get some options and ideas on how to involve your church family in your steps toward better health. For example, perhaps you could ask to bring fruit to the church picnic this year so that you can count on having some health options available. I bet you are not the only church member who would like to make important health changes!"

*Arrange*: "Next time you are here, let's discuss how your religion has helped you make these important health behavior changes we have discussed today."

Although many patients may practice religion and have deep spiritual beliefs, African Americans are a patient population for whom the influence of spirituality on health and health behaviors may be underestimated [99] and should be considered a focus for health-care providers [103].

## Specific Recommendations for Health Behaviors

Substantial and consistent evidence demonstrates that the risk of cancer can be significantly reduced by increasing physical activity, adopting physically active lifestyles, eating healthy foods, not using tobacco, and abstaining from or limiting consumption of alcohol [22, 104, 105].

### *Tobacco and Alcohol Use*

Kushi and colleagues [22] recommend that cancer survivors avoid tobacco use and environmental tobacco smoke to reduce the risk of new cancers. In regard to alcohol consumption, one drink is defined as consuming 12 oz of beer, 5 oz of wine, or 1.5 oz of hard liquor [22]. The ACS [21] recommends that cancer survivors limit their alcohol consumption to no more than two drinks per day for men and one drink per day for women. Cancer survivors at increased risk for cancer recurrence or new cancers may consider abstaining from alcohol [22].

## Physical Activity

Kushi and colleagues [22] summarized the ACS guidelines on physical activity for cancer prevention and cancer recurrence:

- Adults: engage in at least 30 min of moderate to vigorous physical activity, above usual activities, on 5 or more days of the week. Forty-five to sixty minutes of intentional physical activity are preferable.
- Children and adolescents: engage in at least 60 min/day of moderate to vigorous physical activity at least 5 days/week.

The following examples of moderate and vigorous activities are provided by Kushi and colleagues [22] (Table 4.1), along with ways to reduce sedentary behavior (Table 4.2).

## Nutrition

A strong evidence base indicates that consuming a dietary pattern consistent with our current national nutrition guidelines, the *Dietary Guidelines for Americans* [106], is important for cancer prevention. Therefore, the ACS [22] and the World Cancer Research Fund (WCRF) in collaboration with American Institute for Cancer Research (AICR) [56] have issued dietary recommendations for cancer prevention. In contrast, specific dietary advice for secondary cancer prevention and reoccurrence are lacking. Thus, cancer survivors are advised to follow the nutrition

**Table 4.1** Examples of moderate and vigorous intensity physical activities (From Kushi et al. [22]. Copyright John Wiley and Sons. With kind permission)

| | Moderate intensity activities | Vigorous intensity activities |
|---|---|---|
| Exercise and leisure | Walking, dancing, leisurely bicycling, ice skating, roller skating, horseback riding, canoeing, and yoga | Jogging or running, fast bicycling, circuit weight training, aerobic dance, martial arts, jumping rope, and swimming |
| Sports | Volleyball, golfing, softball, baseball, badminton, doubles tennis, and downhill skiing | Soccer, field or ice hockey, lacrosse, singles tennis, racquetball, basketball, and cross-country skiing |
| Home activities | Mowing the lawn, general lawn and garden maintenance | Digging, carrying, masonry, and carpentry |
| Occupational activities | Walking and lifting as part of the job (custodial work, farming, and auto or machine repair) | Heavy manual labor (forestry, construction work, and fire fighting) |

**Table 4.2** American Cancer Society suggestions for reducing sedentary behavior (From Kushi et al. [22]. Copyright John Wiley and Sons. With kind permission)

- Use stairs rather than an elevator.
- If you can, walk or bike to your destination.
- Exercise at lunch with your coworkers, family, or friends.
- Take a 10-min exercise break at work to stretch or take a quick walk.
- Walk to visit coworkers instead of sending an email message.
- Go dancing with your spouse or friends.
- Plan active vacations rather than only driving trips.
- Wear a pedometer every day and watch your daily steps increase.
- Join a sports team.
- Use a stationary bicycle while watching TV.
- Plan your exercise routine to gradually increase the days per week and minutes per session.
- Spend time playing with your kids.

recommendations for cancer prevention which are consistent with our national nutrition guidelines for chronic disease prevention established for the general population [106].

The ACS Guidelines on Nutrition and Physical Activity for Cancer Prevention and the WCRF/AICR Food, Nutrition, Physical Activity, and Cancer Prevention report share many commonalities. Both sets of dietary recommendations encourage consuming a healthy diet with an emphasis on plant sources and choosing foods and beverages in amounts that help achieve and maintain a healthy weight. In addition, individuals are advised to limit intake of red meat, processed meat, and alcoholic drinks [22, 56].

For cancer patients and survivors who are underweight, weakness, fatigue, inferior quality of life, and poorer outcomes are the primary issues [107, 108]. Therefore, the goals of nutrition care for these individuals are to achieve a healthy body weight through positive energy balance, prevent or reverse nutrient deficiencies, preserve lean body mass, and minimize nutrition-related side effects (e.g., nausea, vomiting, swallowing issues, and changes in taste, smell, and oral mucosa function) [65, 109]. For underweight cancer patients and survivors, the ACS recommends consuming energy-dense foods that are easy to chew and swallow and mild in flavor [66].

For cancer patients and survivors who are overweight and obese, current guidelines advocate for moderate weight loss of 1–2 lb/week accomplished through decreasing caloric intake and increasing physical activity upon oncologist approval [22, 66]. To reduce caloric intake, the primary nutrients targeted should be those that provide little or no essential nutrients but are energy-dense, specifically added sugars, saturated fat, *trans* fat, and alcohol. Table 4.3 summarizes detailed recommendations for consuming nutritious foods while maintaining a healthy body weight.

**Table 4.3** Suggestions for following the American Cancer Society Nutrition Guidelines (American Cancer Society Guidelines on Nutrition and Physical Activity for Cancer Prevention: reducing the risk of cancer with healthy food choices and physical activity. CA Cancer J Clin, 56(5), 2006 Sep–Oct, 254–281; quiz 313–314. Copyright [2006, Kushi et al.]. This material is reproduced with permission of John Wiley & Sons, Inc. [22])

- Balance caloric intake with physical activity
- Avoid excessive weight gain throughout the life cycle
- Achieve and maintain a healthy weight
- Become familiar with serving sizes and actual servings consumed by reading food labels
- Eat smaller portions of high-calorie foods
- Substitute fruits, vegetables, and other low-calorie foods and beverages for calorie-dense foods and beverages
- Choose foods low in calories, fat, and sugar and avoid large portions when eating away from home
- Eat five or more servings of fruits and vegetables each day by: including fruits and vegetables at each meal, eating fruits and vegetables for snacks, choosing 100% fruit and vegetable juices, and limiting fried vegetables products (e.g., French fries and chips)
- Choose whole grains in preferences to processed (refined) grains and sugars by choosing whole grain rice, bread, pasta, and cereals and limiting consumption of pastries, sweetened cereals, and other high-sugar foods
- Limit consumption of processed and red meats by choosing fish, poultry, or beans as an alternative to beef, pork, and lamb; select lean cuts and smaller portions of meat; and bake, broil, or poach meat rather than frying or charbroiling

## Summary

The large and growing prevalence of individuals with a personal history of cancer has created new challenges for cancer patients, their families, and in the long-term health care that is available to them. This is a positive problem stemming from the successes of early diagnosis and treatment. As a result, for most people diagnosed with cancer today, it is a chronic condition rather than a life-limiting condition. The challenge to provide quality health care to cancer survivors pertains to their physical and psychosocial well-being, as well as to general health promotion. Given that unhealthy behaviors account for a large number of cancer deaths [24, 85, 104, 105] and that cancer survivors are at increased risk for the development of chronic health conditions including second cancers [110], healthy behaviors (physical activity, balanced diets, nonsmoking, and limited consumption of alcoholic beverages) are an important aspect of quality care.

There are many strategies providers can use to optimize their patients' chances of success in making health behavior changes. Prioritizing steps to take, assessing, and if necessary help modify a patient's confidence and ability to change, and helping patients problem solve through barriers can greatly influence whether or not patients undertake such challenges. Tailoring steps to the individual and the cultural context from which they come is also critical element of quality health care that is still often ignored as well as the active effort to reduce racial/ethnic disparities in cancer survivorship. Providers interested in learning additional strategies for improving cultural competence are encouraged to visit websites such as the US Department of Health and Human Services covering cultural competency and health literacy resources at websites such as: http://www.hrsa.gov/culturalcompetence/.

The challenge is to promote long-term health and motivate patients to care for themselves in order to optimize health, function, and well-being. To achieve this end there is a need for research focused on the development of population-specific health promotion and behavior change strategies for different types of cancer survivors at different stages in their efforts to engage in such health-promoting behaviors. The research needs to focus on better understanding of key obstacles to behavior change and maintenance in this diverse group of cancer survivors who have differing residual or late effects, comorbidities, and time from primary treatment, all of which may impact the self-management of these behaviors. The evidence base this research will provide will form the foundation for the development of more effective health behavior change interventions specific to differences among cancer survivors. This should further improve the long-term quality care of many cancer survivors.

## References

1. Rowland JH, Yancik R. Cancer survivorship: the interface of aging, comorbidity, and quality care. J Natl Cancer Inst. 2006;98(8):504–5.
2. Nord C, Mykletun A, Thorsen L, Bjoro T, Fossa SD. Self-reported health and use of health care services in long-term cancer survivors. Int J Cancer. 2005;114(2):307–16.
3. Reulen RC, Winter DL, Frobisher C, Lancashire ER, Stiller CA, Jenney ME, et al. Long-term cause-specific mortality among survivors of childhood cancer. JAMA. 2010;304(2):172–9.
4. Printz C. Adult survivors of childhood and adolescent cancer have more heart disease. Cancer. 2010;116(11):2507.
5. Shin DW, Nam JH, Kwon YC, Park SY, Bae DS, Park CT, et al. Comorbidity in disease-free survivors of cervical cancer compared with the general female population. Oncology. 2008;74(3–4):207–15.
6. Meacham LR, Chow EJ, Ness KK, Kamdar KY, Chen Y, Yasui Y, et al. Cardiovascular risk factors in adult survivors of pediatric cancer – a report from the childhood cancer survivor study. Cancer Epidemiol Biomark Prev. 2010;19(1):170–81.
7. Hooning MJ, Aleman BM, van Rosmalen AJ, Kuenen MA, Klijn JG, van Leeuwen FE. Cause-specific mortality in long-term survivors of breast cancer: a 25-year follow-up study. Int J Radiat Oncol Biol Phys. 2006;64(4):1081–91.
8. Hoff AO, Gagel RF. Osteoporosis in breast and prostate cancer survivors. Oncology (Williston Park). 2005;19(5):651–8.
9. Mao JJ, Armstrong K, Bowman MA, Xie SX, Kadakia R, Farrar JT. Symptom burden among cancer survivors: impact of age and comorbidity. J Am Board Fam Med. 2007;20(5):434–43.
10. Carver JR, Shapiro CL, Ng A, Jacobs L, Schwartz C, Virgo KS, et al. American Society of Clinical Oncology clinical evidence review on the ongoing care of adult cancer survivors: cardiac and pulmonary late effects. J Clin Oncol. 2007;25(25):3991–4008.

11. McGinnis JM, Foege WH. Actual causes of death in the United States. JAMA. 1993;270(18):2207–12.
12. Coups EJ, Ostroff JS. A population-based estimate of the prevalence of behavioral risk factors among adult cancer survivors and noncancer controls. Prev Med. 2005;40(6):702–11.
13. Centers for Disease Control and Prevention. FASTSTATS – exercise or physical activity. 2009 [cited 2010 Sept 7]. Available from: http://www.cdc.gov/nchs/fastats/exercise.htm.
14. Flegal KM, Carroll MD, Ogden CL, Curtin LR. Prevalence and trends in obesity among US adults, 1999–2008. JAMA. 2010;303(3):235–41.
15. Lewis JE, Soler-Vila H, Clark PE, Kresty LA, Allen GO, Hu JJ. Intake of plant foods and associated nutrients in prostate cancer risk. Nutr Cancer. 2009;61(2):216–24.
16. Zenk SN, Schulz AJ, Israel BA, James SA, Bao S, Wilson ML. Fruit and vegetable access differs by community racial composition and socioeconomic position in Detroit, Michigan. Ethn Dis. 2006;16(1):275–80.
17. Hewitt M, Rowland JH, Yancik R. Cancer survivors in the United States: age, health, and disability. J Gerontol A Med Sci. 2003;58(1):M82–91.
18. National Cancer Institute. Surveillance epidemiology and end results. 2006 [cited 2010 Aug 25]. Available from: http://www.seer.cancer.gov.
19. Deimling GT, Schaefer ML, Kahana B, Bowman K. Racial differences in the health of older adult long-term cancer survivors. Psychooncology. 2002;20(4):71–94.
20. Deimling GT, Bowman KF, Sterns S, Wagner LJ, Kahana B. Cancer-related health worries and psychological distress among older adult, long-term cancer survivors. Psychooncology. 2006;15(4):306–20.
21. American Cancer Society. Cancer Facts & Figures 2010. Atlanta; 2010.
22. Kushi LH, Byers T, Doyle C, Bandera EV, McCullough M, McTiernan A, et al. American Cancer Society Guidelines on Nutrition and Physical Activity for cancer prevention: reducing the risk of cancer with healthy food choices and physical activity. CA Cancer J Clin. 2006;56(5):254–81. quiz 313–4.
23. American Cancer Society. The importance of behavior in cancer prevention and early detection. 2008 [cited 2010 Aug 14]. Available from: http://www.cancer.org/Research/ResearchProgramsFunding/the-importance-of-behavior-in-cancer-prevention-and-early-detection.
24. World Health Organization. Cancer: diet and physical activity's impact. 2010 [cited 2010 Aug 31]. Available from: http://www.who.int/dietphysicalactivity/publications/facts/cancer/en/.
25. National Cancer Institute. Smoking. 2009 [cited 2010 Aug 25]. Available from: http://cip.cancer.gov/cancertopics/smoking.
26. National Cancer Institute. Cancer trends progress report – 2009/2010 update: cancer survivors and smoking. 2010 [cited 2010 Aug 26]. Available from: http://progressreport.cancer.gov/.
27. Emmons KM, Butterfield RM, Puleo E, Park ER, Mertens A, Gritz ER, et al. Smoking among participants in the childhood cancer survivors cohort: the Partnership for Health Study. J Clin Oncol. 2003;21(2):189–96.
28. Burke L, Miller LA, Saad A, Abraham J. Smoking behaviors among cancer survivors: an observational clinical study. J Oncol Pract. 2009;5:6–9.
29. Courneya KS, Friedenreich CM. Physical activity and cancer control. Semin Oncol Nurs. 2007;23(4):242–52.
30. Galvao DA, Newton RU. Review of exercise intervention studies in cancer patients. J Clin Oncol. 2005;23(4):899–909.
31. McTiernan A. Physical activity after cancer: physiologic outcomes. Cancer Investig. 2004;22(1):68–81.
32. Aiello EJ, Yasui Y, Tworoger SS, Ulrich CM, Irwin ML, Bowen D, et al. Effect of a yearlong, moderate-intensity exercise intervention on the occurrence and severity of menopause symptoms in postmenopausal women. Menopause. 2004;11(4):382–8.
33. Segal R, Evans W, Johnson D, Smith J, Colletta S, Gayton J, et al. Structured exercise improves physical functioning in women with stages I and II breast cancer: results of a randomized controlled trial. J Clin Oncol. 2001;19(3):657–65.

34. Pinto BM, Clark MM, Maruyama NC, Feder SI. Psychological and fitness changes associated with exercise participation among women with breast cancer. Psychooncology. 2003;12(2):118–26.
35. Courneya KS, Mackey JR, Bell GJ, Jones LW, Field CJ, Fairey AS. Randomized controlled trial of exercise training in postmenopausal breast cancer survivors: cardiopulmonary and quality of life outcomes. J Clin Oncol. 2003;21(9):1660–8.
36. Courneya KS. Exercise in cancer survivors: an overview of research. Med Sci Sports Exerc. 2003;35(11):1846–52.
37. Schmitz KH, Holtzman J, Courneya KS, Masse LC, Duval S, Kane R. Controlled physical activity trials in cancer survivors: a systematic review and meta-analysis. Cancer Epidemiol Biomark Prev. 2005;14(7):1588–95.
38. Cohen J. Statistical power analysis for the behavioral sciences. 2nd ed. Hillsdale: Lawrence Erlbaum Associates; 1988.
39. Park Y, Hunter DJ, Spiegelman D, Bergkvist L, Berrino F, van den Brandt PA, et al. Dietary fiber intake and risk of colorectal cancer: a pooled analysis of prospective cohort studies. JAMA. 2005;294(22):2849–57.
40. Zhang S, Hunter DJ, Hankinson SE, Giovannucci EL, Rosner BA, Colditz GA, et al. A prospective study of folate intake and the risk of breast cancer. JAMA. 1999;281(17):1632–7.
41. Giovannucci E. The epidemiology of vitamin D and cancer incidence and mortality: a review (United States). Cancer Causes Control. 2005;16(2):83–95.
42. International Agency for Research on Cancer. Fruits and vegetables, vol. 8. Lyon, France: World Health Organization; 2003.
43. Aune D, De Stefani E, Ronco A, Boffetta P, Deneo-Pellegrini H, Acosta G, et al. Legume intake and the risk of cancer: a multisite case-control study in Uruguay. Cancer Causes Control. 2009;20(9):1605–15.
44. Pelucchi C, Bosetti C, Rossi M, Negri E, La Vecchia C. Selected aspects of Mediterranean diet and cancer risk. Nutr Cancer. 2009;61(6):756–66.
45. Rodriguez C, McCullough ML, Mondul AM, Jacobs EJ, Chao A, Patel AV, et al. Meat consumption among Black and White men and risk of prostate cancer in the Cancer Prevention Study II Nutrition Cohort. Cancer Epidemiol Biomark Prev. 2006;15(2):211–6.
46. Chao A, Thun MJ, Connell CJ, McCullough ML, Jacobs EJ, Flanders WD, et al. Meat consumption and risk of colorectal cancer. JAMA. 2005;293(2):172–82.
47. Giovannucci E. Diet, body weight, and colorectal cancer: a summary of the epidemiologic evidence. J Womens Health (Larchmt). 2003;12(2):173–82.
48. Kolonel LN. Fat, meat, and prostate cancer. Epidemiol Rev. 2001;23(1):72–81.
49. Cho E, Smith-Warner SA, Ritz J, van den Brandt PA, Colditz GA, Folsom AR, et al. Alcohol intake and colorectal cancer: a pooled analysis of 8 cohort studies. Ann Intern Med. 2004;140(8):603–13.
50. Lin J, Zhang SM, Cook NR, Rexrode KM, Liu S, Manson JE, et al. Dietary intakes of fruit, vegetables, and fiber, and risk of colorectal cancer in a prospective cohort of women (United States). Cancer Causes Control. 2005;16(3):225–33.
51. Miller PE, Lesko SM, Muscat JE, Lazarus P, Hartman TJ. Dietary patterns and colorectal adenoma and cancer risk: a review of the epidemiological evidence. Nutr Cancer. 2010;62(4):413–24.
52. Miller PE, Lazarus P, Lesko SM, Muscat JE, Harper G, Cross AJ, et al. Diet index-based and empirically derived dietary patterns are associated with colorectal cancer risk. J Nutr. 2010;140(7):1267–73.
53. Giovannucci E, Chan AT. Role of vitamin and mineral supplementation and aspirin use in cancer survivors. J Clin Oncol. 2010;28(26):4081–5.
54. Miller PE, Vasey JJ, Short PF, Hartman TJ. Dietary supplement use in adult cancer survivors. Oncol Nurs Forum. 2009;36(1):61–8.
55. Ferrucci LM, McCorkle R, Smith T, Stein KD, Cartmel B. Factors related to the use of dietary supplements by cancer survivors. J Altern Complement Med. 2009;15(6):673–80.

56. World Cancer Research Fund/American Institute for Cancer Research. Food, nutrition, physical activity and the prevention of cancer: A global perspective, vol. 2. Washington, DC: AICR; 2007.
57. Jacobs EJ, Newton CC, Wang Y, Patel AV, McCullough ML, Campbell PT, et al. Waist circumference and all-cause mortality in a large US cohort. Arch Intern Med. 2010;170(15):1293–301.
58. Parr CL, Batty GD, Lam TH, Barzi F, Fang X, Ho SC, et al. Body-mass index and cancer mortality in the Asia-Pacific Cohort Studies Collaboration: pooled analyses of 424, 519 participants. Lancet Oncol. 2010;11(8):741–52.
59. Geyer SM, Morton LM, Habermann TM, Allmer C, Davis S, Cozen W, et al. Smoking, alcohol use, obesity, and overall survival from non-Hodgkin lymphoma: a population-based study. Cancer. 2010;116(12):2993–3000.
60. Hellmann SS, Thygesen LC, Tolstrup JS, Gronbaek M. Modifiable risk factors and survival in women diagnosed with primary breast cancer: results from a prospective cohort study. Eur J Cancer Prev. 2010;19(5):366–73.
61. Rock CL, Demark-Wahnefried W. Nutrition and survival after the diagnosis of breast cancer: a review of the evidence. J Clin Oncol. 2002;20(15):3302–16.
62. Goodwin PJ, Boyd NF. Body size and breast cancer prognosis: a critical review of the evidence. Breast Cancer Res Treat. 1990;16(3):205–14.
63. Abrahamson PE, Gammon MD, Lund MJ, Flagg EW, Porter PL, Stevens J, et al. General and abdominal obesity and survival among young women with breast cancer. Cancer Epidemiol Biomark Prev. 2006;15(10):1871–7.
64. Dignam JJ, Polite BN, Yothers G, Raich P, Colangelo L, O'Connell MJ, et al. Body mass index and outcomes in patients who receive adjuvant chemotherapy for colon cancer. J Natl Cancer Inst. 2006;98(22):1647–54.
65. Barrera S, Demark-Wahnefried W. Nutrition during and after cancer therapy. Oncology (Williston Park). 2009;23(2 Suppl Nurse Ed):15–21.
66. Doyle C, Kushi LH, Byers T, Courneya KS, Demark-Wahnefried W, Grant B, et al. Nutrition and physical activity during and after cancer treatment: an American Cancer Society guide for informed choices. CA Cancer J Clin. 2006;56(6):323–53.
67. Demark-Wahnefried W, Aziz NM, Rowland JH, Pinto BM. Riding the crest of the teachable moment: promoting long-term health after the diagnosis of cancer. J Clin Oncol. 2005;23(24):5814–30.
68. Mosher CE, Sloane R, Morey MC, Snyder DC, Cohen HJ, Miller PE, et al. Associations between lifestyle factors and quality of life among older long-term breast, prostate, and colorectal cancer survivors. Cancer. 2009;115(17):4001–9.
69. Boyar AP, Rose DP, Loughridge JR, Engle A, Palgi A, Laakso K, et al. Response to a diet low in total fat in women with postmenopausal breast cancer: a pilot study. Nutr Cancer. 1988;11(2):93–9.
70. Thomson CA, Rock CL, Giuliano AR, Newton TR, Cui H, Reid PM, et al. Longitudinal changes in body weight and body composition among women previously treated for breast cancer consuming a high-vegetable, fruit and fiber, low-fat diet. Eur J Nutr. 2005;44(1):18–25.
71. Chlebowski RT, Rose D, Buzzard IM, Blackburn GL, Insull Jr W, Grosvenor M, et al. Adjuvant dietary fat intake reduction in postmenopausal breast cancer patient management. The Women's Intervention Nutrition Study (WINS). Breast Cancer Res Treat. 1992;20(2):73–84.
72. de Waard F, Ramlau R, Mulders Y, de Vries T, van Waveren S. A feasibility study on weight reduction in obese postmenopausal breast cancer patients. Eur J Cancer Prev. 1993;2(3):233–8.
73. Djuric Z, DiLaura NM, Jenkins I, Darga L, Jen CK, Mood D, et al. Combining weight-loss counseling with the weight watchers plan for obese breast cancer survivors. Obes Res. 2002;10(7):657–65.

74. Hebert JR, Ebbeling CB, Olendzki BC, Hurley TG, Ma Y, Saal N, et al. Change in women's diet and body mass following intensive intervention for early-stage breast cancer. J Am Diet Assoc. 2001;101(4):421–31.
75. Loprinzi CL, Athmann LM, Kardinal CG, O'Fallon JR, See JA, Bruce BK, et al. Randomized trial of dietician counseling to try to prevent weight gain associated with breast cancer adjuvant chemotherapy. Oncology. 1996;53(3):228–32.
76. Nordevang E, Callmer E, Marmur A, Holm LE. Dietary intervention in breast cancer patients: effects on food choice. Eur J Clin Nutr. 1992;46(6):387–96.
77. Pierce JP, Newman VA, Flatt SW, Faerber S, Rock CL, Natarajan L, et al. Telephone counseling intervention increases intakes of micronutrient- and phytochemical-rich vegetables, fruit and fiber in breast cancer survivors. J Nutr. 2004;134(2):452–8.
78. Pierce JP, Faerber S, Wright FA, Rock CL, Newman V, Flatt SW, et al. A randomized trial of the effect of a plant-based dietary pattern on additional breast cancer events and survival: the Women's Healthy Eating and Living (WHEL) Study. Control Clin Trials. 2002;23 (6):728–56.
79. Stefanick ML, Mackey S, Sheehan M, Ellsworth N, Haskell WL, Wood PD. Effects of diet and exercise in men and postmenopausal women with low levels of HDL cholesterol and high levels of LDL cholesterol. N Engl J Med. 1998;339(1):12–20.
80. Nieman DC, Brock DW, Butterworth D, Utter AC, Nieman CC. Reducing diet and/or exercise training decreases the lipid and lipoprotein risk factors of moderately obese women. J Am Coll Nutr. 2002;21(4):344–50.
81. Melanson KJ, Dell'Olio J, Carpenter MR, Angelopoulos TJ. Changes in multiple health outcomes at 12 and 24 weeks resulting from 12 weeks of exercise counseling with or without dietary counseling in obese adults. Nutrition. 2004;20(10):849–56.
82. Wood PD, Stefanick ML, Williams PT, Haskell WL. The effects on plasma lipoproteins of a prudent weight-reducing diet, with or without exercise, in overweight men and women. N Engl J Med. 1991;325(7):461–6.
83. Morey MC, Snyder DC, Sloane R, Cohen HJ, Peterson B, Hartman TJ, et al. Effects of home-based diet and exercise on functional outcomes among older, overweight long-term cancer survivors: RENEW: a randomized controlled trial. JAMA. 2009;301(18):1883–91.
84. Boffetta P, Hashibe M. Alcohol and cancer. Lancet Oncol. 2006;7(2):149–56.
85. Centers for Disease Control and Prevention. Cancer fact sheet. 2002 [cited 2010 Aug 14]. Available from: http://www.atsdr.cdc.gov/com/cancer-fs.html.
86. Rollnick S, Mason P, Butler C. Health behavior change: a guide for practioners. New York: Churchill Livingstone; 1999.
87. Pinto BM, Eakin E, Maruyama NC. Health behavior changes after a cancer diagnosis: what do we know and where do we go from here? Ann Behav Med. 2000;22(1):38–52.
88. Park CL, Gaffey AE. Relationships between psychosocial factors and health behavior change in cancer survivors: an integrative review. Ann Behav Med. 2007;34(2):115–34.
89. Feuerstein M, Findley P. The cancer survivor's guide: the essential handbook to life after cancer. New York: Marlowe & Company; 2006.
90. Deimling GT, Bowman KF, Sterns S, Wagner LJ, Kahan B. Cancer-related health worries and psychological distress among older, adult, long-term cancer survivors. Psychooncology. 2006;15:306–20.
91. Mitchell AJ. Pooled results from 38 analyses of the accuracy of distress thermometer and other ultra-short methods of detecting cancer-related mood disorders. J Clin Oncol. 2007;25(29):4670–81.
92. Dabrowski M, Boucher K, Ward JH, Lovell MM, Sandre A, Bloch J, et al. Clinical experiences with the NCCN distress thermometer in breast cancer patients. J Natl Compr Cancer Netw. 2007;5(1):104–11.
93. Glasgow RE, Davis CL, Fennell MM, Beck A. Implementing practical interventions to support chronic illness self-management. Joint Comm J Qual Patient Saf. 2003;29(11):563–74.
94. Fiore MC, Bailey WC, Cohen SJ, Dorfman SF, Goldstein MG, Gritz ER, et al. Treating tobacco use and dependence, Quick Reference Guide for Clinicians. Rockville: Department of Health and Human Services; 2000.

95. Haskell W, Lee I, Pate R, Powell KE, Blair SN, Franklin BA, et al. Physical activity and public health: updated recommendation for adults from the American College of Sports Medicine and the American Heart Association. Med Sci Sports Exerc. 2007;39(8):1423–34.
96. Locke DEC, Cerhan JH, Wu W, Malec JF, Clark MM, Rummans TA, et al. Cognitive rehabilitation and problem-solving to improve quality of life of patients with primary brain tumors: a pilot study. J Support Oncol. 2008;6(8):383–91.
97. Ferraro KF, Albrecht-Jensen CM. Does religion influence adult health? J Sci Study Relig. 1991;30:193–202.
98. Holt CL, Clark E, Kreuter MW, Rubio DM. Spiritual health locus of control and breast cancer beliefs among urban African American women. Health Psychol. 2003;22(3):294–9.
99. Samuel-Hodge CD, Headen SW, Skelly AH, Ingram AF, Keyserling TC, Jackson EJ, et al. Influences on day-to-day self-management of type 2 diabetes among African-American women. Diab Care. 2000;23:928–33.
100. Olson LM, Reis J, Murphy L, Gehm JH. The religious community as a partner in health care. J Community Health. 1988;13(4):249–57.
101. Jackson S. FAME church incorporates exercise in worship experience. Los Angeles Sentinal. 2010 [cited 2010 Mar 9]. Available from: http://www.famechurch.org/event-archive/jul_10/excercise.html.
102. Sbrocco T, Carter MM, Lewis EL, Vaughn NA, Kalupa KL, King S, et al. Church-based obesity treatment for African-American women improves adherence. Ethn Dis. 2005;15(2):246–55.
103. Figueroa LR, Davis B, Baker S, Bunch JB. The influence of spirituality on health care-seeking behaviors among African Americans. ABNF J. 2006;17(2):82–8.
104. Friedenreich CM. Physical activity and cancer prevention: from observational to intervention research. Cancer Epidemiol Biomark Prev. 2001;10(4):287–301.
105. Friedenreich CM, Orenstein MR. Physical activity and cancer prevention: etiologic evidence and biological mechanisms. J Nutr. 2002;132(11 Suppl):3456S–64.
106. U.S. Department of Health and Human Services and U.S. Department of Agriculture. Dietary guidelines for Americans, 2005. 6th ed. Washington, DC: U.S. Government Printing Office; 2005.
107. Hofman M, Ryan JL, Figueroa-Moseley CD, Jean-Pierre P, Morrow GR. Cancer-related fatigue: the scale of the problem. Oncologist. 2007;12 Suppl 1:4–10.
108. Muscaritoli M, Molfino A, Gioia G, Laviano A, Rossi Fanelli F (2010). The "parallel pathway": a novel nutritional and metabolic approach to cancer patients. Intern Emerg Med. 2010. doi: 10.1007/s11739-010-0426-1.
109. Toles M, Demark-Wahnefried W. Nutrition and the cancer survivor: evidence to guide oncology nursing practice. Semin Oncol Nurs. 2008;24(3):171–9.
110. Brown JK, Byers T, Doyle C, Coumeya KS, Demark-Wahnefried W, Kushi LH, et al. Nutrition and physical activity during and after cancer treatment: an American Cancer Society guide for informed choices. CA Cancer J Clin. 2003;53(5):268–91.

# Chapter 5
# Rehabilitation in the Context of Cancer Survivorship

**Julie K. Silver and Laura S. Gilchrist**

## Introduction

It is widely understood that people treated for cancer often feel much better before their therapy begins than they do when it has concluded. Novelist Wilfred Sheed wrote of his cancer experience in his memoir, *In Love With Daylight: A Memoir of Recovery* [1]. Sheed noted,

> As the radiologist (radiation oncologist) reads off the list of possible side- and after-effects, to run concurrently and forever, it's awfully hard to remember that this guy is supposed to be on your side. There he is, about to kill off thousands of your favorite cells, adding up to a large tract of the body that brought you this far, and they call this man a healer! Talk about bombing villages in order to liberate them; talk about napalming whole forests on suspicion. For all anyone knew, I might not even *have* cancer at this stage. But bomb we must. One can't be too careful. (p. 234)

In her memoir, *A Season in Hell*, Marilyn French who was diagnosed with esophageal cancer wrote this about physicians, "Simply to treat cancer means they must violate the primary tenet of their code: First, do no harm" [2] (p. 60).

The dilemma of prolonging life without causing so much suffering that the quality of life is irreparably harmed is something that every oncology healthcare professional considers. Indeed, there are no easy answers, but acknowledging this potentially catastrophic dilemma – that may result in undertreating a patient and thus not prolonging her life or over-treating a patient and thus insuring that she lives with far more disability than necessary – is one that is necessary to understand what happens when acute cancer treatment has finished.

The Institute of Medicine (IOM) investigated the issue of survivorship care and released a pivotal report titled *From Cancer Patient to Cancer Survivor: Lost in Transition*. This report documented the many unmet needs of those who finish acute oncology treatment and then are left to struggle with a number of concerns including the toxic side effects of treatment that often leave survivors unnecessarily

J.K. Silver (✉)
Harvard Medical School, Boston, MA, USA
e-mail: Julie_silver@hms.harvard.edu

M. Feuerstein and P.A. Ganz (eds.), *Health Services for Cancer Survivors*,
DOI 10.1007/978-1-4419-1348-7_5, © Springer Science+Business Media, LLC 2011

disabled, or at the very least, able to function but not at an optimal level [3]. Indeed, pain, profound fatigue, and deconditioning, loss of range of motion of joints due to surgery, chemotherapy and radiation treatments, and many other lingering side effects of treatment can be managed with a variety of rehabilitation services, though few survivors get them. Interestingly, the IOM report listed ten key recommendations, including creating cancer survivorship as a distinct phase of cancer care (Table 5.1). One can assume that oncology rehabilitation would play a major role in this new phase of cancer care, though the report did not explicitly state this.

**Table 5.1** Ten key recommendations for cancer survivorship from the Institute of Medicine with recommendations about oncology rehabilitation as they pertain to the IOM report (Adapted from Hewitt and Ganz [3]). *These are the authors' recommendations (Silver & Gilchrist)

| |
|---|
| Recommendation 1 |
| Establish cancer survivorship as a distinct phase of cancer care |
| *This should include raising the awareness of the need for oncology rehabilitation and a concerted effort to ensure the delivery of appropriate rehabilitation interventions to survivors |
| Recommendation 2 |
| Provide a comprehensive care summary and follow-up plan (survivorship care plan) to survivors |
| *The survivorship care plan should have recommendations regarding rehabilitation assessments and interventions |
| Recommendation 3 |
| Use evidence-based clinical practice guidelines, assessment tools, and screening instruments to identify and manage late effects of cancer and its treatment |
| *These measures should include those that identify and help guide the rehabilitation treatment of cancer survivors |
| Recommendation 4 |
| Develop quality of care measures that pertain specifically to cancer survivors and implement quality assurance programs to monitor/improve the care that all survivors receive |
| *The quality of care measures that are developed and implemented should include oncology rehabilitation |
| Recommendation 5 |
| Test models of interdisciplinary survivorship care in diverse patient populations and across systems of care |
| *This testing should include oncology rehabilitation |
| Recommendation 6 |
| Develop comprehensive cancer control plans that include survivorship care and promote the implementation, evaluation, and refinement of existing state cancer control plans |
| *These comprehensive cancer control plans should also include oncology rehabilitation |
| Recommendation 7 |
| Expand and coordinate efforts to educate healthcare providers so that they may be equipped to address the health care and quality of life issues facing cancer survivors |
| *Rehabilitation healthcare professionals should receive ongoing education in oncology rehabilitation in order for them to optimally treat cancer survivors. Oncology healthcare professionals should be educated about the benefits of rehabilitation medicine and the best ways to interface with rehabilitation professionals |

(continued)

**Table 5.1** (continued)

| |
|---|
| Recommendation 8 |
| Act to eliminate discrimination and minimize adverse effects of cancer on employment, while supporting cancer survivors with short-term and long-term disabilities that affect work |
| *Rehabilitation may enable more survivors to return to work and to function at the highest level possible |
| Recommendation 9 |
| Act to ensure that all cancer survivors have access to adequate and affordable health insurance with help from insurers and healthcare payors |
| *Rehabilitation interventions are part of conventional medicine and thus generally covered by health insurance and healthcare payors |
| Recommendation 10 |
| Increase funding support of survivorship research in order to better guide effective survivorship care |
| *Oncology rehabilitation research should be emphasized in both oncology and rehabilitation medicine |

There is no doubt that cancer treatments are toxic and can cause significant disability. Major problems with activities of daily living (ADLs) occur in 15% of prostate cancer survivors, 35% of colon cancer survivors, and 40% of lung cancer survivors [4]. In one study that assessed 96 cancer patients' symptoms at admission and on discharge from an acute rehabilitation hospital, researchers found that the most intense symptoms both on admission and discharge were poor appetite and fatigue. Discharge evaluations revealed significant improvements in appetite, fatigue, pain, constipation, anxiety, sense of well-being, and insomnia [5]. The significant disability that cancer survivors face may last many years or even a lifetime. For example, elderly breast cancer survivors who were 5 years out from acute treatment demonstrated significantly more problems with ADLs than did age-matched controls [6].

In a systematic review of 64 studies on employment and work-related issues in cancer survivors, the rate of employment or return to work in cancer survivorship was 63.5% [7]. The presence of fatigue and physical symptoms was a barrier for returning to work. Among adult survivors of childhood cancer, the functional limitations may be quite profound. One study evaluated more than 11,000 people who were treated before age 21 for a variety of cancer diagnoses and compared them to siblings [8]. Compared to their siblings, the childhood cancer survivors were more likely to report performance limitations that included restrictions in personal care skills, routine activities, and the ability to work and/or attend school. Among the most disabled were survivors of brain cancer and bone cancer. Hodgkin's survivors also had many limitations. Survivors who had undergone radiation treatment were more likely to report significant limitations when compared to the surgery-only group. Neurologic late effects were highly prevalent among survivors, with more than 40% reporting neurologic problems. Chronic pain in the trunk or extremities was the most commonly reported problem. Leg and arm weakness were also frequent neurological sequelae. In this study, the researchers concluded that, "Adult survivors of childhood cancer are at risk for performance limitations and should be monitored for functional loss throughout their lives and referred for appropriate rehabilitation services when indicated."

It is not unusual to see oncology rehabilitation either not represented or under-represented when it comes to survivorship care. Oncology rehabilitation recommendations are typically not included because the type of services and expected outcomes are not well understood by the healthcare community. In addition, it takes time, a level of training, and community awareness to structure rehabilitation services for cancer survivors and work out the details of reimbursement for rehabilitation services in this emerging area. These are some of the reasons why oncology rehabilitation, though potentially a critical part of survivorship as a distinct phase of cancer care, is often underdeveloped – even in comprehensive cancer centers.

## Overview of Rehabilitation Services and Integration with Other Health Professionals/Services

The IOM report missed an opportunity to highlight the importance of the role of rehabilitation in survivorship care. This maybe in part because few cancer centers or hospitals offer comprehensive interdisciplinary oncology rehabilitation services [9], and thus the concept of oncology-specific rehabilitation is not well integrated in either oncology or rehabilitation culture. Indeed, it is not uncommon to see that even institutions that have a major commitment to creating survivorship services may leave out or implement fragmented oncology rehabilitation services when they put together their survivorship programs. If this level of service is infrequently available to the patient at a comprehensive cancer center, it is even more unlikely that the patients treated in smaller settings receive any specific oncology rehabilitation services. Perhaps, in the past, rehabilitation was not viewed as a realistic option given the extent of disability and mortality that was observed even just a decade ago. Currently, more and more cancer patients are living longer and are looking to improve levels of function. In addition, recent research has focused on the young adult and the 20–65-year-old survivors demonstrating that functional limitations are often associated with cancer and its treatment leading healthcare providers to ask how can we prevent and treat these issues. Rehabilitation services are appropriate for this patient population and are attempting to address this need.

Rehabilitation medicine focuses on a multi- or interdisciplinary team approach. Not all services are third-party-payor-reimbursable, but typically the core services are covered (e.g., physician evaluations and follow-up visits by physiatrists, physical/occupational/speech evaluations, and treatment interventions). Many professionals may individually provide various oncology rehabilitation services to help optimize functional outcomes (listed in Table 5.2), though most rehabilitation teams will not have all of these professionals represented.

**Table 5.2** Rehabilitation Service Providers

| |
|---|
| Physiatrists |
| Physical therapy assistants |
| Occupational therapy assistants |
| Speech/language pathology assistants |
| Rehabilitation nurses |
| Psychologists |
| Social workers |
| Prosthetists/orthotists |
| Recreational therapists |
| Vocational counselors |

The interdisciplinary rehabilitation approach to many illnesses is very consistent with the important aspects of quality cancer survivorship care. Thus, we suggest that:

1. Every institution that provides comprehensive cancer services should offer oncology rehabilitation services with an interdisciplinary team approach.
2. Every survivor care plan should address oncology rehabilitation so that patients know where they can find resources that will help them function at the highest possible level.

## Specific Impairments and Limitations in Cancer Survivors

While some cancer survivors are able to maintain high levels of function both during and after cancer treatment, other survivors of cancer are at risk for having lasting impairments and functional limitations as well as late effects that can impact multiple body systems [6, 8, 10, 11]. One area for improving survivorship care is for common impairments and limitations to be identified by primary healthcare providers and make the appropriate referrals to rehabilitation professionals. In this section and in Table 5.3, we review a few of the most frequent impairments and limitations found in cancer survivors and suggest screening tools to assist in referral. If left undetected, these changes in body structure and function can lead to progressive limitations in physical function.

### *Pain and Musculoskeletal Concerns*

Pain is one of the most common side effects of cancer and its treatment [11–14] and is often feared by patients. Although acute pain during treatment is generally well managed, cancer survivors may suffer from ongoing pain even after treatment is

**Table 5.3** Frequent impairments in cancer survivors and screening suggestions

| Impairment | Specific cancer groups impacted | Suggested screening |
|---|---|---|
| Pain | Many | Ask about pain and discomfort, even distant from the tumor location |
| Impaired arm mobility | Breast cancer, head and neck cancer | Ask patients to raise both arms overhead and to reach behind their back |
| Impaired lower extremity mobility | Childhood cancers, lower extremity bone tumors | Have patients walk on their heels or lift their toes off the floor when standing. Ask about functional mobility including stairs, curbs, and uneven ground |
| Decreased balance and falls risk | Brain tumors, any cancer where the patient received neurotoxic chemotherapy, especially breast cancer and childhood cancers | Ask patients if they have had recent falls or have fear of falling. Have patients stand on one foot for 10 s or rise from a chair five times without the use of arms (more than 12.9 s indicates falls risk) |
| Deconditioning | Many cancers – if have documented cardiotoxicity or cardiopulmonary structure involvement may need a graded exercise test | Ask about ability to tolerate mild exercise, such as walking a mile |
| Fatigue | Breast cancer, lymphoma | Ask about unrelenting sense of tiredness |
| Lymphedema | Breast cancer, pelvic cancers | Difference of 2 cm in extremity girth, presence of pitting or hardened swelling |
| Speech and swallowing difficulties | Head and neck cancers, brain tumors | Note speech difficulty and ask about difficulty swallowing including different textures (liquids vs. solid foods) |

completed. In a large study of symptom burden in cancer survivors, it was found that 34% of adult survivors had recurrent pain compared to 17% of the control group [15]. Cancer-related pain can be quite complex as it can stem from multiple sources. Pain may arise from muscular complications such as contracture formation, skeletal morbidity such as compression fractures or osteonecrosis, or neuropathic pain as a result of nerve compression or chemotherapy-induced peripheral neuropathy. Each of these types of pain will need to be managed differently, and thus the assessment process is especially important for the best clinical management. The quality of pain may be quite informative in determining the underlying cause and determining the appropriate management. Referral to a pain specialist is warranted when pain cannot be easily managed or it interferes with the patient's function even when managed.

Other musculoskeletal problems can exist in cancer survivors that can greatly impact functional abilities. One area that has received much attention in breast cancer survivors is arm disability. Altered movement patterns have been demonstrated in female survivors of breast cancer that correlates with pain and functional disability [16]. Such changes are likely widespread among breast cancer survivors and often are not adequately addressed. In one study of arm morbidity 6–12 months after breast cancer surgery, 50% of women were found to have range of motion deficits on the surgical side, although few discussed this issue with healthcare professionals [17, 18]. Less work has been completed in other types of cancers, but survivors of head and neck cancers [19] and childhood cancer survivors [20] have also been shown to have both range of motion restrictions and strength deficits, making it likely that these issues are broadly shared among many cancer types. Evidence is mounting that physical therapy interventions are effective in remediating these mobility deficits and that early intervention is important in avoiding the range of motion deficits specifically in patients treated for breast cancer [21–24]. Oncologists and primary healthcare providers can easily ask patients about their overall function and screen major joint motions through functional movements. For example, simply asking patients to raise their arms overhead can demonstrate unilateral deficits in shoulder function. Likewise, if a person cannot walk on their heels, they may have an ankle range of motion deficit, muscle weakness, or balance dysfunction. Each may require the attention of a physical therapist.

## *Balance and Falls*

There is evidence that cancer survivors are at increased risk of functional decline, but little attention has been placed on the increased risk of falls and fractures in the cancer survivor population. An increased falls risk has been demonstrated in men undergoing androgen-deprivation therapy for prostate cancer [25] and female survivors of breast cancer [26]. Cancer survivors often have multiple risk factors for falls including decreased lower extremity strength [27], decreased sensation and reflexes due to chemotherapy-induced peripheral neuropathy (CIPN) [28, 29], and decreased static and dynamic balance control [28]. When paired with decreased bone mineral density found in both adult [26] and pediatric cancer survivors [30–33] this could lead to an increased risk of fall-related fractures.

Impairments in balance control in cancer survivors have been infrequently investigated, but research in breast cancer [28] and leukemia [34] survivors indicates that subtle, yet important changes in balance control exist after completion of cancer treatment. Because of the subtlety of the changes in balance, measuring postural control in challenging positions can be important in order to detect deficits [35] and improve balance.

Another issue in the detection of balance-related deficits has been the underappreciation of CIPN by healthcare professionals [29]. Currently, there is no standard evaluation for CIPN, although a number of clinical and patient reported measures have been developed. Rehabilitation professionals, specifically physical therapists and physiatrists, are well educated to evaluate and treat balance-related disorders arising from a multitude of conditions. While the efficacy of cancer-specific balance rehabilitation is lacking, numerous trials have been conducted on improving postural control in those at risk of falls demonstrating the effectiveness of this approach in other populations [36–39]. By focusing on decreasing the impact of balance disorders and increasing bone mineral density through specific exercise programs, rehabilitation professional could make an important contribution to improving the overall health and well-being of cancer survivors.

Screening for fall risk can be as simple as asking about recent falls and even inquiring about fear of falling as it has been demonstrated that individuals who are afraid of falling are at increased risk for fall-related fractures [40]. Certain groups are likely to have a greater risk of balance impairment such as patients treated for brain tumors [8] and patients treated with neurotoxic chemotherapies such as taxanes and vinca alkaloids [28, 34]. More objective tests that can help providers detect some of these problems include having the survivor stand up from a chair without the use of their arms to test for functional lower extremity strength (five times sit-to-stand test with a score >12.9 s indicating falls risk) [41] or asking the person to stand on one leg with eyes open to assess static balance control (less than 10 s indicating falls risk) [42]. Referral to a physiatrist or physical therapist would be indicated if physical impairments such as weakness, loss of sensation, or incoordination appear to be contributing to their decreased balance control and increased falls risk and overall functional limitations.

## *Deconditioning and Fatigue*

Decreased exercise tolerance and reduced cardiorespiratory fitness have been well documented for both cancers that directly impact the cardiopulmonary systems (e.g., primary or metastatic lung cancers [43]) as well as for other types of cancer such as breast and prostate cancer [44]. The decline in exercise capacity is likely multifactorial. For cancers involving the lung, surgical removal of lung tissue of course directly limits oxygen diffusing capacity and thus exercise capacity. Yet other surgeries may also acutely impact cardiovascular fitness due to bed-rest and deconditioning. Both radiation therapy involving the chest wall and pharmacological management of cancers can also impact exercise tolerance. For example, if a patient has radiation treatment to the chest wall for left-sided breast cancer, she may develop lasting fibrosis of the chest wall and heart, and myocardial perfusion can be decreased [45]. Additionally, chemotherapy may impact the cardiopulmonary system. Specifically, anthracyclines can induce permanent cardiac toxicity [46] and bleomycin may result in pulmonary fibrosis [47].

In addition to decreased exercise tolerance, cancer survivors may be impacted by cancer-related fatigue that reduces their participation in physical activity. Fatigue occurs in the vast majority of patients who receive treatment for cancer [48], and in many survivors this fatigue does not resolve upon the completion of cancer treatment [49]. The National Comprehensive Cancer Network (NCCN) generally defines cancer-related fatigue (CRF) as a "distressing persistent, subjective sense of tiredness or exhaustion related to cancer or cancer treatment that is not proportional to recent activity and interferes with usually functioning." There are clinical guidelines for CRF that have been developed by the NCCN [50].

Are there interventions for the reduced exercise capacity and increased levels of fatigue in this population? Exercise training has been shown to improve cardiovascular capacity and reduce fatigue in cancer survivors without serious adverse events [44, 51–54]. Exercise has been studied most extensively in the female breast cancer population [55]. Both aerobic conditioning and strength training have been found to produce positive results in breast cancer survivors [55–57]. In a meta-analysis on the effects of exercise on breast cancer survivors, McNeely et al. found that exercise leads to statistically significant improvements in quality of life, physical functioning, peak oxygen consumption, and reduction of fatigue symptoms [58].

The concern that strength training might promote the development of lymphedema or worsen existing symptoms in breast cancer survivors has been addressed by recent research. The trend in developed countries has been to utilize sentinel lymph node biopsy (SLNB) rather than axillary lymph node dissection in many women with early stage breast cancer. SLNB is a less invasive procedure that generally results in reduced morbidity [56, 57]. Also, there is increasing evidence that strength training does not promote the onset or progression of lymphedema [59].

Because of the potential for cardiotoxicity and other toxicities of treatment, there may be circumstances when unsupervised exercise is not appropriate. For example, women who develop cardiac complications from chemotherapy (e.g., doxorubicin/Adriamycin) will require a graded exercise test to determine the appropriate parameters and supervision for exercise. Survivors who are severely deconditioned will also benefit from specific guidance of a physical therapist. In addition to improving strength and cardiovascular conditioning, exercise has been shown to have significant psychosocial benefits on mood and quality of life [60, 61]. Exercise has also been shown to have a significant impact on improving cancer-related fatigue in this population [62].

Whether exercise prevents cancer recurrence is controversial, but the breast cancer literature suggests that it might, and offers some insights as to the possible mechanisms including a reduction in body fat, positive changes in metabolic and growth factors (e.g., lower insulin and insulin like growth factors such as IGF-1), effects on sex hormones (e.g., decreased estrogen), and/or inflammation (e.g., C-reactive protein) [63].

## *Lymphedema*

Lymphedema is a chronic disorder where lymphatic fluids accumulate in a region of the body leading to the feeling of heaviness or pressure in the impacted region and swelling that is not usually relieved by elevation. Secondary lymphedema, caused by injury to the lymphatic system, is fairly common after certain cancer treatments due to surgical disruption of the lymphatic system and radiation effects. While lymphedema can occur after treatment for many types of cancer such as breast, prostate, ovarian, skin, and head and neck cancers, it has been best studied in the breast cancer survivor population. The incidence of lymphedema is reported to be between 15% and 30% in female survivors of breast cancer [64]. Lymphedema in any form can result in both pain and functional morbidity.

Generally lymphedema is diagnosed in breast cancer survivors when there is a difference of 2 cm in arm girth between sides [65]. Lymphedema cannot be cured, but it can be successfully managed by rehabilitation specialists using decongestive massage, specialized garments, and exercise. Although the benefit of different forms of rehabilitation on lymphedema has been demonstrated in a number of clinical trials [66–69], high quality evidence is still needed to better inform practitioners on the specific interventions and parameters [70, 71]. The treatment of lymphedema is generally not an entry-level skill for most rehabilitation professionals, and thus advanced training in the treatment of lymphedema is needed by both physical and occupational therapists that treat this disorder. Though preoperative assessment and specific follow-up care for breast cancer patients has been shown to decrease the incidence and severity of this disorder [72], it is important for healthcare practitioners to understand that the onset of lymphedema may occur years after the cancer treatment.

## *Speech and Swallowing*

Speech and swallowing issues may be found in several cancer survivor populations but perhaps the most affected are the head and neck cancer survivors. The treatment of head and neck cancers typically involves surgery, especially in the early stages when removal of the tumor is possible. Radiation therapy is often used as well. Surgery and radiation may both be potentially curative while chemotherapy by itself is usually palliative. Plastic surgery for reconstruction is often needed as well.

Comprehensive or "radical" neck dissection involves the removal of lymph nodes, cranial nerve XI, the internal jugular vein, and the sternocleidomastoid muscle. There are different types of "modified" neck dissections, which means that at least some of the structures that are normally sacrificed in the comprehensive neck dissection are spared.

The treatment of head and neck cancers often results in significant problems with vital functions such as speech, breathing, chewing, swallowing, shoulder dysfunction, and loss of cervical range of motion. Hearing may be impacted as well. Lymphedema may result from lymph node removal, and cosmesis is also an issue for many patients.

The treatment team for head and neck cancers often involves not only medical, surgical, and radiation oncologists but also dental, speech, swallowing, auditory, and nutritional evaluations. The rehabilitation of the head and neck cancer survivor may be very complicated and involve interventions for speech, swallowing, breathing, pain, fatigue, cervical and shoulder dysfunction, psychosocial sequelae, and more.

Though it is clear that rehabilitation interventions are needed in this patient population, there is not enough research available to specifically guide treatment. For example, in a systematic review of 15 studies on head and neck cancers, the authors had two goals: (1) to identify the negative side effects of concomitant chemotherapy and/or radiation therapy on mouth opening, pain and quality of life before and after treatment in head and neck cancer patients; and (2) to identify evidence-based rehabilitation options to ameliorate these side effects [73]. When it came to the second goal, identifying evidence-based rehabilitation strategies, the authors noted that only 2 of the 15 studies mentioned rehabilitation and there were very little available data to assess rehabilitation interventions.

In one study, the strongest predictors of reduced Health-Related Quality Of Life (HRQOL) among head and neck cancer survivors 6 months posttreatment included lower body mass index (BMI), depression, younger age, gastrostomy, history of radiation therapy, and higher education [74]. Quality of life and survival in head and neck cancer survivors are being studied, with one study suggesting that quality of life may help predict survival [75].

A study from the United Kingdom noted that while some patients receive PT immediately after surgery in the inpatient hospital setting, they are often not referred to outpatient PT until much later, when they have developed significant shoulder pain and dysfunction [76]. A primary goal is identifying the rehabilitation needs of cancer survivors along the continuum of care and referring them appropriately. A breakdown in care often occurs with outpatient rehabilitation so that patients receive intervention only after they present with significant disability at a later date. Unfortunately, for many patients this means a less optimal outcome in terms of impairments and disability. The head and neck cancer population is particularly vulnerable because they have so many rehabilitation and psychosocial needs. It is extremely important for the entire interdisciplinary team to work in a coordinate manner throughout the care continuum.

Sometimes, assistive devices are needed to help with breathing or swallowing. A prosthodontist may be able to make prostheses to replace missing dental or facial anatomy to improve function or cosmesis or both. Temporary or permanent tracheostomy and gastrostomy may be an option for some survivors to offer alternate ways to breathe or provide nutrition, respectively.

Speech and language pathologists can be instrumental in helping to rehabilitate the head and neck cancer survivor as both speech and swallowing tend to be major factors in quality of life and greatly affect survivors' ability to function at home, at work, and in the community. For patients at risk for dysphagia, early referral to a speech and language pathologist is important so that they may assess which patients may need further testing and to generate a treatment plan to ensure adequate and safe nutrition. The role of swallowing therapy in treating dysphagia includes postural techniques, sensory techniques, motor exercises, swallowing maneuvers, and changes in diet [77].

## Interventions

Initially, the primary healthcare provider will need to determine if referral to a physiatrist, physical therapist, occupational therapist, speech and language pathologist (or other member of the rehabilitation team) is the best course of action. When a survivor has multiple rehabilitation needs (such as pain, lymphedema, fatigue, and a swallowing disorder), an initial referral to a physiatrist or interdisciplinary cancer rehabilitation clinic is the best choice. If the patient has primarily one complaint, such as an increased falls risk or lymphedema, often referral to a therapist with advanced training in cancer rehabilitation is appropriate.

Every rehabilitation professional will start their encounter with an examination of the functional limitations and a determination of the underlying anatomical or physiological impairments. They will also take a history of the cancer treatment in order to determine what potential side effects of treatment or late effects may be anticipated so that they provide appropriate monitoring.

In general, rehabilitation professionals will use a combination of exercise, adaptive and therapeutic equipment (canes, compressive garments, electrical stimulation), and education to address the individual patients' needs. Programming should be individually tailored for each patient's needs, although sometimes exercise may be done in a group setting. Patients should be prepared to be active participants in their rehabilitation. Even if a therapist uses a passive technique, such as decongestive massage to reduce lymphedema, this will only be a portion of the rehabilitation of the patient, and the survivor will indeed learn how to independently manage this condition with exercise and compression garments. Rehabilitation will also be targeted at increasing the independence of the individual while decreasing their symptoms. Thus rehabilitation is oriented toward patient goals with the intent of improving the patient's overall quality of life.

For some individuals with moderate to severe neurologic insults, such as patients who have been treated for brain or spinal cord tumors, rehabilitation may occur in inpatient units much like rehabilitation for a stroke or traumatic brain injury. Other patients may have received rehabilitation services while in the acute care hospital for cancer treatments, yet often rehabilitation for survivors back living in the community is limited.

## Current Status and Future Trends

Currently, rehabilitation services are not a common aspect of survivorship health care. This can result in a level of physical limitations that can either be prevented or improved with physical rehabilitation. Outpatient rehabilitation needs of cancer survivors are often the most underserved with one study demonstrating that patients are approximately 100 times more likely to receive rehabilitation care as an inpatient than as an outpatient [78]. At least from the survivors' perspective, problems in the area of physical function are common. In one study, researchers surveyed community-dwelling outpatients in order to estimate the prevalence of rehabilitation and symptom control problems among the participants and determine whether patient-identified problems were documented in the oncology clinic notes [79]. Nearly 250 patients filled out questionnaires and identified a total of 875 self-reported "needs." Of the 875 self-reported needs, just over 47% were functional problems. More than 65% of patients reported functional problems.

There are many barriers to rehabilitation [80]. One of the most problematic barriers is a lack of training in the subcategory of oncology rehabilitation for those providers who specialize in rehabilitation medicine. Indeed, most physiatrists receive very little training in oncology rehabilitation. The same is true for other rehabilitation professionals including physical and occupational therapists as well as speech and language pathologists. Becoming a skilled and effective provider of oncology rehabilitation care can pose a daunting task for those already in practice who may feel overwhelmed by the knowledge they must accumulate to expertly treat cancer patients. As the prevalence of survivors continues to increase and more is learned about the incidence and impact of physical limitations, we will see an increased level of attention both in terms of training and service related to this underserved area of quality care.

Another barrier is the sometimes nonexistent or often weak interface between oncology and rehabilitation healthcare providers. The rehabilitation and oncology departments are often physically separated in hospitals, and rehabilitation does not exist at all in many cancer centers. The professionals who work in these two specialties need to come together in order to develop a cancer rehabilitation team. Providers in both medical specialties need to identify patients with rehabilitation needs and then refer them for appropriate services. Of course, these services need to be developed in many hospitals, cancer centers, and outpatient facilities.

There are many other barriers as well – some dependent on individual institutions or people within the institutions who support (or do not support) oncology rehabilitation. There is a clear need for well-controlled outcome studies of the impact of specific rehabilitation services with specific functional limitations. The evidence base, while present in other disorders, needs to be created related to cancer survivors.

At this time, survivorship care is viewed favorably by many patients, doctors, nurses, administrators, hospital supporters, and the community [81]. Oncology rehabilitation can provide an important missing element in the health care of many who survive cancer but experience symptoms of pain and or functional limitations that interfere with a life well lived. Imagine a future where every cancer survivor has the opportunity to heal as well as possible and function optimally.

## References

1. Sheed W. In love with daylight: a memoir of recovery. New York: Simon & Schuster Inc.; 1995.
2. French M. A season in hell. New York: Alfred A. Knopf Inc.; 1998.
3. Hewitt M, Ganz P. From cancer patient to cancer survivor: lost in transition. Washington, DC: The National Academies Press; 2006.
4. Ganz PA, Haskell M. Cancer treatment. Philadelphia, PA: Saunders; 1990.
5. Guo Y, Young BL, Hainley S, Palmer JL, Bruera E. Evaluation and pharmacologic management of symptoms in cancer patients undergoing acute rehabilitation in a comprehensive cancer center. Arch Phys Med Rehabil. 2007;88(7):891–5.

6. Sweeney C, Schmitz KH, Lazovich D, Virnig BA, Wallace RB, Folsom AR. Functional limitations in elderly female cancer survivors. J Natl Cancer Inst. 2006;98(8):521–9.
7. Mehnert A. Employment and work-related issues in cancer survivors. Crit Rev Oncol Hematol [Online] 2010. [Accessed 5 Aug 2010]. Available from: http://www.ncbi.nlm.nih.gov/pubmed/20117019.
8. Ness KK, Hudson MM, Ginsberg JP, Nagarajan R, Kaste SC, Marina N, et al. Physical performance limitations in the Childhood Cancer Survivor Study cohort. J Clin Oncol. 2009;27(14):2382–9.
9. Tesauro GM, Rowland JH, Lustig C. Survivorship resources for post-treatment cancer survivors. Cancer Pract. 2002;10:277–83.
10. Yabroff KR, Lawrence WF, Clauser S, Davis WW, Brown ML. Burden of illness in cancer survivors: findings from a population-based national sample. J Natl Cancer Inst. 2004;96(17):1322–30.
11. Reitman JS, Dijkstra PU, Debreczeni R, Geertzen JH, Robinson DP, De Vries J. Impairments, disabilities and health related quality of life after treatment for breast cancer: a follow-up study 2.7 years after surgery. Disabil Rehabil. 2004;26:78–84.
12. Cleeland CS, Gonin R, Hatfield AK, Edmonson JH, Stewart JA, Pandya KJ. Pain and its treatment in outpatients with metastatic cancer. N Engl J Med. 1994;3(330):592–6.
13. Tasmuth T, von Smitten K, Hietanen P, Kataja M, Kalso E. Pain and other symptoms after different treatment modalities of breast cancer. Ann Oncol. 1995;6:453–9.
14. Teunissen SC, Wesker W, Kruitwagen C, de Haes HC, Voest EE, de Graeff A. Symptom prevalence in patients with incurable cancer: a systematic review. J Pain Symptom Manage. 2007;34:94–104.
15. Mao JJ, Armstrong K, Bowman MA, Xie SX, Kadakia R, Farrar JT. Symptom burden among cancer survivors: impact of age and comorbidity. J Am Board Fam Med. 2007;20(5):434–43.
16. Shamley D, Srinaganathan R, Oskrochi R, Lascurain-Aguirrebeña I, Sugden E. Three-dimensional scapulothoracic motion following treatment for breast cancer. Breast Cancer Res Treat. 2009;118(2):315–22.
17. Thomas-Maclean RL, Hack T, Kwan W, Towers A, Miedema B, Tilley A. Arm morbidity and disability after breast cancer: new directions for care. Oncol Nurs Forum. 2008;35(1):65–71.
18. Merchant CR, Chapman T, Kilbreath SL, Refshauge KM, Krupa K. Decreased muscle strength following management of breast cancer. Dis Rehabil. 2008;30(15):1098–105.
19. Güldiken Y, Orhan KS, Demirel T, Ural HI, Yücel EA, Değer K. Assessment of shoulder impairments after functional neck dissection: long term results. Auris Nasus Larynx. 2005;32(4):387–91.
20. Hartman A, van den Bos C, Stijnen T, Pieters R. Decrease in peripheral muscle strength and ankle dorsiflexion as long-term side effects of treatment for childhood cancer. Pediatr Blood Cancer. 2008;50(40):833–7.
21. Chan DN, Lui LY, So WK. Effectiveness of exercise programmes on shoulder mobility and lymphoedema after axillary lymph node dissection for breast cancer: a systematic review. J Adv Nurs [Online] 2010 [Accessed 5 Aug 2010]. Available from: http://www.ncbi.nlm.nih.gov/pubmed/20626480.
22. McNeely ML, Campbell K, Ospina M, Rowe BH, Dabbs K, Klassen TP, et al. Exercise interventions for upper-limb dysfunction due to breast cancer treatment. Cochrane Database Syst Rev. 2010;6:CD005211.
23. Lee SA, Kang JY, Kim YD, Kim SW, Kim YS, Lim JY. Effects of a scapular-oriented exercise programme on upper limb dysfunction in breast cancer survivors: a randomized controlled pilot trial. Clin Rehabil. 2010;24:600–13.
24. van der Molen L, van Rossum MA, Burkhead LM, Smeele LE, Rasch CR, Hilgers FJ. A randomized preventive rehabilitation trial in advanced head and neck cancer patients treated with chemoradiotherapy: feasibility, compliance, and short-term effects. Dysphagia [Online] 2010 [Accessed 5 Aug 2010]. Available from: http://www.ncbi.nlm.nih.gov/pubmed/20623305.

25. Bylow K, Dale W, Mustian K, Stadler WM, Rodin M, Hall W, et al. Falls and physical performance deficits in older patients with prostate cancer undergoing androgen deprivation therapy. Urology. 2008;72(2):422–7.
26. Winters-Stone KM, Nail L, Bennerr JA, Schwartz A. Bone health and falls: fracture risk in breast cancer survivors with chemotherapy-induced amenorrhea. Oncol Nurs Forum. 2009;36:315–25.
27. Simmonds MJ. Physical function in patients with cancer: psychometric characteristics and clinical usefulness of a physical performance battery. J Pain Symptom Manage. 2002;24(4):404–14.
28. Wampler MA, Topp KS, Miaskowski C, Byl NN, Rugo HS, Hamel K. Quantitative and clinical description of postural instability in women with breast cancer treated with taxane chemotherapy. Arch Phys Med Rehabil. 2007;88(8):1002–8.
29. Markman M. Chemotherapy-induced peripheral neuropathy: underreported and underappreciated. Curr Pain Headache Rep. 2006;10:275–8.
30. Hu MI, Gagel RF, Jimenez C. Bone loss in patients with breast or prostate cancer. Curr Osteoporos Rep. 2007;5:170–8.
31. Wasilewski-Masker K, Kaste SC, Hudson MM, Esiashvili N, Mattano LA, Meacham LR. Bone mineral density deficits in survivors of childhood cancer: long-term follow-up guidelines and review of the literature. Pediatrics. 2008;121:e705–13.
32. Chlebowski RT, Tagawa T. Early breast and prostate cancer and clinical outcomes (fracture). Oncology. 2009;23(14 Suppl 5):S16–20.
33. Mussa A, Bertorello N, Porta F, Galletto C, Nicolosi MG, Manicone R, et al. Prospective bone ultrasound patterns during childhood acute lymphoblastic leukemia treatment. Bone. 2010;46(4):1016–20.
34. Wright MJ, Galea V, Barr RD. Proficiency of balance in children and youth who have had acute lymphoblastic leukemia. Phys Ther. 2005;85(8):782–90.
35. Gilchrist LS, Galantino ML, Wampler M, Marchese VG, Morris GS, Ness KK. A framework for assessment in oncology rehabilitation. Phys Ther. 2009;89(3):286–306.
36. Volger CM, Sherrington C, Ogle SJ, Lord SR. Reducing risk of falling in older people discharged from hospital: a randomized controlled trial comparing seated exercises, weight-bearing exercises, and social visits. Arch Phys Med Rehabil. 2009;90(8):1317–24.
37. Burke TN, Franca FJ, de Meneses SR Ferreira, Cardoso VI, Marques AP. Postural control in elderly persons with osteoporosis: efficacy of an intervention program to improve balance and muscle strength: a randomized controlled trial. Am J Phys Med Rehabil. 2010;89(7):549–56.
38. Forster A, Lambley R, Young JB. Is physical rehabilitation for older people in long-term care effective? Findings from a systematic review. Age Aging. 2010;39(2):169–75.
39. Piva SR, Gil AB, Almeida GJ, DiGioia 3rd AM, Levison TJ, Fitzgerald GK. A balance exercise program apprears to improve function for patients with total knee arthroplasty:a randomized clinical trial. Phys Ther. 2010;90(6):880–94.
40. Luukinen H, Koski K, Laippala P, Kivela SL. Factors predicting fractures during falling impacts among home-dwelling older adults. J Am Geriatr Soc. 1997;45(11):1302–9.
41. Khazzani H, Allali F, Bennani L, Ichchou L, El Mansouri L, Abourazzak FE, et al. The relationship between physical performance measures, bone mineral density, falls and the risk of peripheral fracture: a cross-sectional analysis. BMC Public Health. 2009;9:297.
42. Muir SW, Berg K, Chesworth B, Klar N, Speechley M. Balance impairment as a risk factor for falls in community-dwelling older adults who are high functioning: a prospective study. Phys Ther. 2010;90(3):338–47.
43. Travers J, Dudgeon DJ, Amjadi K, McBride I, Dillon K, Laveneziana P, et al. Mechanisms of exertional dyspnea in patients with cancer. J Appl Physiol. 2008;104(1):57–66.
44. Jones LW, Eves ND, Haykowsky M, Freedland SJ, Mackey JR. Exercise intolerance in cancer and the role of exercise therapy to reverse dysfunction. Lancet Oncol. 2009;10(6):598–605.
45. Marks LB, Yu X, Prosnitz RG, Zhou SM, Hardenbergh PH, Blazing M, et al. The incidence and functional consequences of RT-associated cardiac perfusion defects. Int J Radiat Oncol Biol Phys. 2005;63(1):563–70.

46. Ewer MS, Lippman SM. Type II chemotherapy-related cardiac dysfunction: time to recognize a new entity. J Clin Oncol. 2005;23(13):2900–2.
47. Ginsberg SJ, Comis RL. The pulmonary toxicity of antineoplastic agents. Semin Oncol. 1982;9(1):34–51.
48. Ahlberg K, Ekman T, Gaston-Johansson F, Mock V. Assessment and management of cancer-related fatigue in adults. Lancet. 2003;362(9384):640–50.
49. Bower J, Ganz P, Desmond K. Fatigue in breast cancer survivors: occurrence, correlates, and impact on quality of life. J Clin Oncol. 2000;18(4):743–53.
50. Mock V, Atkinson A, Barsevick AM, Berger AM, Cimprich B, Eisenberger MA, et al. Cancer-related fatigue. Clinical practice guidelines in oncology. J Natl Compr Canc Netw. 2007;5:1054–78.
51. Cramp F, Daniel J. Exercise for the management of cancer-related fatigue in adults. Cochrane Database Syst Rev. 2008;2:CD006145.
52. Kuchinski AM, Reading M, Lash AA. Treatment-related fatigue and exercise in patients with cancer: a systematic review. Medsrug Nurs. 2009;18(3):174–80.
53. Roine E, Roine RP, Rasanen P, Vuori I, Sintonen H, Saarto T. Cost-effectiveness of interventions based on physical exercise in the treatment of various diseases: a systematic literature review. Int J Technol Assess Health Care. 2009;25(4):427–54.
54. Spence RR, Heesch KC, Brown WJ. Exercise and cancer rehabilitation: a systematic review. Cancer Treat Rev. 2010;36(2):185–94.
55. Silver JK. Rehabilitation in women with breast cancer. Phys Med Rehabil Clin N Am. 2007;18(3):521–37.
56. Haid A, Köberle-Wührer R, Knauer M, Burtscher J, Fritzsche H, Peschina W, et al. Morbidity of breast cancer patients following complete axillary dissection or sentinel node biopsy only: a comparative evaluation. Breast Cancer Res Treat. 2002;73(1):31–6.
57. Schulze T, Mucke J, Markwardt J, Schlag P, Bembenek A. Long-term morbidity of patients with early breast cancer after sentinel lymph node biopsy compared to axillary lymph node dissection. J Surg Oncol. 2006;93(2):109–19.
58. McNeely M, Campbell K, Rowe B, Klassen T, Mackey J, Courneya K. Effects of exercise on breast cancer patients and survivors: a systematic review and meta-analysis. CMAJ. 2006;175(1):34–41.
59. Cheema B, Gaul CA, Lane K, Fiatarone Singh MA. Progressive resistance training in breast cancer: a systematic review of clinical trials. Breast Cancer Res Treat. 2008;109(1):9–26.
60. Bicego D, Brown K, Ruddick M, Storey D, Wong C, Harris SR. Effects of exercise on quality of life in women living with breast cancer: a systematic review. Breast J. 2009;15(1):45–51.
61. Valenti M, Porzio G, Aielli F, Verna L, Cannita K, Manno R, et al. Physical exercise and quality of life in breast cancer survivors. Int J Med Sci. 2008;5(1):24–8.
62. Hewitt JA, Mokbel K, van Someren KA, Jewell AP, Garrod R. Exercise for breast cancer survival: the effect on cancer risk and cancer-related fatigue (CRF). Int J Fertil Womens Med. 2005;50(5 pt 1):231–9.
63. Irwin ML. Physical activity interventions for cancer survivor. Br J Sports Med. 2009;43(1):32–8.
64. Kwan W, Jackson J, Weir LM, Dingee C, McGregor G, Olivotto IA. Chronic arm morbidity after curative breast cancer treatment: prevalence and impact on quality of life. J Clin Oncol. 2002;20(20):4242–8.
65. Harris SR, Hugi MR, Olivotto IA, Levine M. Steering committee for clinical practice guidelines for the care and treatment of breast cancer. CMAJ. 2001;164(2):191–9.
66. Andersen L, Hojris I, Erlandsen M, Andersen J. Treatment of breast-cancer-related lymphedema with or without manual lymphatic drainage – a randomized study. Acta Oncol. 2000;39:399–405.
67. Williams AF, Vadgama A, Franks PJ, Mortimer PS. A randomized controlled crossover study of manual lymphatic drainage in women with breast cancer-related lymphoedema. Eur J Cancer Care. 2002;11(4):254–61.

68. McNeely ML, Magee DJ, Lees AW, Bagnall KM, Haykowsky M, Hanson J. The addition of manual lymph drainage to compression therapy for breast cancer related lymphedema: a randomized controlled trial. Breast Cancer Res Treat. 2004;86(2):95–106.
69. Didem K, Ufuk YS, Serdar S, Zumre A. The comparison of two different physiotherapy methods in treatment of lymphedema after breast surgery. Breast Cancer Res Treat. 2005;93(1):49–54.
70. Badger C, Preston N, Seers K, Mortimer P. Physical therapies for reducing and controlling lymphoedema of the limbs. Cochrane Database Syst Rev. 2004;4:CD003141.
71. Moseley AL, Carati CJ, Pillner NB. A systematic review of common conservative therapies for arm lymphoedema secondary to breast cancer treatment. Ann Oncol. 2007;18:639–46.
72. Gergich NL, Pfalzer LA, McGarvey C, Springer B, Gerber LH, Soballe P. Preoperative assessment enables the early diagnosis and successful treatment of lymphedema. Cancer. 2008;112(12):2809–19.
73. van der Molen L, van Rossum MA, Burkhead LM, Smeele LE, Hilgers FJ. Functional outcomes and rehabilitation strategies in patients treated with chemoradiotherapy for advanced head and neck cancer: a systematic review. Eur Arch Otorhinolaryngol. 2009;266(6):901–2.
74. Rogers LQ, Rao K, Malone J, Kandula P, Ronen O, Markwell SJ, et al. Factors associated with quality of life in outpatients with head and neck cancer 6 months after diagnosis. Head Neck. 2009;31(9):1207–14.
75. Karvonen-Gutierrez CA, Ronis DL, Fowler KE, Terrell JE, Gruber SB, Duffy SA. Quality of life scores predict survival among patients with head and neck cancer. J Clin Oncol. 2008;26(16):2754–60.
76. Lauchlan DT, McCaul JA, McCarron T. Neck dissection and the clinical appearance of post-operative shoulder disability: the post-operative role of physiotherapy. Eur J Cancer Care Engl. 2008;17(6):542–8.
77. Murphy BA, Gilbert J. Dysphagia in head and neck cancer patients treated with radiation: assessment, sequelae, and rehabilitation. Semin Radiat Oncol. 2009;19(1):35–42.
78. Cheville AL, Troxel AB, Basford JR, Kornblith AB. Prevalence and treatment patterns of physical impairments in patients with metastatic breast cancer. J Clin Oncol. 2008;26(16):2621–9.
79. Cheville AL, Beck LA, Petersen TL, Marks RS, Gamble GL. The detection and treatment of cancer-related functional problems in an outpatient setting. Support Care Cancer. 2009;17(1):61–7.
80. Silver J, Mayer RS. Barriers to pain management in the rehabilitation of the surgical oncology patient. J Surg Oncol. 2007;95(5):427–35.
81. Hewitt ME, Bamundo A, Day R, Harvey C. Perspectives on post-treatment cancer care: qualitative research with survivors, nurses, and physicians. J Clin Oncol. 2007;25(16):2270–3.

# Chapter 6
# Long-Term Psychological Well-Being: Strategies for Assessment and Intervention

**Anne Coscarelli, Christopher Recklitis, and Kauser Ahmed**

## Introduction

A cancer diagnosis typically precipitates a health crisis as patients cope with the shock of a life-threatening illness, and face cancer treatments that can be physically and emotionally arduous. Patients' social, family, and economic functioning are usually disrupted; at the same time, they find themselves facing fears of death or disability. Not surprisingly, many patients show signs of psychological distress or acute stress reactions at some point during their treatment [1–3]. The clinical literature has focused largely on the diagnosis and treatment phases of cancer care, and comparatively less is known about the psychological adaptation of cancer survivors after completion of therapy. Given the substantial burdens experienced by cancer patients during treatment, it is a testament to human resilience, and the quality of care and support patients receive, that most adapt to these challenges and are able to establish positive psychological outcomes. Most studies of long-term cancer survivors indicate that the vast majority do not suffer from severe psychological distress, and may be no more prone to psychiatric disorders than those never affected by cancer [2, 4–7]. At the same time, there is a sizable minority of cancer survivors whose lives will be significantly disrupted by the health challenges of cancer, and these survivors report significant psychological distress requiring additional support and psychological treatment. The focus of this chapter is on understanding the psychological challenges that arise for survivors in the posttreatment period, the risk factors associated with distress, and the role of professionals in identifying and addressing these issues.

With two out of three Americans expected to face cancer in their lifetime, and two-thirds of those expected to survive 5 years or more after diagnosis [5, 8], there can be little doubt that the psychosocial needs of cancer survivors constitute a significant and growing subset of health-care concerns. Moreover, with more than

A. Coscarelli (✉)
University of California, Los Angeles, CA, USA
e-mail: acoscarelli@mednet.ucla.edu

M. Feuerstein and P.A. Ganz (eds.), *Health Services for Cancer Survivors*,
DOI 10.1007/978-1-4419-1348-7_6, 

12 million cancer survivors in the USA [9], the diversity of survivor experiences and associated psychological issues can be only touched on in a brief treatment of the subject. Our focus in this chapter is on understanding the most common psychological challenges facing survivors who have completed treatment. We choose this focus, not because other phases of care are less important, but because patients who have completed active treatment have fewer visits with their medical providers, making it harder for providers to monitor psychological adjustment, even as new issues of "life after cancer" emerge. Since most cancer patients are adults at the time of diagnosis, we emphasize research and clinical care relevant to these survivors and make efforts to point out the special needs of younger cancer survivors where appropriate.

## Studies of Psychological Adjustment After Cancer

A review of the literature on psychological adjustment after cancer found that prevalence estimates for psychological distress in long-term survivors range from 0% to 58% [7]. This lack of consensus underscores the great variability in how psychological distress has been defined and measured, and the different populations studied. Characterizing distress in any population is complicated by several factors. First, the words "depression," or "anxiety" can describe normal transient variations in mood, lasting and potentially pathological mood states, as well as psychiatric disorders characterized by multiple symptoms associated with significant impairment. Depending on which meaning is intended, and how it is operationalized and measured, the prevalence will vary considerably. In addition, in medically involved groups like cancer survivors, psychological symptoms overlap with symptoms of medical conditions and medication side effects, making it difficult to differentiate between psychological and medical factors. Finally, some psychiatric symptoms are common in the general population, so reports of these disorders or related symptoms in a medically involved group may only reflect the background level of disorders expected in the general population. Understanding these limitations is important in both the assessment of individual survivors, as well as in considering the research on depression after completion of cancer therapy.

Population-based studies comparing long-term survivors to controls or normative reference groups on self-report symptom measures report an increased prevalence of psychological distress in long-term cancer survivors [5, 10–12]. For example, using data from the National Health Interview Survey, Hoffman et al. [5] found 5.6% of long-term survivors reported symptoms of serious psychological distress compared to only 3.0% of matched non-cancer controls. Similarly, in a survey of Medicare beneficiaries, Baker et al. [10], found cancer survivors as a group had poor emotional as well as physical quality-of-life functioning compared to unaffected individuals. Furthermore, in a 2-year follow-up study [13], these differences were found to persist, indicating that they did not reflect transient difficulties associated with short-term adaptation to cancer. Reeve et al. [14] also reported a decline in mental health–related quality of life following a cancer diagnosis in a similar study of Medicare beneficiaries. Two studies that used depression-specific ratings across cancer groups also reported significantly elevated rates of depressive symptoms, even in survivors 4–8 years after diagnosis [11, 12]. Costanzo et al. [12], for example, found that symptoms of depression and anxiety were increased in survivors utilizing a unique data set that allowed for a comparison of survivors' post-cancer symptom ratings with ratings made prior to their cancer. Studies of long-term survivors of pediatric cancers using data from the Childhood Cancer Survivor Study have similarly reported higher levels of psychological distress in survivors compared to sibling controls including symptoms of anxiety and depression [15].

Evidence of increased prevalence of psychological distress after cancer can also be found in epidemiological studies from several Scandinavian countries reporting elevated rates of suicide in persons with a history of cancer [16–18]. A recent registry study conducted in the USA [19] similarly reported that among persons diagnosed with cancer, 31.4 suicides occur for every 100,000 person-years of follow-up – almost twice the rate of the general population (16.7 suicides for every 100,000 person-years). Prior registry studies have typically focused on suicides occurring within the first 2–5 years of cancer diagnosis, but this study and at least one other show that rates of suicide remain elevated in cancer survivors as long as 8–10 years following diagnosis [20]. Studies have also found some form of suicidal ideation was reported to be present in 8% of ambulatory cancer patients [21], and a study of childhood cancer survivors reported by Recklitis et al. [22] found suicidal ideation was more prevalent in survivors than in controls, even though most of the survivors were more than 15 years from diagnosis.

Taken together, these studies provide some of the strongest evidence that prevalence of psychological symptoms is increased in cancer survivors. However, it is important to note that results have been quite different when studies have been limited to a single disease or survivor population. For example, studies of colorectal survivors have reported higher levels of depressive symptoms, but similar studies of breast and testicular survivors have not [23–26].

Similarly, it should be noted that the preponderance of studies of psychological late effects of cancer have examined the prevalence of symptoms of *distress* and not *psychiatric disorders*. For example, many studies report cancer survivors are at risk for depression, but almost none have examined whether cancer survivors are at increased risk for the psychiatric diagnosis of major depressive disorder (MDD) rather than symptoms of depression. This is an important distinction because MDD is a major mental illness that negatively impacts mental, physical, and functional status. Using data from a large epidemiological study that used structured diagnostic interviews to specifically assess MDD, Pirl et al. [6] found no difference in the rate of MDD between cancer survivors and controls. They interpret these findings as indicating that long-term cancer survivors are at increased risk for depressive symptoms, but not necessarily a diagnosis of MDD. This finding is similar to several studies examining posttraumatic stress disorder (PTSD) after cancer, which have found a high prevalence of posttraumatic stress symptoms (PTSS), but not necessarily elevated rates of fully diagnosable psychiatric disorders [27, 28].

This raises an important question as to why cancer survivors may experience more symptoms of distress but not the mental disorders defined in the psychiatric nosology. Criteria for a psychiatric diagnosis typically include a minimum number of key symptoms that endure for a minimum amount of time, and are associated with at least some amount of impairment [29]. Some survivors with symptoms of distress that are not sufficiently severe or not associated with sufficient impairments to qualify for a particular diagnosis, and may be appropriately considered cases of "subthreshold," or "subclinical" distress. Other survivors may have symptoms that simply do not coincide with the patterns derived from studies of mental illness – but these symptoms may be severe and cause significant impairment.

## Beyond Psychiatric Diagnoses: Defining the Continuum of Distress

Using psychiatric definitions and measures is important in clinical evaluation and research, but these diagnostic criteria were not developed to reflect the cancer survivor experience; the study of psychological adaptation to cancer or supportive interventions for survivors should not be limited to addressing psychiatric disorders. Following conventions used in studies of cancer patients and survivors [4, 30], as well as recommendations from the National Comprehensive Cancer Network (NCCN) [31–33], in this chapter we address the concerns of cancer survivors and focus broadly on the psychological and behavioral symptoms that cause either *subjective distress* or *impairment in functioning*, not only those that meet criteria for psychiatric diagnoses.

As noted in a report from the NCCN [31], the term "distress" may be relatively free of stigma, an important consideration in cancer survivorship. Also, it encompasses the full continuum of responses that individuals may experience from normal reactions of worry to disabling psychiatric conditions, making it particularly useful to describe the range of symptoms and adaptive problems that survivors may experience. The distress may be experienced in the years immediately after treatment as individuals grapple with trying to recover normal functioning or years later as they continue to experience the fear of recurrence. The distress may be short-lived and "subclinical," or, in conjunction with other stressors, it could become the pathway to a clinical psychiatric diagnosis. Lastly, we chose the word distress because we believe that it also communicates that the experience is amenable to change and can be shaped by appropriate, timely, and collaborative interventions between survivors and health professionals, as well as survivor advocacy and community organizations. In the following sections, we provide a framework for understanding and addressing survivors' psychosocial distress as it typically presents in the primary care setting. Highlighted in Fig. 6.1, we address both common factors that can place survivors at high risk for significant distress as well as periods of vulnerability during which distress may be heightened. The subsequent sections, Assessment and Interventions, aim to assist clinicians in having useful conversations with their

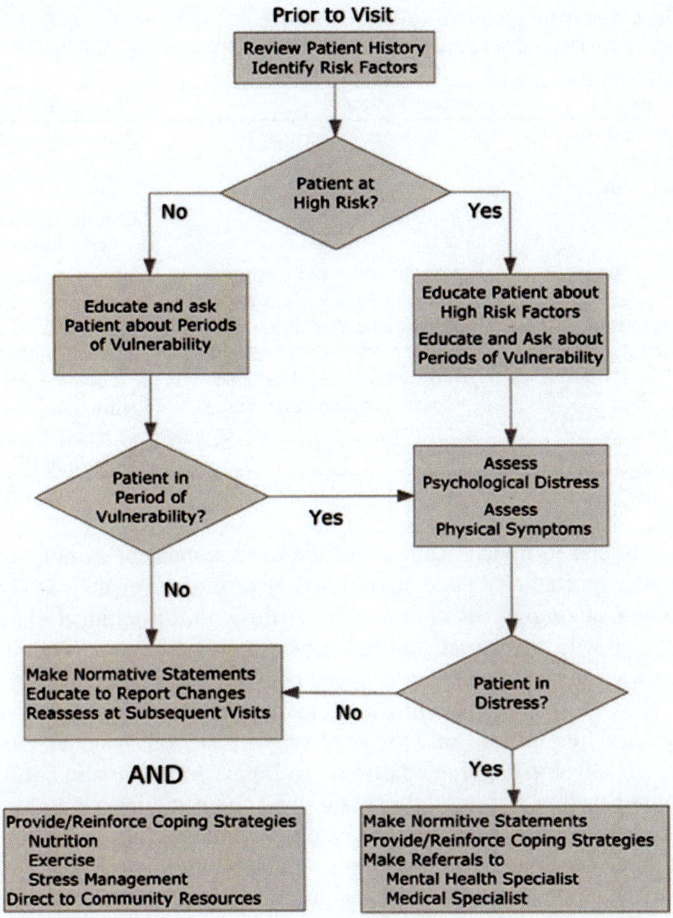


**Fig. 6.1** Assessing and intervening in psychosocial distress

survivor patients about the kinds of issues they may be facing and directing them to treatment and support strategies that may be beneficial in addressing their psychosocial needs.

## *Risk Factors for Psychological Distress After Cancer*

Psychological challenges are part of life. As Erikson so wisely demonstrated [34] in tracing the "crises of development" from infancy to adulthood, the specific challenges change and change us as individuals, but they are ongoing throughout life. For Erikson, the normative challenges of adulthood provide opportunities for reworking past unresolved issues as well as the danger that failure to master a

**Table 6.1** Risk factors for psychological distress after cancer (Reprinted, with permission, from Oncology (Williston Park) 22(11 Suppl Nurse Ed):11–20, 2008. Copyright 2008, CMP Healthcare Media, LLC)

| Personal factors | Disease factors | Physical factors |
|---|---|---|
| Preexisting conditions– Mental illness, functional limits | Residual disease/recurrence | Poor health status |
| Economic hardship | High risk for relapse | Chronic medical conditions |
| Lack of social support | Prolonged or intense treatment (e.g., bone marrow transplant) | Pain or disfigurement |
| Life stressors (e.g., divorce, unemployment) | Problems adjusting or adhering to treatment (e.g., medication noncompliance, substance abuse, extreme emotional distress) | Functional limitations (e.g., ambulation, communication) |
| Disability | | Difficulties in self-care (e.g., dressing, eating, bathing) |

challenge may end in maladaptation and the development of symptoms. Cancer, though not an expected challenge, may similarly result in growth as well as maladjustment. Generalizing across cancers can be difficult, but clinical experience as well as research with cancer patients and survivors suggest that several factors may predispose a cancer survivor to have ongoing psychological problems (see Table 6.1 [5, 7, 12, 15, 35–39]). Understanding the role of these risk factors can be helpful in identifying survivors in need of additional support as well as understanding why some survivors develop ongoing emotional problems and others do not.

Background factors or preexisting conditions about the individual survivor are important to consider – psychiatric history, other conditions, lack of resources such as low income, lack of adequate housing or transportation – as these are known or suspected to be associated with poor outcomes after cancer or other stresses and suggest increased vulnerability to future psychological distress. Similarly, extreme emotional or behavioral reactions that occurred during treatment should be considered risk factors for ongoing emotional distress. Several aspects of the cancer diagnosis and its treatment may also be associated with future emotional distress. Specifically, poor prognosis, cancer relapse, treatments of long duration and high intensity may all increase the likelihood of later emotional distress.

Perhaps most important in understanding the likelihood for psychological problems are the individual's *health and functional status* after completion of treatment. Survivors who have *chronic conditions* (e.g., heart disease, diabetes, COPD), and especially those with multiple chronic conditions, or chronic pain may be particularly vulnerable. In particular, physical symptoms that lead to loss of important aspects of individual identity – sexual dysfunction, problems with bladder or bowel control, as well as disfigurement, fatigue, and cognitive changes – can be particularly burdensome and lead to increased psychological distress. Similarly, the loss of independence associated with not being able to return to work or other previous activities or any condition that limits independence should be considered a likely risk factor.

Risk factors can be an important guide to assessing and monitoring survivors, and very useful in identifying those survivors who are most likely to develop psychological distress. However, it is important to appreciate that the course of cancer survivorship is dynamic and individuals who may initially present with no risk factors still require ongoing monitoring and evaluation.

## *Periods of Vulnerability/Psychosocial Stressors in Cancer Survivorhood*

In addition to the factors which may place *some* individuals at greater risk for distress, there are other stressors (periods of vulnerability) in cancer survivorhood which can potentially impact any survivor and can precipitate psychological distress, which are detailed in Table 6.2. These are stressors that can occur early or late in the survivorhood trajectory and impact all survivors, including those who appear to have had a sustained period of healthy recovery and good psychosocial adjustment. Psychological adjustment to cancer survivorhood, like physical adjustment, generally improves with time but there can remain some vulnerabilities that do not ever abate. These vulnerabilities are largely triggered by anxieties about cancer recurrence.

Thoughts about cancer recurrence can lead to the unexpected onset of sadness, anxiety, and fear. These emotions, and their corollary behavioral disruptions in sleep, appetite, concentration, or mood, can be triggered by both predictable and unanticipated events. Routine scans or the anniversary of the date of diagnosis can

**Table 6.2** Periods of vulnerability

*New events or triggers*

- New symptoms of unknown origin
  - Workup of symptoms
  - Awaiting results of workup/watch and reassess
- Diagnosis of late effects
- Secondary cancer
- New primary
- New onset of other health problems
- Scientific findings altering treatment strategies for future patients
- Recurrence of cancer
- Diagnosis friends/family
- Notable cancer-related media events

*Ongoing*

- Bothersome continuing symptoms
- Regular medical follow-up/surveillance

*Transitions*

- End of treatment
- Transitions in adjuvant treatment (e.g., transition on/off trastuzumab, hormonal therapy)
- Career and health insurance changes
- Reproduction initiation

often be the catalyst that generates acute worry, and re-experiencing traumatic memories of treatment. Similarly, unexpected events such as the onset of new physical symptoms or exams to work up suspicious findings are also significant triggers that can spike preoccupation with symptoms and fears of dying. Outside environmental stressors such as learning of a peer's recurrence or even the death of a celebrity due to cancer, someone personally unknown but whose death creates ongoing media exposure about cancer, can have a similar impact. Such events can jar an individual from an otherwise healthy adjustment and normal functioning into a period of acute, symptomatic distress with prominent feelings of worry, difficulty concentrating, weepiness, trouble sleeping, and other disruptions [40, 41].

While some distress may take place when individuals first begin to transition from active treatment to survivorhood, the experience of loss may not be fully absorbed for some time. For example, treatment effects that lead to infertility may not be immediately felt until the survivor finds a mate and wants to begin a family. The loss of the ability to bear children may give rise to a new level of distress which is rooted in the earlier experience of cancer. Similarly, late effects that diminish functioning and persist into the second year or beyond may affect career or lifestyle choices, such as retirement and travel. The losses may not be fully appreciated until one evaluates the ways in which cancer may have derailed occupational success or enjoyment of long-cherished plans. Losses that have a larger impact on ongoing identity may not be experienced in the immediacy of the end of treatment, but rather as the individual hits changing developmental milestones and must negotiate them as a cancer survivor.

The episodes of distress created by any of these periods of vulnerabilities or triggers can be brief, lasting a few days or weeks, or given other risk factors, they can persist and worsen, cascading toward clinical depression or anxiety. Survivors may present in their primary care physicians' office with complaints of physical symptoms, requests for more aggressive or frequent testing, or unspecified anxiety. It can be very useful for physicians to ask about psychosocial stressors as part of their routine monitoring of the cancer survivor patient. Acknowledgment by the health-care team of these feelings of sadness or anxiety around stressful life events and periods of life transition can be enormously powerful in destigmatizing the emotional distress and help survivors to normalize their reactions as an expected part of the late effects of their cancer treatment.

## Assessment

Given the various sources of psychosocial distress that cancer survivors can experience, how best can their psychological concerns be evaluated in the primary care setting? There are two approaches to assessing the psychological well-being and needs of survivors. The first approach is an organic process that evolves in the primary care environment and requires clinicians to develop some knowledge of the kinds of problems that survivors might expect as outlined in Table 6.3 as well as understanding the risk factors and periods of vulnerability described in Tables 6.1 and 6.2.

**Table 6.3** Categories of survivor psychological distress/well-being

*Depression*
- Mild
- Major depressive episode
- Suicidal ideation

*Anxiety*
- Fear of recurrence
- Heightened sense of vulnerability
  - Distress associated with reduction in contact/treatment
  - Other things can go wrong
- Post-traumatic stress symptoms
  - Intrusive thoughts and worries
  - Memories and psychological distress exacerbated by exposure to
    - Others with cancer in environment or media
    - Medical environment, tests, procedures
    - Anniversaries of diagnosis, treatments, end of treatment
    - Screening tests
    - Workup for specific findings/symptoms

*Distress/loss associated with post-treatment physical health (delayed or immediate)*
- Fertility
- Changes in sexual functioning
- Lymphedema
- Cognitive impairment/changes
- Sleep disruptions and changes
- Bodily function impairments/changes
- Weight gain
- Menopause
- Fatigue and energy
- Pain
- Performing physical activity such as exercise
- Secondary cancers

*Relational stressors*
- Impact on intimate relationships
- Impact on children
- Fear for others (e.g., children, siblings)
  - Due to cancer history
  - Genetic mutations

*Economic and vocational/educational/employment concerns*
- Returning to work or school
- Changes in job, promotion, accomplishment
- Changes in drive
- Health insurance maintenance

*Spiritual/existential*
- Meaning of experience
- Meaning of life
- Challenges to faith
- Reordering of life priorities
- Positive growth

(continued)

**Table 6.3** (continued)

| |
|---|
| *Other life stressors* |
| • Divorce |
| • Loss of spouse/partner |
| • Parenting struggles |
| • Loss of family of origin |
| • Caregiving responsibilities for others |
| • Health concerns/comorbid illness |
| • Loss of employment |
| • Spiritual and existential crises |

**Table 6.4** Menu of psychosocial assessment questions in the medical/primary care environment

- What is it like for you coming back to the medical environment now that your treatment is over?
- Do you find yourself thinking about what happened to you or about the future frequently? Do these thoughts interfere with your sense of pleasure, sleep, daily functioning?
- Are you having any ongoing concerns regarding symptoms, issues with your family, work, mood, sex, or spiritual needs that you would like to talk about?
- Have you ever received any counseling or support for these difficulties?
- Would you like to have someone to talk to about these experiences?
- Who do you talk to when you have worries or concerns about being a cancer survivor?
- Do you have concerns about your health because of your cancer? For example, do you worry about late effects of treatment or your cancer coming back?
- Are you having difficulties with your mood, sleep, pain or other areas that do not seem to be getting better or might be getting worse?
- Have you noticed any positive or negative effects on your relationships with children or partner [support system]?
- Do you worry that your cancer may have implications for your children? Do you have concerns about cancer history, genetic issues, or screening for members of your family?
- Are there any new stressors in your life? Do you feel like you need assistance with any of these?
- Do you have concerns that you are not doing everything you can to keep the cancer from returning? How much distress does this create?

An educated clinician can initiate questions around the potential areas of distress as part of a clinical assessment and communicate both knowledge of the survivorhood trajectory and an openness to hear the survivor's experiences. Table 6.4 presents examples of these types of questions. With these tools as guides, providers can begin ongoing dialogues with their survivor patients in order to understand their patients' evolving needs. As suggested in the flowchart presented in Fig. 6.1, this informal assessment allows provider and patient to easily address a number of concerns and consider a variety of interventions that might otherwise be missed.

Cancer survivors are often interested in talking about these issues, but often wait for providers to "start the conversation [42–44]." For some individuals, reassurance from their physician that their experience is normal may be sufficient to help maintain psychological well-being. Table 6.5 presents a menu of examples of supportive/normative statements as illustrations of this process. For others,

**Table 6.5** Menu of supportive normative statements

| |
|---|
| • It is common for patients to feel more vulnerable when treatment ends and there is less intense contact with the medical team. If you feel this and are worried about symptoms, come in and let us evaluate what you are experiencing. |
| • Many survivors worry about cancer coming back. It can be helpful to develop some strategies to manage anxiety such as relaxation and mindfulness, but if you are worried about symptoms or recurrence, we should evaluate what is going on with you. |
| • I know that when we do these scans, it is likely to bring back feelings of worry and anxiety about your original diagnosis or even the possibility of the cancer returning. This is perfectly normal. I want to minimize the impact of this stress on you. I will get the results back to you as soon as possible. You should contact me in "*X*" number of days. |
| • When these late effects arise, years later, it often brings back a lot of feelings of loss and sadness about having been diagnosed with cancer. |
| • Sometimes survivors of cancer have an increased sense of well-being, positive changes or personal growth as a result of what they learned through the process. |
| • Many people who have had cancer report that it has affected their relationships with their friends and family members. |
| • Fatigue or reduced energy is a common experience for cancer survivors. It usually gets better with time, but sometimes it can take longer than you might expect or want. It is important to give yourself room to heal. Healthy nutrition and regular exercise, starting slowly and increasing your time in a walking program can have physical and psychological benefits. |
| • Sometimes survivors have feelings of loss or sadness associated with changes in their body image, bodily function, or sexuality after a cancer diagnosis. It is sometimes helpful to have someone to talk to about these areas. |
| • Survivors often benefit from a consultation with a health psychologist [other mental health professional] to talk about the changes they have experienced as a result of their cancer diagnosis and treatment. The psychologist can help you problem-solve how to best manage some of the symptoms you are experiencing. |
| • Survivors often feel frightened by the information they find on the Internet about their cancer or treatment. Sometimes it is helpful to address your concerns here with me [your doctor] rather than searching on the web. |
| • Many survivors find that they need support in figuring out how to manage the stresses of returning to their regular life. There are different kinds of resources to help you with this. |
| • Even though you won't be having so much contact with me, there are other people in the health-care community who are trained to assist you as you move through the phases of recovery and into long-term survivorship. I'm happy to assist you in identifying what might be helpful to you. |
| • Many survivors find benefit from learning a stress management technique such as mindfulness, yoga, or relaxation training. |
| • Many survivors make lifestyle changes or begin utilizing complementary medicine such as vitamins, acupuncture, and supplements in an effort to make themselves as cancer unfriendly as possible. I would like you to keep me informed about the choices you are making. |

recommendations for self-care strategies may be beneficial. For those indicating more distress, formal referral to other professionals such as psychologists, psychiatrists, social workers and mental health nurses may be warranted. Education and monitoring of psychosocial stressors can be helpful to all survivors, and should be incorporated into routine survivor follow-up care, thus, communicating to survivors that their psychosocial well-being is important and will be attended to if they begin to experience difficulties at a later date.

A second approach which may be more easily adapted in some settings than others requires using formalized assessment tools that include items addressing emotional health, economic, social, and functional status in a nursing assessment or review of systems checklist completed by survivors at the time of their office visit. Self-report assessment has the advantage of being simple to incorporate into each visit and presenting relatively little burden to providers and survivors. It also insures that these topics are addressed, and "primes" survivors and providers to discuss these issues. At a minimum, these items would include six to ten questions about general emotional functioning including depressed mood, anxiety, feelings of hopelessness and suicidal thoughts, as well as other symptoms or functional limitations. Self-report rating scales that have been previously validated can also be important tools for screening cancer survivors, and many specialized survivor clinics use some form of symptom checklist for routine assessment of psychological functioning. Validated rating scales have the advantage of being standardized so that information can be compared to some normative data that facilitate interpretation and comparison with the general population.

To be practical for clinical settings and minimize survivor burden, brief measures (< 20 items) including the Hospital Anxiety and Depression Scale (HADS) [45], the Brief Symptom Inventory-18 (BSI-18) [46], the Distress Thermometer [47], and the Patient Health Questionnaire-9 (PHQ-9) [48] have been favored [49]. Short measures can have limited scope, however, meaning that only one or two symptom domains (e.g., fatigue, pain, depression) can be covered. In addition, very brief scales (less than five items) can have limited psychometric properties, and longer scales may be more successful at differentiating between significant and nonsignificant levels of distress [49]. The one-item distress thermometer has been widely used in cancer patients, but reports of its sensitivity to clinical distress have varied across populations with a recent review suggesting that longer measures may be more accurate and advantageous than the distress thermometer and other very brief scales [49–51]. Whenever self-report rating scales are applied to cancer survivors, it is important to carefully evaluate how these instruments may operate. It is well known that the reliability and validity of tests will vary in different populations, and several studies have indicated that previously validated tests may operate differently or require different cutoff scores to be used in cancer patients or survivors [52–54].

In selecting a self-report screening measure, providers should consider instruments that focus on problems likely to be most relevant to their particular population. In many survivor groups, depression and anxiety will be common concerns and because studies show cancer survivors are at higher risk for suicidal thoughts and behaviors, some consideration should be given to including feelings of hopelessness and suicidal thoughts. The HADS, BSI-18, as well as the more recently developed Psychosocial Screen for Cancer have been used to address symptoms of depression and anxiety after cancer, and several other measures such as the Beck Anxiety Inventory, Zung depression scales, and PHQ-9 and CES-D assess either depression or anxiety alone (see Vodermaier et al. for review) [49]. In some survivor groups, other symptom areas such as cognitive problems or substance abuse may be important to address. Using the published literature on screening for psychological distress in cancer patients [49, 55] can help identify candidate screening measures, though caution should be exercised in generalizing the application of these same measures to cancer survivors. Until research on cancer survivors has provided specific validation of the instrument and clinical cutoff scores in cancer survivors, clinicians should carefully consider how to interpret both negative and positive screening information and should work closely with a mental health consultant familiar with clinical screening tools to select and implement this kind of screening in a clinical environment.

Whatever written assessment is used, reviewing screening responses and discussing them directly with the survivor is essential. By way of introduction, a provider may simply ask: "When you completed the questions about mood and emotional functioning, did any of those questions seem to apply to you?" The provider can then quickly scan the responses to the self-report items and inquire about any that were endorsed. Assuming that no significant emotional issues were raised, a final question, such as, "Is there anything else about how you are feeling emotionally, getting along at home or at work that we should talk about?," may help encourage reticent survivors to bring up any other emotional concerns, or to close the topic and provide a segue to the next area for discussion.

Depending on the survivor population, between 10% and 30% of survivors can be expected to indicate they are experiencing some significant symptoms of depression, and they will require further assessment and/or, referral to a mental health or medical professional. In talking with survivors about their symptoms, it is important to acknowledge that everyone experiences normal variation in mood. Since medical visits can be a source of anxiety, it is important that providers distinguish between anxiety related to a follow-up visit versus anxiety that is more lasting and potentially impairing a survivor's functioning. Assessment should focus on symptoms that are lasting, cause distress or impaired functioning, or that are associated with other key symptoms like poor sleep or appetite. Because survivors of some cancers may have persistent fatigue, it is important to try to differentiate this from depression. Although it may be difficult to tease apart depression and fatigue, depression generally has more psychological symptoms such as sadness and inability to experience pleasure. Evaluation of depression, anxiety, and other psychological symptoms in survivors must include an investigation of medical conditions or medications that may be contributing. Cancer treatments may have medical late effects affecting hormonal, cardiac, pulmonary, and neurological functioning, and effects of these systems may be associated with psychological symptoms. Treatment for an underlying condition that may be causing emotional symptoms (e.g., thyroid dysfunction) may significantly improve emotional health. Similarly, many commonly prescribed medications may cause symptoms of depression or anxiety, and a careful medication history may reveal possible associations with medications.

## Interventions That Can Help Promote Well-Being

Estimates suggest that at most 10% of cancer patients receive psychosocial interventions to ameliorate the difficulties they face during treatment. Studies examining the utility of specific psychosocial intervention modalities for individuals going through cancer have not led to consistent recommendations, due to the heterogeneity of study designs and participants [56]. There is even less evidence-based data regarding interventions within the cancer survivor population. Nonetheless, reviews of existing literature provide reason to believe that psychosocial interventions have the ability to help individuals with cancer cope better, improve their affective states, decrease negative effects of treatment, and to positively increase their quality of life [57–59, 83].

Table 6.6 lists strategies that can be employed both for prevention of psychosocial distress and as coping strategies for managing psychosocial distress. Whenever possible, these recommendations are based on empirical evidence including cognitive behavioral therapy to reduce cancer-related depression [60], supportive expressive group therapies for providing emotional support and facilitating psychosocial adjustment [2, 61, 62], yoga and exercise for reducing cancer-related

**Table 6.6** Prevention/coping strategies

| Education and information |
|---|
| Mind–body strategies<br>• Mindfulness<br>• Relaxation training<br>• Yoga<br>• Qigong |
| Cognitive behavioral interventions<br>• Anxiety management<br>• Depression management<br>• Stress management<br>• Sleep disorders<br>• Relationship/intimacy distress |
| Psychotropic medication evaluation |
| Communication with health-care team |
| Healthy lifestyle changes<br>• Nutrition<br>• Exercise<br>• Complementary and alternative medicine (integrative medicine) |
| Enlisting social support<br>• Communication with family, friends<br>• Connection with survivors<br>• Support groups<br>• Advocacy |

fatigue [63], relaxation/guided imagery to assist patients in managing anxiety as well as physical symptoms [64]. These skills can help anchor patients during the course of their treatment and assist them in taking an active role in their care. While we await more systematic research, there is limited risk and potentially great benefit in utilizing the modalities that have shown promise for relieving distress among cancer survivors. Case 1 presents a clinical example.

**Case 1** Thirty-five-year-old male, diagnosed with non-Hodgkin's lymphoma treated with radiation to the pelvic region one year ago. Recent scans and blood work indicate disease is still in remission. Survivor seen by PCP for follow-up for resolving upper respiratory virus. PCP asks about fatigue since cancer treatment and how it has affected other aspects of life. Survivor acknowledges he is not sleeping well due to some pelvic pain, has not fully resumed normal work, and social activities have been limited. Survivor expresses some worry about recurrence while waiting for test results and recent illness has triggered additional worries which disrupt his sleep and increase fatigue.

**Interventions**

- Discussion with primary care doctor about persistence of symptoms
- Development of schedule for next screening tests with reassurance about current results
- Instruction provided about walking program with incremental increases and additional exercise as tolerated
- Plan developed for reengagement with social network
- Assessment and ruling out depression, with recommendations for sleep hygiene
- Referral for mind/body relaxation stress management class
- Education about variations in survivorhood trajectory and normalization of physical symptoms and psychological distress
- Assess and treat pain

The intervention recommendations that we propose are in three broad areas: (1) basic psychoeducation that health-care practitioners can provide to all cancer survivors as a framework for what to expect in the survivorhood trajectory and for normalizing some of the distresses that are part of the process; (2) self-care tools (yoga, meditation, support groups), nutrition and exercise guidelines that practitioners can recommend to survivors to maintain well-being and to address symptoms of mild to moderate distress; and (3) recommendations for situations that may warrant further consultation and referral to mental health practitioners.

## *Psychoeducation in Survivorship*

We advocate that health-care practitioners in the primary care setting be educated to understand the nature of the long-term "survivorhood trajectory" so that they can appropriately educate their patients and properly facilitate comprehensive care. Recent studies in Canada and the USA [65, 66] indicate that primary care physicians feel unprepared to address the complex needs of cancer survivors in their practices and look for additional educational programs and practice guidelines to assist them.

As cancer survivors leave the world of active treatment with frequent contact with their oncology care team, they require a "roadmap" of the course ahead; one that must be updated as the journey extends in time. Survivors need realistic expectations of how long the process of recovery from treatment can take and ways of understanding the milestones and hurdles that exist in the years ahead. Appropriate education delivered by their physician can offset the distress that may manifest as shame, demoralization, and anxiety of not feeling "back to normal" for patients that are experiencing normative limitations and are unable to function at their pre-diagnosis capacity. A psychosocial "roadmap" of what may happen could also assist survivors in having important conversations with loved ones and with employers about their evolving needs. Survivors do not exist in a vacuum; their adaptation is very much influenced by their ability to manage the various relational, social, and occupational contexts in which they live. Facilitation of this process may well allow survivors to communicate

**Table 6.7** Survivor community resources

| |
|---|
| Lance Armstrong Foundation<br>http://www.livestrong.org |
| National Coalition for Cancer Survivorship<br>http://www.canceradvocacy.org |
| American Cancer Society<br>http://www.cancer.org |
| CancerCare<br>http://www.cancercare.org |
| Fertile Hope (A Live**STRONG**™ Initiative)<br>http://www.fertilehope.org |
| Cancer Survivors Network<br>http://www.csn.org |
| American Psychosocial Oncology Society<br>http://www.apos-society.org |
| National Cancer Institute: Office of Cancer Survivorship<br>http://dccps.nci.nih.gov/ocs |
| American Society of Clinical Oncology<br>http://www.Cancer.net |
| National Cancer Survivors Day Foundation<br>http://www.ncsdf.org |
| OncoLink: Live**STRONG**™ Care Plan<br>http://www.oncolink.org/oncolife |
| Planet Cancer for Young Adults (A Live**STRONG**™ Initiative)<br>http://www.planetcancer.org/ |

better, and develop better social support, rather than becoming isolated. While this chapter focuses on the psychosocial needs of cancer survivors who are a year or more beyond active treatment, it is suggested that some of the distress that individuals experience in later survivorhood could be mitigated by timely psychoeducation as they cross the "threshold" to survivor care. Such education can be supplemented by written materials found on survivor-specific websites and referrals to support resources, examples of which are included in Table 6.7. Most importantly, the initiation of communication about survivor psychosocial concerns by their health-care practitioner signals to survivors that their emotional concerns are valid and their physician is receptive to addressing them.

## *Health Improvement Strategies: Nutrition, Exercise, Stress Management*

In the period after treatment, many survivors begin searching in earnest for tools that can help them stay "cancer free." The reasons stem from both sound medical reasoning – current literature suggests that there may be value to making appropriate diet and exercise changes as part of developing a healthy survivorhood plan – and also from a need to manage the psychological distress that comes with completing treatment. Many survivors state that once they are no longer being actively treated for cancer, they feel vulnerable to the risk of recurrence and singularly responsible for doing all that they can to stay well [67]. Survivors are bombarded with a myriad of information from the popular press, family, and friends about not only the correct diet or complementary treatments to stay cancer-free, but also about the correct psychological attitude to have toward stress and worry to make sure that cancer does not return because of their "negativity." Empowering survivors to work at improving their physical and emotional well-being can be important to promoting survivors' positive adaptation. Leaving survivors to struggle alone with their feelings that they may be to "blame" for cancer recurrence or complications of therapy can only increase their stress and deny them needed opportunities to confront genuine feelings of sadness and disappointment tied to their survivorship experiences, and also limit their ability to access resources that could enhance their functioning.

Survivors need specific tools for managing the ongoing and bumpy transition from being a patient treated for cancer to a healthy survivor. These tools need to address the fact that survivorship can be an inherently anxiety-provoking state. Survivors can benefit from recommendations from their health-care team about effective forms of self-care strategies including yoga, mindfulness, relaxation and exercise for maintaining well-being and for managing periods of heightened stress, such as in the weeks before upcoming scans or around cancer-related anniversaries. In a study conducted by Saxe et al. [68], among individuals with a cancer diagnosis who received a form of mindfulness training, mindfulness-based stress reduction (MBSR), those in the remission phase of treatment showed greater benefit than those in active treatment. Qualitative reports also indicated that in addition to improved quality of life, individuals using MBSR reported more openness to new experiences, greater ability to tolerate strong emotions, and more appreciation for life [68]. Similarly, information about the role of evidence-based nutrition can be essential to survivors in committing to healthier dietary practices, and for curbing anxiety about doing what they can to prevent a cancer recurrence. Fatigue, a common and sometimes persistent problem for survivors, is both physically and psychologically taxing; however, regularly scheduled exercise has been shown to target aerobic capacity and improve muscle strength that has been diminished by cancer treatment [69]. Taken in conjunction with ongoing psychoeducation and normalization about the survivorhood trajectory provided by their health-care provider, many individuals may find these strategies sufficient to negotiate the challenges of this period.

## *Psychosocial Support and Psychotropic Medication*

Some individuals, particularly those who may be at high risk for psychosocial distress, those who experience multiple episodes of stressors, or those who are experiencing significant distress due to changes in sleep, fatigue, pain, or mood due to late effects of treatments, may require referrals for more comprehensive assessment and treatment. Case 2 is just such an example. Preferably, these referrals will be made to practitioners with a knowledge base of cancer survivorship. Knowledgeable mental health practitioners are able to provide the appropriate evidence-based cognitive behavioral and supportive therapies to assist with managing depression, anxiety, sleeplessness, relationship/intimacy issues, and loss. Additionally, they can be instrumental in assisting individuals who are struggling with reprioritizing their lives after cancer and want to stay committed to a greater sense of meaning that they experienced during their treatment. Individuals with significant symptoms of depression, anxiety, PTSD, menopausal symptoms, as well as debilitating fatigue and/or sleeplessness can benefit enormously from a consultation for medication management with a knowledgeable psychiatrist. Effective and timely psychological/psychiatric care can be critical for remaining on the path toward healthy survivorhood.

Psychologists and psychiatrists need some specialized training to appreciate the unique presentation of distress and the specific interventions that can be helpful to cancer survivors. Psychiatrists need to know what psychotropic medications may be contraindicated for survivors. For example, selective serotonin reuptake inhibitors (SSRI) medications have been found to limit the effectiveness of tamoxifen, a frequent adjunctive treatment for breast cancer survivors in the first five years after primary treatment [70]. In addition, psychiatrists must treat symptoms of depression or anxiety that may be complicated by medically induced factors such as fatigue, sleep disturbance, pain or hormonal changes. Standard treatments and dosages are not necessarily most effective for these individuals who may have persistent symptoms that are functionally impairing, but do not fall into DSM-IV-R [29] categories. Likewise, psychotherapists within the community are often not equipped to understand and readily address the specific cancer-related losses and anxieties that propel the distress in cancer survivorhood (as outlined in Table 6.2). These concerns highlight the importance of addressing psychosocial distress within the medical context in which survivors receive their care and not as a separate, tangential set of concerns to refer out. We advocate for the integration of psychologists, psychiatrists, and social workers within the workings of primary care.

**Case 2** Fifty-year-old female diagnosed with stage II breast cancer and treated with lumpectomy, radiation, and chemotherapy followed by plan for five years of tamoxifen. High functioning manager in busy office setting, married with two school-age children. Minimal difficulties during active treatment, seen in follow-up one year after primary treatment for regular checkup. Survivor appears in good spirits until PCP asks about how she is functioning in her work and family life. Survivor wells-up with tears and reports significant cognitive difficulties including problems with short-term memory, word retrieval, and inability to multitask. When PCP asks about mood, survivor also notes new onset of mood changes such as lability, weepiness, and irritability as well as difficulties sleeping, hot flashes, and weight gain. She notes that she feels far worse now than at the end of treatment. She has expectations that she should be well and feels like she is disappointing her family and boss. Survivor expresses a sense of loss about who she is now and hopelessness about what she can look forward to.

**Interventions**

- Psychiatry consultation for medication evaluation for mood and menopausal symptoms leading to a trial on venlafaxine (an antidepressant that does not appear to interfere with tamoxifen)
- Development of strategies for managing cognitive changes that aid in memory, organization, and executive functioning
- Development of reconditioning and exercise program with spouse and children such as hikes, swimming, nightly walks, and strength training
- Short-term counseling with health psychologist focused on reevaluation of life priorities, esteem building, acceptance of loss, and valuation of gains and strengths

## *Community Resources*

Throughout this chapter we have highlighted the various needs of cancer survivors which can and should be addressed in the context of their medical treatment. As the numbers of survivors increase and hopefully, live long into healthy survivorhood, it is also necessary to recognize the role that community resources outside of a medical setting play in meeting patient needs, and to strengthen those resources that provide optimal support.

A community resource that is a fact of modern life is the Internet. Current figures indicate that up to 58% of patients with cancer utilize Internet resources for support and information [71] and that 28% of all Americans participate in online support groups related to medical or personal problems [72]. The growing literature in this area suggests that the Internet can serve to increase social support, a sense of community, increase coping and decrease levels of depression, loneliness, and anxiety [73–75]. These forms of support can be invaluable to individuals who are in regionally remote areas or are physically unable to attend live meetings. The medium, however, comes with significant limitations; information found on the Internet can be intimidating, confusing, and frightening, particularly to individuals coping with a life-threatening illness or vague symptoms [76]. Survivors who use online boards may find themselves interacting with a self-selecting population of individuals who are having the most distress, physically and psychologically, and may become demoralized by the content of the news they hear.

Nonetheless, technologically mediated social interaction is increasingly becoming the norm within the general population, particularly for younger individuals. Exploration of the most effective means of delivering support, information, and networking through the Internet is needed. One of the best examples may be through the work of UCLA Live **STRONG**™ Survivorship Center for Excellence, "Healthy Lives After Cancer" program for young adult survivors in which a trained coordinator uses web-based networking to promote live educational and supportive events for young adults about relevant topics including how to obtain or maintain health insurance and the use of creative art forms as expressions of survivorship that offer healing [77]. Just as importantly, these events are held in community settings including libraries, art galleries, and not in the hospital environment. For survivors, there is added benefit in providing needed resources outside of medical settings so that individuals who want to "move past cancer as the defining feature of my life" can take advantage of survivorhood-supportive resources in a noninstitutional forum and away from their treatment site. This is especially relevant for the needs of pediatric cancer survivors who may have had treatment a decade or more ago and do not feel that they belong in a hospital or outpatient clinic. The benefits of these strategies have not yet been fully documented.

Many intervention modalities can and should be incorporated into community settings. Meditation, yoga, mindfulness, and nutrition classes that exist within community centers can be modified to meet the needs of cancer survivors. Practitioners in these disciplines can be certified with appropriate training to understand and meet the unique needs of survivors. For example, initiative between the Lance Armstrong Foundation and 10 YMCAs across the nation created wellness programs for cancer survivors, called "Exercise and Thrive" which assists cancer survivors to rebuild muscle strength, increase fitness and flexibility, and obtain health and wellness coaching. This endeavor comes out of a growing literature that suggests physical and psychological benefits to both behavioral and physical activity interventions [78]. As the numbers of cancer survivors grow, currently at 10% of the population and perhaps soon to be beyond, it can only be beneficial from a public health policy perspective for the communities to develop the resources necessary to achieve and maintain healthy survivorhood.

## Looking to the Future

Survivorship care begins at the point of diagnosis with special attention paid to the threshold when patients move from active treatment to surveillance. The health care team must recognize that difficulties arise throughout the survivorhood journey and often involve both physical symptoms and their concomitant psychological sequelae. Practitioners need to assess from both perspectives and provide survivors with appropriate education and referrals. Several examples exist at our institutions that utilize this multidisciplinary approach in different ways. At UCLA we have evolved models where patients are seen by a mental health specialist and their physician in specific clinics including the UCLA – Live**STRONG**™ Survivorship Center for Excellence [79] and a specialized follow-up program for patients with breast cancer in the UCLA/Revlon Breast Center. Both of these clinics are staffed by mental health providers (specifically a psychologist) from the Simms/Mann – UCLA Center for Integrative Oncology [80]. Both clinics provide the opportunity for all survivors to be interviewed and assessed at the time of their medical visit by a mental health professional, usually as the first contact, and the medical team. The psychologist helps tease out the psychological needs for intervention from the medically specific interventions as well as provide a normative experience for the patient with guidance about their individual survivor trajectory. We envision this model being extended to the primary care environment where a health psychologist might be available to assess cancer survivors and make interventions in the medical setting, rather than designating them "psychologically impaired" and referring to an outside mental health clinic. This builds upon our premise of the normative experiences. Patients who are experiencing more extreme levels of distress might receive referrals for ongoing care or a few individualized sessions. In our setting patients can see the psychologist for several follow-up sessions or another member of the Simms/Mann Center team.

While these approaches represent an ideal level of integration of medical and psychosocial care, they may not be feasible in many medical settings and may not be efficient in populations of survivors where psychosocial distress is low. For these settings, an alternative model based on ensuring that psychosocial assessment is integrated into routine medical care and that mental health professionals actively consult to medical providers and survivors whenever problems are identified has been implemented in survivor clinics at the Dana-Farber Cancer Institute [81]. In this model (Fig. 6.2), survivors' psychosocial needs are evaluated by patient report on medical history forms, by completing self-report symptoms checklists, and in direct assessment from the medical provider (as described above). In this model the

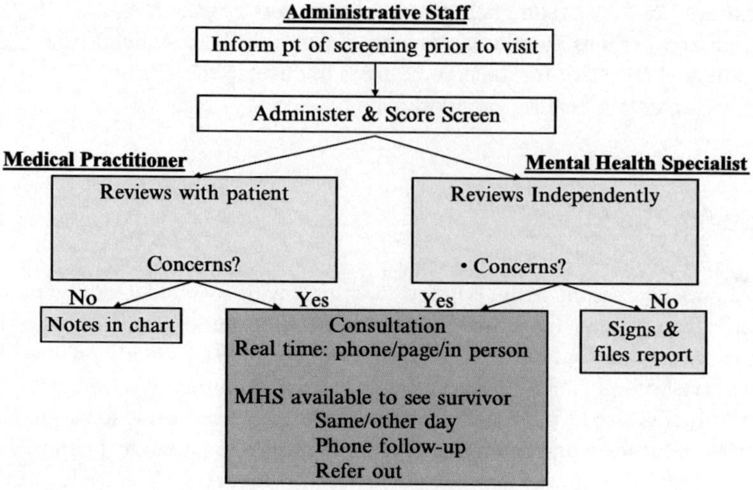


**Fig. 6.2** Integrating psychosocial screening in survivor care

psychologist and medical provider share responsibility for selecting the psychosocial assessment domains and measures and working with administrative staff to insure they are implemented in routine practice. The administrative staff is responsible for informing the survivors about the availability of psychosocial services and for administering the self-report measures to the survivors and getting the survivors' responses to the medical and psychology providers in real time for their independent review. The medical provider has primary responsibility for reviewing the survivor's responses to evaluate their psychosocial functioning as part of their clinical evaluation. The psychologist independently reviews the information at the time of the survivor's clinic visit, but does not directly evaluate the survivor unless some significant issues are raised. In that case, when either the medical provider or psychologist identifies an indicator of significant psychosocial concerns, or whenever the survivors directly request it, a psychosocial consultation is made available. In many cases, this may take the form of a team consultation of the medical and psychology provider seeing the patient together or referring the survivor for a psychology visit which may be a routine, urgent, or emergent visit depending on the survivor's concerns.

An important part of implementing successful survivorship care is a broad-based training program for existing mental health providers and primary care doctors in recognizing the "survivorhood trajectory" and knowing how to normalize the experience and intervene rapidly in the kinds of distress that are likely to arise for a majority of patients, for example, worries and fear of recurrence, coping with loss, reexperiencing symptoms. At a policy level, continuing education for primary care physicians, oncologists, nurses, and mental health professionals could include mandatory training in working with individuals with cancer and cancer survivorship in the way that mandatory training exists for many health professionals in child abuse, elder abuse, human sexuality, and more recently in pain and palliative care. National standards could be established that would address the continuum of cancer care through survivorship with both awareness of the issues and specific suggestions about particular interventions that cross-disciplines. In many ways, making these programs cross-disciplinary would be particularly helpful and might lead to greater cross talk among the different professions. What if psychologists, physicians, nurses, and social workers were all required to complete 10 hours of continuing education in cancer survivorship before renewal of their licenses and these trainings were required to include representatives from these disciplines as trainers?

Ongoing research in this domain is clearly an important piece of the puzzle. Research developing instrumentation for assessment, programmatic evaluation of interventions, and assessment of the multidisciplinary model would add to our knowledge base and help reshape this care. That being said, we are struck by the words of a leading psychological researcher summarizing the current state of psychosocial oncology care for survivors: "In the last 30 years, hundreds of randomized psychologic interventions trials have shown mental health improvements for cancer patients in comparison with those in control conditions, although dissemination of interventions to the 1.4 million cancer patients diagnosed annually remains a goal rather than a reality [82]." We need to strive toward a reality of care that incorporates what we currently know, and expand upon it as that knowledge base changes. We cannot fail to act now on behalf of cancer survivors; a truly multidisciplinary commitment to integrate our already existing knowledge, skills, and tools is all that is needed to make a substantial improvement in the well-being of survivors today.

## References


1. Massie MJ, Gagnon P, Holland JC. Depression and suicide in patients with cancer. J Pain Symptom Manage. 1994;9:325–40.
2. Stanton AL. Psychosocial concerns and interventions for cancer survivors. J Clin Oncol. 2006;24:5132–7.
3. Iconomou G, Mega V, Koutras A, Iconomou AV, Kalofonos HP. Prospective assessment of emotional distress, cognitive function, and quality of life in patients with cancer treated with chemotherapy. Cancer. 2004;101:404–11.
4. Kornblith AB. Psychosocial adaptation of cancer survivors. In: Holland JC, editor. Psycho-oncology. New York: Oxford University Press; 1998. p. 223–54.
5. Hoffman KE, McCarthy EP, Recklitis CJ, Ng AK. Psychological distress in long-term survivors of adult-onset cancer: results from a national survey. Arch Intern Med. 2009;169:1274–81.
6. Pirl WF, Greer J, Temel JS, Yeap B, Gilman S. Major depressive disorder in long-term cancer survivors: Analysis of the National Comorbidity Survey-Replication. J Clin Oncol. 2009;27:4130–4.
7. Stein KD, Syrjala KL, Andrykowski MA. Physical and psychological long-term and late effects of cancer. Cancer. 2008;112(11 Suppl):2577–92.

8. Center for Disease Control. Cancer survivorship – United States, 1971–2001. MMWR Wkly. 2004;53:526–9.
9. National Cancer Institute. The nation's investment in cancer research: connecting the cancer community. Washington, DC: National Institutes of Health, US Department of Health and Human Services; 2008.
10. Baker F, Haffer S, Denniston M. Health-related quality of life of cancer and noncancer patients in Medicare managed care. Cancer. 2003;97:674–81.
11. Polsky D, Doshi JA, Marcus S, Oslin D, Rothbard A, Thomas N, et al. Long-term risk for depressive symptoms after a medical diagnosis. Arch Intern Med. 2005;165:1260–6.
12. Costanzo ES, Ryff CD, Singer BH. Psychosocial adjustment among cancer survivors: findings from a national survey of health and well-being. Health Psychol. 2009;28:147–56.
13. Baker F, Denniston M, Haffer SC, Liberatos P. Change in health-related quality of life of newly diagnosed cancer patients, cancer survivors, and controls. Cancer. 2009;115:3024–33.
14. Reeve B, Potosky A, Smith A, Han P, Hays R, Davis W, et al. Impact of cancer on health-related quality of life of older Americans. J Natl Cancer Inst. 2009;101:860–8.
15. Zeltzer LK, Recklitis C, Buchbinder D, Zebrack B, Casillas J, Tsao JC, et al. Psychological status in childhood cancer survivors: a report from The Childhood Cancer Survivor Study. J Clin Oncol. 2009;27:2396–404.
16. Bjorkenstam C, Edberg A, Ayoubi S, Rosen M. Are cancer patients at higher suicide risk than the general population? Scand J Public Health. 2005;33:208–14.
17. Hem E, Loge JH, Haldorsen T, Ekeberg Ø. Suicide risk in cancer patients from 1960 to 1999. J Clin Oncol. 2004;22:4209–16.
18. Yousaf U, Christensen ML, Engholm G, Storm HH. Suicides among Danish cancer patients 1971–1999. Br J Cancer. 2005;92:995–1000.
19. Misono S, Weiss NS, Fann JR, Redma M, Yueh B. Incidence of suicide in persons with cancer. J Clin Oncol. 2008;26:4731–8.
20. Schairer C, Brown LM, Chen BE, Howard R, Lynch CF, Hall P, et al. Suicide after breast cancer: an international population-based study of 723, 810 women. J Natl Cancer Inst. 2006;98:1416–9.
21. Walker J, Waters RA, Murray G, Swanson H, Hibberd CJ, Rush RW, et al. Better off dead: suicidal thoughts in cancer patients. J Clin Oncol. 2008;26:4725–30.
22. Recklitis CJ, Diller LR, Li X, Najita J, Robison LL, Zeltzer L. Suicide ideation in adult survivors of childhood cancer: a report from the childhood cancer survivor study. J Clin Oncol. 2010;28:655–61.
23. Ramsey SD, Berry K, Moinpour C, Giedzinski A, Andersen MR. Quality of life in long term survivors of colorectal cancer. Am J Gastroenterol. 2002;97:1228–34.
24. Arndt V, Merx H, Stegmaier C, Ziegler H, Brenner H. Quality of life in patients with colorectal cancer 1 year after diagnosis compared with the general population: a population based study. J Clin Oncol. 2004;22:4829–36.
25. Ganz PA, Rowland JH, Meyerowitz BE, Desmond KA. Impact of different adjuvant therapy strategies on quality of life in breast cancer survivors. Recent Results Cancer Res. 1998;152:396–411.
26. Dahl AA, Haaland CF, Mykletun A, Bremnes R, Dahl O, Klepp O, et al. Study of anxiety disorder and depression in long-term survivors of testicular cancer. J Clin Oncol. 2005;23:2389–95.
27. Cordova MJ, Andrykowski MA, Kenady DE, McGrath PC, Sloan DA, Redd WH. Frequency and correlates of posttraumatic-stress-disorder-like symptoms after treatment for breast cancer. J Consult Clin Psychol. 1995;63:981–6.
28. Green BL RJ, Krupnick JL, Krupnick JL, Epstein SA, Stockton P, Stern NM, et al. Prevalence of posttraumatic stress disorder in women with breast cancer. Psychosomatics. 1998;39:102–11.
29. American Psychiatric Association. Diagnostic and statistical manual of mental disorders. 4th ed. Washington, DC: American Psychiatric Association; 1994.
30. Jacobsen P. Screening for psychological distress in cancer patients: challenges and opportunities. J Clin Oncol. 2007;25:4526–7.
31. National Comprehensive Cancer Network. Distress management clinical practice guidelines. J Natl Compr Cancer Netw. 2003;1:344–74.

32. Holland J, Andersen B, Breitbart WS, Dabrowski M, Dudley MM, Fleishman S. Distress management. J Natl Compr Cancer Netw. 2007;5:66–98.
33. Holland JC, Breitbart WS, Compas B, Dudley MM, Fleishman S, Fulcher CD, et al. NCCN Distress Management Panel: distress management. J Natl Compr Cancer Netw. 2010;8:448–85.
34. Erikson EH. Identity: youth and crisis. Oxford, England: Norton & Co; 1968.
35. Deimling GT, Kahana B, Bowman KF, Schaefer ML. Cancer survivorship and psychological distress in later life. Psychooncology. 2002;11:479–94.
36. Kornblith AB, Ligibel J. Psychosocial and sexual functioning of survivors of breast cancer. Semin Oncol. 2003;30:799–813.
37. Derks W, de Leeuw RJ, Hordijk GJ, Winnubst JA. Quality of life in elderly patients with head and neck cancer one year after diagnosis. Head Neck. 2004;6:1045–52.
38. de Graeff A, de Leeuw JR, Ros WJ, Hordijk GJ, Blijham GH, Winnubst JA. Pretreatment factors predicting quality of life after treatment for head and neck cancer. Head Neck. 2000;22:398–407.
39. Lueboonthavatchai P. Prevalence and psychosocial factors of anxiety and depression in breast cancer patients. J Med Assoc Thai. 2007;90:2164–74.
40. Gill KM, Mishel M, Belyea M, Germino B, Germino LS, Porter L, et al. Triggers of uncertainty about recurrence and long-term treatment side effects in older African American and Caucasian breast cancer survivors. Oncol Nurs Forum. 2004;31:633–9.
41. Lee-Jones C, Humphris G, Dixon R, Hatcher MB. Fear of cancer recurrence – a literature review and proposed cognitive formulation to explain exacerbation of recurrence fears. Psychooncology. 1997;6:95–105.
42. Lance Armstrong Fund. LIVESTRONG poll finds nearly half of people living with cancer feel their non-medical needs are unmet by their healthcare system. Austin: Lance Armstrong Foundation; 2004.
43. Detmar SB, Aaronson NK, Wever LDV, Muller M, Schornagel JH. How are you feeling? Who wants to know? Patients' and oncologists' preferences for discussing health-related quality-of-life issues. J Clin Oncol. 2000;18:3295–301.
44. Greenberg DB. Barriers to the treatment of depression in cancer patients. J Natl Cancer Inst Monogr. 2004;32:127–35.
45. Zigmond AS, Snaith RP. The hospital anxiety and depression scale. Acta Psychiatr Scand. 1983;67:361–70.
46. Derogatis L. BSI 18: brief symptom inventory 18: administration, scoring, and procedure manual. Minneapolis: NCS Pearson; 2001.
47. Roth AJ, Kornblith AB, Batel-Copel L, Peabody E, Scher HI, Holland JC. Rapid screening for psychologic distress in men with prostate carcinoma: a pilot study. Cancer. 1998;82:1904–8.
48. Kroenke K, Spitzer RL, Williams JB. The PHQ-9: validity of a brief depression severity measure. J Gen Intern Med. 2001;16:606–13.
49. Vodermaier A, Linden W, Siu C. Screening for emotional distress in cancer patients: a systematic review of assessment instruments. J Natl Cancer Inst. 2009;21:1464–88.
50. Recklitis CJ, Licht I, Ford J, Oeffinger K, Diller L. Screening adult survivors of childhood cancer with the distress thermometer: a comparison with the SCL-90-R. Psychooncology. 2007;16:1046–9.
51. Mitchell AJ. Pooled results from 38 analyses of the accuracy of distress thermometer and other ultra-short methods of detecting cancer-related mood disorders. J Clin Oncol. 2007;25:4670–81.
52. Johnson LC, Murphy SA, Dimond M. Reliability, construct validity, and subscale norms of the Brief Symptom Inventory when administered to bereaved parents. J Nurs Meas. 1996;4:117–27.
53. Zabora J, BrintzenhofeSzoc K, Jacobsen P, Curbow B, Piantadosi S, Hooker C, et al. A new psychosocial screening instrument for use with cancer patients. Psychosomatics. 2001;42:241–6.
54. Recklitis CJ, Rodriguez P. Screening childhood cancer survivors with the brief symptom inventory-18: classification agreement with the symptom checklist-90-revised. Psychooncology. 2007;16:429–36.

55. Mitchell AJ. Short screening tools for cancer-related distress: a review and diagnostic validity meta-analysis. J Natl Compr Cancer Netw. 2010;8:487–94.
56. Newel SA, Sanson-Fisher RW, Savolainen NJ. Systematic review of psychological therapies for cancer patients: overview and recommendations for future research. J Natl Cancer Inst. 2002;8:558–84.
57. Fawzy FI. Psychosocial interventions for patients with cancer: what works and what doesn't. Eur J Cancer. 1999;11:1559–64.
58. Meyer TJ, Mark MM. Effects of psychosocial interventions with adult cancer patients: a meta-analysis of randomized experiments. Health Psychol. 1995;14:101–8.
59. Sheard T, Maguire P. The effect of psychological interventions on anxiety and depression in cancer patients: results of two meta-analyses. Br J Cancer. 1999;80:1770–80.
60. Antoni MH, Lehman JM, Kilbourn KM, Boyers AE, Culver JL, Alferi SM, et al. Cognitive-behavioral stress management intervention decreases the prevalence of depression and enhances benefit finding among women under treatment for early-stage breast cancer. Health Psychol. 2001;20:20–32.
61. Cella DF, Yella SB. Cancer support groups: the state of the art. Cancer Pract. 1993;1:56–61.
62. Samarel N, Fawcett J, Krippendorf K, Piacentino JC, Eliasof B, Hughes P, et al. Women's perceptions of group support and application to breast cancer. J Adv Nurs. 1998;28: 1259–68.
63. Bower JA, Woolery A. Yoga for cancer patients and survivors. Cancer Control. 2005;12:165.
64. Spiegel D, Moore R. Imagery and hypnosis in the treatment of cancer patients. Oncology. 1997;11:1179–89.
65. Del Giudice M, Grunfeld E, Harvey B, Piliotis E, Verma S. Primary care physicians' views of routine follow up care of cancer patients. J Clin Oncol. 2009;20:3338–45.
66. Bober SL, Recklitis CJ, Campbell EG, Park ER, Kutner JS, Najita JS, et al. Caring for cancer survivors. Cancer. 2009;115:4409–18.
67. Costanzo ES, Lutegendorf SK, Roeder SL. Common-sense beliefs about cancer and health practices among women completing treatments for breast cancer. Psychooncology. 2011;20:53–61.
68. Saxe G, Hebert J, Carmody J, Kabat-Zinn J, Rosenzweig P, Jarzobski D, et al. Can diet in conjunction with stress reduction affect the rate of increase in prostate-specific antigen after biochemical recurrence of prostate cancer? J Urol. 2001;166:2207.
69. Vanweert E, Hoekstra-Weebers J, Otter R, Postema K, Sandeman R, van der Schans C. Cancer related fatigue: predictors and effects of rehabilitation. Oncologist. 2006;11:184–96.
70. Stearns V, Johnson MD, Rae JM, Morocho A, Novielli A, Bhargava P, et al. Active tamoxifen metabolite plasma concentrations after coadministration of tamoxifen and the selective serotonin reuptake inhibitor paroxetine. J Natl Cancer Inst. 2003;95:1758–64.
71. Monnier J, Laken M, Carter CL. Patient and caregiver interest in Internet-based cancer services. Cancer Pract. 2002;10:305–10.
72. Internet. The mainstreaming of online life. Pew Internet Project. Trends 2005. http://pewresearch.org/assets/files/trends2005-internet.pdf. Accessed March 9, 2011.
73. Fogel J, Albert SM, Schnabel F, Ditkoff BA, Neugut AI. Internet use and social support in women with breast cancer. Health Psychol. 2002;21:398–404.
74. Madara E, White BJ. Online mutual support: the experience of self help clearinghouse. Inf Referral J Alliance Inf Referral Syst. 1997;19:91–107.
75. Lieberman MA, Golant M, Giese-Davis J, Winzleberg A, Benjamin H, Humphreys K, et al. Electronic support groups and breast carcinoma: a clinical trial of effectiveness. Cancer. 2003;97:920–5.
76. Penson RT, Benson RC, Parles K, Chabner BA, Lynch TJ. Virtual connections: Internet health care. Oncologist. 2002;7:555–68.
77. UCLA- Live**STRONG**™ Survivorship Center for Excellence. Available from http://www.cancer.ucla.edu/Index.aspx?page=833. Accessed March 9, 2011.
78. Duijts SF, Faber MM, Oldenburg HS, van Beurden M, Aaronson NK. Effectiveness of behavioral techniques and physical exercise on psychosocial functioning and health-related quality of life in breast cancer patients and survivors-a meta-analysis. Psychooncology. 2011;20:115–126.

79. Shapiro CL, McCabe MS, Syrjala KL, Friedman D, Jacobs LA, Ganz PA, et al. The LIVESTRONG Survivorship Center of Excellence Network. J Cancer Surviv. 2009;3:4–11.
80. Simms/Mann – UCLA Center for Integrative Oncology. http://www.simmsmanncenter.ucla.edu/. Accessed March 8, 2011.
81. Perini Family Survivors' Center at Dana-Farber Cancer Institute. http://www.dana-farber.org/pat/surviving/default.html. Accessed March 9, 2011.
82. Andersen BL, Yang H, Farrar WB, Golden-Kreutz DM, Emery CF, Thornton LJ, et al. Psychological intervention improves survival for breast cancer patients: a randomized clinical trial. Cancer. 2008;113:3450–8.
83. Osborn R, Demoncada A, Feuerstein M. Psychosocial interventions for depression, anxiety, and QOL in cancer survivors: Meta-analyses. International Journal of Psychiatry and Medicine. 2006;36:13–34.

# Chapter 7
# Disparities in Care for Cancer Survivors

**Jacqueline Casillas and John Z. Ayanian**

## Introduction

People who have survived cancer face distinctive health problems for the rest of their lives after their primary cancer diagnosis. Morbidity and mortality for cancer survivors can occur due to the development of chronic health conditions, called late effects, as a result of previous cancer therapy [1, 2]. Examples of late effects include infertility, cardiopulmonary disease, endocrine dysfunction, renal impairment, and subsequent malignancies [3, 4]. Recurrences of primary cancers or the development of secondary cancers, such as breast cancer after radiation therapy for Hodgkin's disease, are the most common causes of late mortality in adult survivors of childhood cancer [5]. The incidence of secondary and even tertiary cancers is increasing after initial diagnoses of cancer in adults [6]. Cancer prevention, ongoing screening and surveillance, and early detection of late effects of cancer treatment are, therefore, essential components of survivorship care. Racial/ethnic and socioeconomic disparities in these components of high-quality survivorship care are crucial to evaluate and address.

Describing the often complex and fragmented care cancer survivors receive is an important first step to define and understand the possible etiologies for disparities in cancer survivorship care. In 2005, an Institute of Medicine (IOM) report, *Lost in Transition*, highlighted the need to recognize survivorship care as a unique phase of cancer care and the concomitant need for formalized survivorship care planning because of the special risks faced by cancer survivors (Fig. 7.1) [7]. A variety of health-care delivery models are utilized by cancer survivors across the USA, including the provision of care by primary care physicians, medical oncologists, radiation oncologists, and surgeons practicing in community settings, as well as providers practicing in regional cancer centers [8]. Across all community or academic settings, however, the lack of effective coordination of care can result in disparities in access to high-quality survivorship care, particularly for vulnerable populations [9]. In this

J. Casillas (✉)
Jonsson Comprehensive Cancer Center, University of California, Los Angeles, CA, USA
e-mail: jcasillas@mednet.ucla.edu

M. Feuerstein and P.A. Ganz (eds.), *Health Services for Cancer Survivors*,
DOI 10.1007/978-1-4419-1348-7_7, © Springer Science+Business Media, LLC 2011

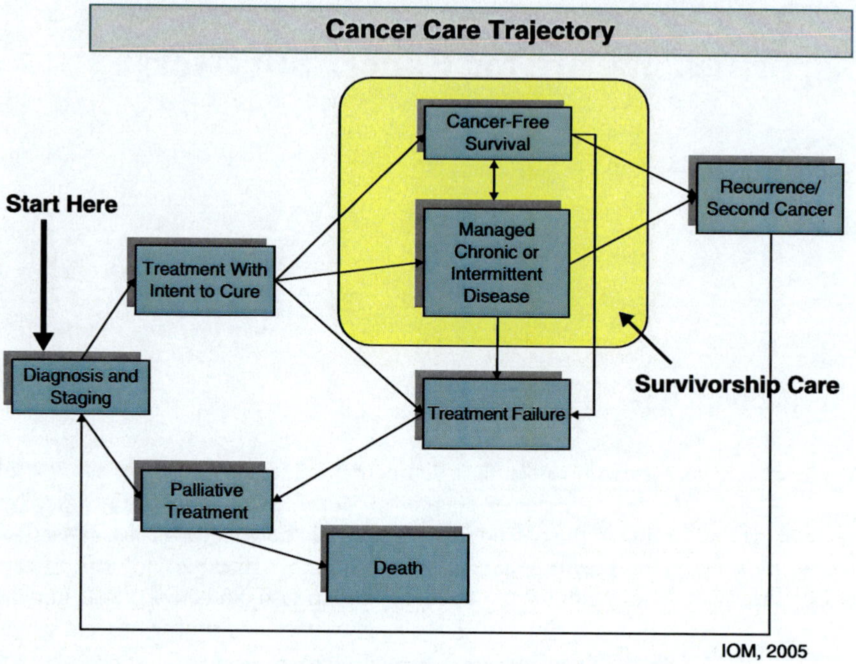


**Fig. 7.1** The cancer treatment trajectory with special identification of the posttreatment survivorship care phase [7] (Reprinted with permission from the National Academies Press, Copyright 2006, National Academy of Sciences)

chapter, we review the literature on (1) disparities in access to care for cancer survivors; (2) disparities in the quality of survivorship care; (3) clinical interventions and recent national policy changes which may reduce these disparities; and (4) future directions to eliminate disparities in care for cancer survivors.

## Disparities in Access to Care for Cancer Survivors

Access to care is important across the continuum of cancer care, including the survivorship period (Fig. 7.2). For newly diagnosed cancer patients, the detection of early-stage disease is associated with improved disease-free survival [10–13]. The goal of posttreatment surveillance in survivorship care is to screen and identify late effects of cancer treatment with the expectation that health promotion and early detection of disease will prevent greater morbidity and mortality. However, there is limited research on access to survivorship care by different populations and the impact this care has on the health outcomes of cancer survivors, possibly due to challenges in quantifying survivorship care visits and long-term follow-up care received by survivors who receive care in a variety of health-care settings.

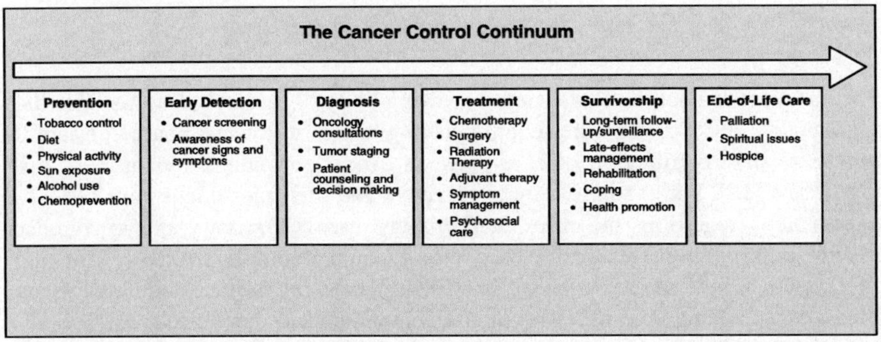


**Fig. 7.2** The cancer control continuum [7] (Reprinted with permission from National Academies Press, Copyright 2006, National Academy of Sciences)

## *Access to Care for Survivors of Childhood Cancer*

For the growing number of young adult cancer survivors [4], health insurance benefits have often been lost in these high-risk patients when they age out of public insurance coverage or their parents' insurance plans [14]. The Childhood Cancer Survivor Study (CCSS), the largest national cohort of long-term survivors, has evaluated the utilization of health care among survivors and found that 88.8% of survivors reported receiving some form of medical care, but only 31.5% reported care that focused on their prior cancer (defined as survivor-focused care), and 17.8% reported survivor-focused care that included advice or discussion about risk reduction for late effects or the ordering of screening tests. Disparities were found for survivors who were older, male, black, or uninsured as they were less likely to report survivor-focused care with risk reduction counseling or screening. Conversely, survivors with chronic morbidities, including pain and anxiety, were more likely to report risk-based, survivor-focused care. Another CCSS study assessing health-care utilization in minority adult survivors of childhood cancer found Hispanic survivors to have lower rates of cervical cancer screening despite equitable access to cancer-related care [15].

CCSS has also examined factors associated with the lack of health insurance coverage and its impact on access to care. Cancer treatment variables, specifically younger age at diagnosis and the receipt of cranial radiation placed survivors at higher risk for being uninsured. Socioeconomic variables associated with the lack of health insurance coverage included less education, lower family income, and being unmarried [16]. Another study exploring barriers to survivorship care for the high-risk population of childhood brain tumor survivors surveyed the national clinical trials group of pediatric oncology centers, the Children's Oncology Group [17]. This study also found that lack of health insurance was an important barrier to accessing survivorship care.

## *Access to Care for Survivors of Cancer in Adulthood*

For survivors of adult malignancies, a growing body of research demonstrates that high-quality survivorship care requires having access to a usual source of care to maximize the coordination of care between cancer specialists and primary care physicians [18]. For example, cancer survivors and their physicians have different expectations regarding the roles that primary care physicians and oncologists assume in providing survivorship care, which can lead to deficiencies in care [19]. In Canada, a randomized trial of survivorship care for women with early-stage breast cancer found no differences in clinical outcomes or health-related quality of life between patients who continued to receive care at their regional cancer center and those who primarily saw their local family physicians [20]. Another potential approach to improve access to quality survivorship care has been the proposed "shared-care model" for cancer survivors in which both the treating oncologist and primary care physician have defined roles and ongoing scheduled time points for communication regarding the care of cancer survivors [21].

Longitudinal research in breast cancer survivors has shown that survivors who visit both a primary care physician and an oncology specialist are more likely to receive preventive care (influenza vaccination, cholesterol screening, bone densitometry) and cancer screening (colorectal screening, mammograms) [22]. In a study of more than 20,000 colorectal survivors using the SEER-Medicare database, survivors who visited a primary care physician and an oncology specialist were most likely to receive preventive care [23]. Racial/ethnic differences were found in the frequency of primary care versus oncology care. African American survivors had more visits to primary care physicians than non-Hispanic white survivors but fewer visits to other providers than non-Hispanic white survivors and other racial and ethnic groups.

The burden of comorbid illness among cancer survivors is another factor to consider when evaluating their access to care. In a large, population-based sample of more than 15,000 cancer patients between the ages of 40 and 84 years, 68.7% reported at least one comorbidity and 32.6% had two or more comorbid conditions [24]. A higher frequency of comorbid conditions was reported among the elderly, African Americans (particularly women), and those with lower socioeconomic status. For cancer survivors, these differences in comorbid illness noted during active cancer therapy may lead to a significantly greater burden of late effects that result from multimodal cancer therapy.

Qualitative research among African American breast cancer survivors has explored the impact of financial barriers faced during long-term survivorship care [25]. In this study, focus group participants reported that being uninsured or underinsured resulted in delayed treatment or fewer treatment options. The significant financial burden associated with active cancer therapy did not end at the completion of treatment but instead persisted into the survivorship period. The financial impact of survivorship care is particularly important for cancer survivors who will require medications to prevent cancer recurrence. To evaluate the economic consequences of adjuvant hormonal treatments for breast cancer among women of lower socioeconomic status, one study examined financial hardship associated with the relationship between adjuvant hormonal therapies (tamoxifen or aromatase inhibitors), given that the latter agents are much more expensive [26]. Breast cancer survivors with no drug coverage or partial drug coverage were significantly more likely to experience financial difficulty than those survivors with full coverage, particularly if using aromatase inhibitors. Importantly, lack of drug coverage was the main factor associated with the likelihood that the survivor did not switch to the recommended regimen of adjuvant hormonal therapy with an aromatase inhibitor. These data highlight the significant effect that cost sharing may have on the receipt of evidence-based survivorship care, particularly for low-income survivors.

A large study used the National Health Interview Survey (NHIS) from 2003 through 2006 to examine the prevalence of forgoing health-care services due to cost among cancer survivors compared to a nationally representative, population-based sample of US adults (>18 years of age) [27]. Prevalence estimates of forgoing or delaying medical care due to cost for cancer survivors, stratified by ethnic group are shown in Fig. 7.3. They found that the prevalence of forgoing medical care and forgoing the purchase of prescription medications due to cost was higher among cancer survivors when compared to the general US population. They also found that non-elderly cancer survivors were more likely to forgo all types of medical care when compared to adults without a history of cancer. As the authors discuss, this finding is particularly concerning as younger adult survivors are at risk for late effects and require long-term follow-up care for disease prevention and health maintenance. Hispanic and African American survivors were also identified as a

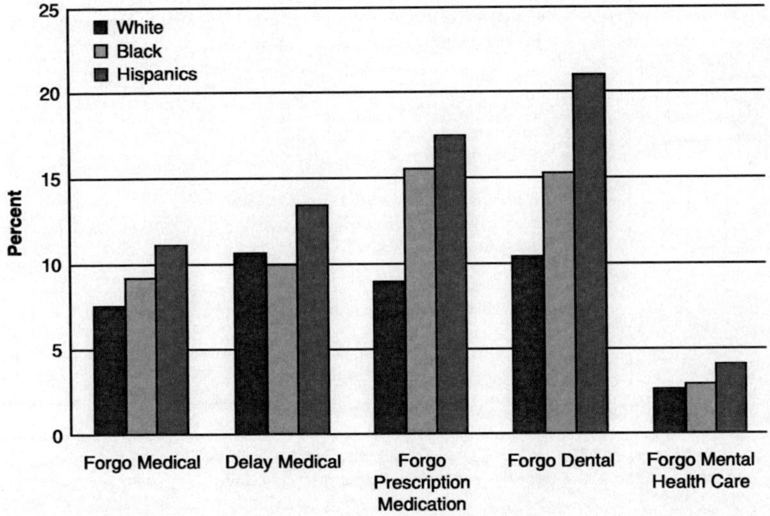


**Fig. 7.3** The prevalence of forgoing or delaying medical care because of cost for cancer survivors is shown by race/ethnicity [27] (Reprinted with permission from John Wiley and Sons)

high-risk population for forgoing prescription medications and dental care when compared to non-Hispanic white survivors. The adjusted models suggested that these observed disparities were largely due to socioeconomic status and lack of health insurance coverage. These data highlight the significant effect that cost can play in the receipt of survivorship care.

## Disparities in Quality of Care for Cancer Survivors

### *Operational Definition of Quality Survivorship Care*

Donabedian's model of quality assessment provides an important conceptual framework to understand the main components of quality of care (structure, process, and outcomes of care) and to observe disparities in these components (Fig. 7.4) [28]. The measurement of structure includes providers' training for survivorship care, the organizations in which survivorship care is provided, and the different populations of survivors to be served. The measurement of processes of survivorship care includes the coordination of survivorship care in diverse practice settings and the use of appropriate screening, surveillance, and diagnostic tests and evidence-based therapies by health-care providers. Lastly, the measurement of outcomes of survivorship care includes survival, late effects, health-related quality of

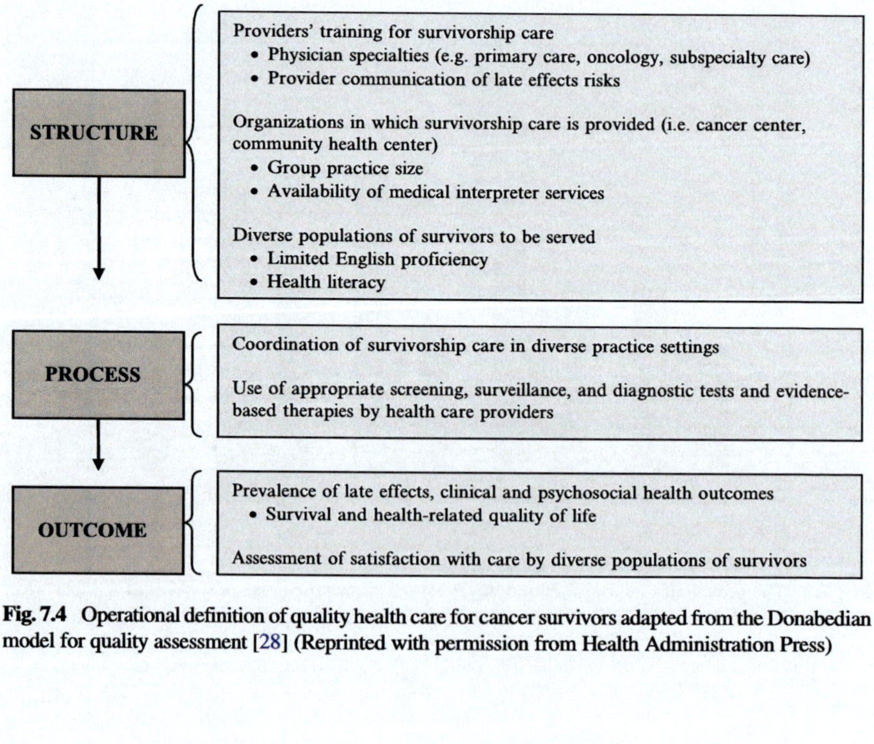


**Fig. 7.4** Operational definition of quality health care for cancer survivors adapted from the Donabedian model for quality assessment [28] (Reprinted with permission from Health Administration Press)

life including psychosocial outcomes, and satisfaction with care. In the following sections, we review the available literature on the major factors of structure, process, and outcomes associated with disparities in the quality of survivorship care.

## *Structure Variables in the Assessment of Quality*

The specialties of physicians who provide services to cancer survivors represent a structural factor that may impact the management of late effects and the delivery of cancer screening and other preventive services. Studies have demonstrated that the further survivors are from their cancer diagnosis the more likely they are to receive their care in the primary care setting and less likely to be seen in the oncology setting [23, 29]. In a study of colon cancer survivors, 5 years after the completion of cancer treatment, 62% of survivors saw only a primary care physician, 21% saw both a primary care physician and an oncologist, and 4% saw only an oncologist [23].

Although survivorship research on the impact of group practice size is limited, small practices (defined as less than or equal to five physicians) provide a substantial proportion of primary care in the USA. These practices face a significant challenge in serving patients with limited English proficiency if their physicians and staff are not fluent in the primary languages of their patients [30]. Research has also shown that the training of health-care providers serving ethnic minority patients with cancer may be inadequate to overcome language and cultural barriers existing between them and their patients [31].

A lack of well-trained interpreters can be another barrier to cancer education for diverse populations of survivors. According to US Census data, approximately 21 million people report limited English proficiency. Interpretive services are therefore an important structural component to provide quality survivorship counseling to those with limited English proficiency [30]. The availability of medical interpreter services and bilingual providers is associated with positive effects on patient satisfaction, quality of care received, and outcomes for those with limited English proficiency [32]. However, the costs of interpreter services and translation of health educational materials can be substantial and are often not reimbursed by health insurers [33]. There may also be an imbalance between available interpreters in the workforce and the number of patients to be served [34]. Survivorship research in colorectal cancer has demonstrated more frequent problems with care reported by non-English-speaking survivors indicating that language barriers may be an important contributor to disparities in care for cancer survivors [35]. A review of national demonstration projects directed at improving language access services has underscored the importance of developing cost-effective ways to provide these services [36].

Low health literacy may also be an important risk factor for disparities in outcomes among cancer survivors [37]. Health literacy not only impacts patients' understanding of cancer-related information but can also impact their shared decision-making with health-care providers. Limited understanding and misperceptions of cancer risk have been found for minority populations, even when patients have a satisfactory literacy score [38]. A study of African American men with adequate health literacy found they had limited understanding about their prostate cancer risk. The men in this study identified the need for community-based health education on cancer risk in churches or by word of mouth from other African Americans. Future research can evaluate the effectiveness of greater community participation to improve awareness of survivorship care for diverse communities.

Qualitative research exploring physicians' perceptions and experiences with patient diversity has suggested that their approach is to remain socially and culturally neutral because the sociocultural background of patients can raise tensions between the patient and provider [39]. This approach, however, may not be the best model to provide patient-centered communication in cancer care [40, 41]. Qualitative research among Spanish-speaking cancer survivors found that difficulty discussing their cancer diagnosis/treatment in English was a significant barrier to seeking cancer information from sources such as the National Cancer Institute's (NCI) Cancer Information Service [42]. These data highlight important cultural and language barriers that providers should recognize when delivering survivorship care to diverse populations.

## *Process Variables in the Assessment of Quality*

Coordination of care is an important process variable in the assessment of quality of care for cancer survivors. Differences in this domain have been found to be an important predictor of cancer survivors' views of the quality of their health care [35, 43]. A survey of colon cancer survivors approximately 9 months after diagnosis demonstrated significant disparities by race, ethnicity, and language in cancer survivors' views of the quality of care [35]. Problems with coordination of care and access to care were significantly more common for African Americans, Asian/Pacific Islanders, and non-English-speaking whites (Fig. 7.5). Hispanics also tended to report more problems with their coordination of care. In all racial/ethnic, and language groups, experiences with coordination of care were most highly correlated with patients' overall ratings of care.

Coordination of care is also highly relevant for long-term survivors of other cancers. For example, survivors of lymphoma, breast cancer, or sarcoma who are exposed to anthracycline chemotherapeutic agents can develop cardiac late effects particularly as they age [44]. It is critical for these at-risk survivors to know which physicians are in charge of their cardiac care issues so opportunities for preventive counseling, screening, and timely evaluation of cardiac-related symptoms are not missed.

Research in breast cancer survivors has demonstrated a lower rate of cancer screening in the elderly population [22, 45]. In a study evaluating the quality of health maintenance among elderly breast cancer survivors enrolled in Medicare, elderly African American survivors experienced significant disparities in receipt of colorectal cancer screening, as well as influenza vaccination, lipid testing, and bone

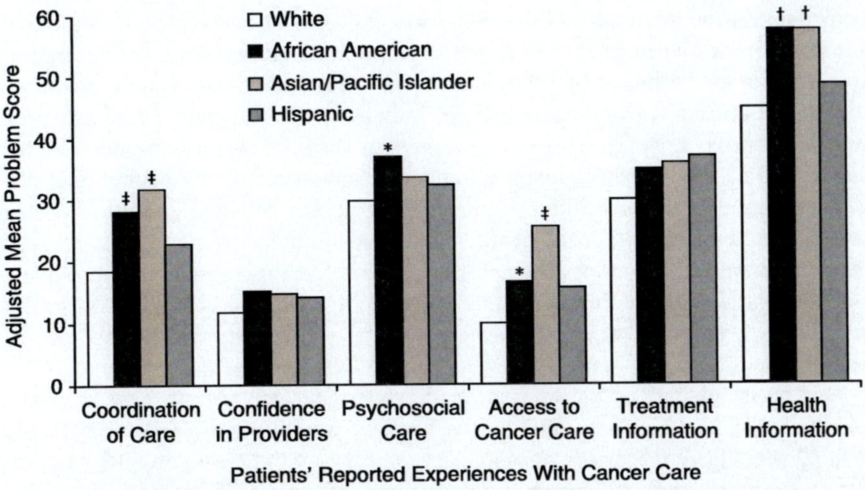


**Fig. 7.5** Adjusted mean problem scores by race and ethnicity for patients' experiences with cancer care. Statistical significance relative to white patients is denoted by *symbols over the bars*: (*) $0.01 < P \leq 0.05$; (†) $0.001 < P \leq 0.01$; (‡) $P \leq 0.001$. Linear regression was used to adjust for demographic characteristics, cancer stage, comorbid conditions, and health-related quality of life (Reprinted with permission. © 2008 American Society of Clinical Oncology. All rights reserved. Ayanian J et al.: J Clin Oncol 23(27), 2005: 6576–86 [35])

densitometry [46]. Another study of elderly breast cancer survivors found lower rates of mammography use in African American women [45]. A third study evaluated the underuse of surveillance mammography among breast cancer survivors and found that women who were older, African American, unmarried or living in certain regions of the USA (specifically Utah, San Jose, Los Angeles, and New Mexico) were less likely to receive surveillance mammography [47]. The rates of mammography were higher for those who continued to receive care by an oncologist, radiation oncologist, or surgeon. Adjusting for visits with providers, however, did not explain the lower rates based on age, race/ethnicity, marital status, and geographic region. Research has shown that cancer decision-making can vary by age, which may be one explanation for the age-related differences found in these survivorship studies [48].

## *Outcome Assessment of Quality*

Over 11 million cancer survivors reside in the USA, with the majority being age 65 or older [49]. Studies evaluating the health outcomes of older adults are therefore important as their risk of late effects from cancer treatment and their vulnerability to health problems associated with aging can contribute to significant disparities in outcomes. In a study of elderly breast, prostate, and colorectal cancer survivors, nearly 40% of respondents had at least one symptom attributed to cancer or its treatment [50]. Reported symptoms included pain, vision, numbness, memory, swelling, urinary incontinence, weakness, balance, hair loss, constipation, diarrhea, bowel incontinence, infection, nausea, pain with urination, and skin burns. Disparities were observed in African American survivors as they reported significantly greater numbers of symptoms, greater functional difficulties, greater perceived illness impact, and poorer self-rated health. Women also reported more comorbid health conditions, more current symptoms, and greater perceptions of illness impact. Given these findings, health-care providers must recognize the additional vulnerability to late effects and chronic health problems for elderly cancer survivors, particularly for those who are women or minorities.

On the other end of the age spectrum, over 300,000 people have survived cancer during childhood in the USA, with approximately two-thirds being older than 20 years [14]. Recurrent or secondary cancers are the most common cause of late mortality in adult childhood cancer survivors [5]. A CCSS analysis evaluating long-term health outcomes in adult childhood cancer survivors found the late mortality rate (6.5%) and 15-year cumulative incidence of secondary cancer (3.5%) to be similar across all racial groups. However, additional long-term follow-up is required to assess the interaction of comorbidities with the late effects of cancer treatment at a young age. New CCSS investigations are exploring the impact that genetic factors, lifestyle factors, and older age may have on treatment-related late effects in different populations of childhood cancer survivors [51].

## Reducing Disparities: Clinical Interventions and National Health Care Policy

### *Clinical Interventions*

Survivorship care plans are an important clinical tool proposed to improve the coordination of care for cancer survivors [18, 52]. Templates for survivorship care plans and treatment summaries have been developed by different national organizations including the American Society of Clinical Oncology (ASCO) [53], the Children's Oncology Group (COG) (Passport for Care) [54], the LIVESTRONG Care Plan in partnership with OncoLink, [55] and Journey Forward (created through a collaboration between the National Coalition for Cancer Survivorship, UCLA Survivorship Center, Wellpoint, and Genentech) [56]. For example, the LIVESTRONG Care Plan is available on the Web and allows for the survivor to input the cancer treatments received in order to generate a care plan. Survivor-initiated care planning is an important consideration for racial/ethnic minorities and non-English-speaking survivors as African American, Asian-Pacific Islanders, and non-English-speaking whites report more problems with knowledge of health and treatment information than white survivors [35]. Young adult survivors of childhood cancers have also been shown to have low knowledge regarding their previous treatment information [57]. Additionally, language may also serve as a barrier to survivor-initiated care planning for diverse populations.

Currently, the LIVESTRONG Care Plan and Journey Forward are available in Spanish. The COG has also made efforts to provide survivorship information to the Latino community of childhood cancer survivors by making some of their materials (Health Links) available in Spanish [58]. These health educational materials for pediatric, adolescent, and young adult survivors are available online (http://www.survivorshipguidelines.org) and cover 42 survivorship topics, with five available in Spanish.

The ASCO template for breast cancer survivorship care plans has been evaluated qualitatively for its effectiveness in minority survivors [59]. The minority survivors in this study reported that although the care plans were useful to facilitate the transition from the oncology to the primary care setting, they viewed the content as being too technical. Minority breast cancer survivors also reported that the care plans did not include enough information on self-help resources and wellness guidelines.

A recent survey of long-term cancer survivors demonstrated important racial and socioeconomic disparities in their ability to obtain high-quality cancer information [60]. While the need for cancer information did not differ significantly by race, ethnicity, education, or income, African American men and low-income men and women reported more barriers to obtaining desired cancer information. In addition, African American women reported receiving a lower quality of cancer information. Thus, further evaluation of the information needs of minority, low income, and non-English-speaking cancer survivors may help ensure they are well informed and improve the coordination of their survivorship care.

Patient navigation is an emerging intervention to improve the quality of survivorship care. Trained individuals guide survivors through the barriers to care they experience. For example, the Lance Armstrong Foundation has opened the LIVESTRONG patient navigation center in Austin, Texas. The goal of this center is to serve as a primary centralized resource in this community for individuals with cancer to access needed services in a timely manner [61]. A qualitative study among African American breast cancer survivors used focus groups to explore their ideas on how their unmet needs could be improved through the use of patient navigation services [62]. Some of the major themes included the need for patient navigation to address access to quality survivorship care, the need for patient navigation to be available across the continuum of cancer care (from diagnosis through cancer survivorship), and the importance of families in the cancer survivorship experience. A second qualitative study among Latino adolescent and young adult survivors and parents explored barriers to accessing recommended survivorship care. The study also reported the significant role that families play in helping survivors navigate their care [63]. The family roles included appointment scheduling and providing psychosocial support related to late effects of cancer treatment.

### *Decreasing Disparities in Survivorship Care Through National Policy Changes*

The Patient Protection and Affordable Care Act signed by President Obama in March, 2010 included three important reforms that have the potential to reduce racial and ethnic disparities in care for cancer survivors: (1) allowing young adults to remain on their parents' health-care plan through the age of 26; (2) eliminating exclusions for coverage of preexisting health conditions; and (3) expanding Medicaid to cover all adults with incomes up to 133% of the Federal poverty level [64]. These national policy changes will make it easier for cancer survivors to obtain or change insurance coverage. These policies may also affect the availability of employment opportunities and career options for cancer survivors. Because minority Americans are substantially more likely than whites to be uninsured and are more likely to have low incomes [65], they may benefit substantially from the expansion of Medicaid in the new health-care reform law.

Despite potential improvements in health-care access for some minority cancer survivors, the current policy changes will leave many immigrants who are cancer survivors without insurance coverage. Specifically, undocumented immigrants will not be covered, and legal residents may be reluctant to enroll in government programs such as Medicaid. Many of these cancer survivors thus will remain reliant on safety-net providers such as public hospitals and community health centers that are financially distressed in many communities.

## Conclusions and Future Directions

Cancer survivors in racial and ethnic minority groups experience disparities in access to survivorship care and the quality of this care due to several factors, including being uninsured, having limited English proficiency, and having greater burdens of chronic disease. Disparities in survivorship care can place them at higher risk for future morbidity and mortality as they face late effects of cancer treatment, including cardiopulmonary disease, endocrine dysfunction, and secondary cancers [66–69].

Recent national quality improvement efforts in survivorship care are beginning to focus on the dissemination of survivorship care plans to improve the coordination of care. These survivorship care plans focus on ensuring regular cancer surveillance, early detection of disease, and effective care of late effects of cancer treatment. Future research must assess the impact these survivorship care plans have on outcomes for different populations of cancer survivors, including those with advanced age, limited English proficiency, and a high burden of chronic disease.

Recent federal reforms in health insurance and health-care delivery may improve access to high-quality survivorship care for minority cancer survivors who are often socioeconomically disadvantaged. Health services research exploring the impact of this expanded health insurance coverage on observed disparities will be a critical priority for the next decade as the number of cancer survivors continues to increase. Given the strong association between being uninsured and disparities in care for cancer survivors, the impact of continuous health insurance coverage on the access to and quality of survivorship care will be an important area for future research. The impact of cost sharing, through copayments and deductibles, on recommended survivorship screening, must also be a research priority given the current economic climate, particularly for those who are underinsured and have limited financial means.

In conclusion, future survivorship research must have a sound conceptual model, building upon the currently identified factors for disparities in quality survivorship care, including the impact of race/ethnicity, culture, language, socioeconomic factors, comorbid illnesses, and age. Over the next decade, survivorship research should identify, and address key factors that will promote equitable access to high-quality survivorship care for all individuals affected by cancer.

## References

1. Committee on Cancer Survivorship: Improving Care and Quality of Life, National Cancer Policy Board. The medical and psychological concerns of cancer survivors after treatment. In: Hewitt M, Greenfield S, Stovall E, editors. From cancer patient to cancer survivor: lost in transition. Washington, DC: The National Academies Press; 2005. p. 66–186.
2. Board National Cancer Policy. Late effects of childhood cancer. In: Hewitt M, Weiner SL, Simone JV, editors. Childhood cancer survivorship: improving care and quality of life. Washington, DC: The National Academies Press; 2003. p. 49–89.
3. Ganz PA. Survivorship: adult cancer survivors. Prim Care. 2009;36(4):721–41.
4. Oeffinger KC, Hudson MM, Landier W. Survivorship: childhood cancer survivors. Prim Care. 2009;36(4):743–80.
5. Mertens AC, Liu Q, Neglia JP, Wasilewski K, Leisenring W, Armstrong GT, et al. Cause-specific late mortality among 5-year survivors of childhood cancer: the Childhood Cancer Survivor Study. J Natl Cancer Inst. 2008;100(19):1368–79.
6. Curtis RE, Freedman DM, Ron E, Ries LAG, Hacker DG, Edwards BK, et al. New malignancies among cancer survivors: SEER cancer registries, 1973–2000. NIH Publ No 05-5302 [serial on the Internet]. 2006. Available from: http://seer.cancer.gov/publications/mpmono/MPMonograph_complete.pdf, March 14, 2011.
7. Committee on Cancer Survivorship: Improving Care and Quality of Life, National Cancer Policy Board. In: Hewitt M, Greenfield S, Stovall E, editors. From cancer patient to cancer survivor: lost in transition. Washington, DC: The National Academies Press; 2005.
8. Klabunde CN, Ambs A, Keating NL, He Y, Doucette WR, Tisnado D, et al. The role of primary care physicians in cancer care. J Gen Intern Med. 2009;24(9):1029–36.
9. Nathan PC, Greenberg ML, Ness KK, Hudson MM, Mertens AC, Mahoney MC, et al. Medical care in long-term survivors of childhood cancer: a report from the childhood cancer survivor study. J Clin Oncol. 2008;26(27):4401–9.
10. Ayanian JZ. Racial disparities in outcomes of colorectal cancer screening: biology or barriers to optimal care? J Natl Cancer Inst. 2010;102(8):511–3.
11. Lannin DR, Mathews HF, Mitchell J, Swanson MS, Swanson FH, Edwards MS. Influence of socioeconomic and cultural factors on racial differences in late-stage presentation of breast cancer. JAMA. 1998;279(22):1801–7.

12. Lantz PM, Mujahid M, Schwartz K, Janz NK, Fagerlin A, Salem B, et al. The influence of race, ethnicity, and individual socioeconomic factors on breast cancer stage at diagnosis. Am J Public Health. 2006;96(12):2173–8.
13. Le H, Ziogas A, Lipkin SM, Zell JA. Effects of socioeconomic status and treatment disparities in colorectal cancer survival. Cancer Epidemiol Biomark Prev. 2008;17(8):1950–62.
14. National Cancer Policy Board. Childhood cancer survivorship: improving care and quality of life. Hewitt M, Weiner SL, Simone JV, editors. Washington, DC: The National Academies Press; 2003.
15. Castellino SM, Casillas J, Hudson MM, Mertens AC, Whitton J, Brooks SL, et al. Minority adult survivors of childhood cancer: a comparison of long-term outcomes, health care utilization, and health-related behaviors from the childhood cancer survivor study. J Clin Oncol. 2005;23(27):6499–507.
16. Park ER, Li FP, Liu Y, Emmons KM, Ablin A, Robison LL, et al. Health insurance coverage in survivors of childhood cancer: the Childhood Cancer Survivor Study. J Clin Oncol. 2005;23(36):9187–97.
17. Bowers DC, Adhikari S, El-Khashab YM, Gargan L, Oeffinger KC. Survey of long-term follow-up programs in the United States for survivors of childhood brain tumors. Pediatr Blood Cancer. 2009;53(7):1295–301.
18. Ganz PA, Casillas J, Hahn EE. Ensuring quality care for cancer survivors: implementing the survivorship care plan. Semin Oncol Nurs. 2008;24(3):208–17.
19. Cheung WY, Neville BA, Earle CC. Associations among cancer survivorship discussions, patient and physician expectations, and receipt of follow-up care. J Clin Oncol. 2010;28(15):2577–83.
20. Grunfeld E, Levine MN, Julian JA, Coyle D, Szechtman B, Mirsky D, et al. Randomized trial of long-term follow-up for early-stage breast cancer: a comparison of family physician versus specialist care. J Clin Oncol. 2006;24(6):848–55.
21. Oeffinger KC, McCabe MS. Models for delivering survivorship care. J Clin Oncol. 2006;24(32):5117–24.
22. Snyder CF, Frick KD, Peairs KS, Kantsiper ME, Herbert RJ, Blackford AL, et al. Comparing care for breast cancer survivors to non-cancer controls: a five-year longitudinal study. J Gen Intern Med. 2009;24(4):469–74.
23. Snyder CF, Earle CC, Herbert RJ, Neville BA, Blackford AL, Frick KD. Trends in follow-up and preventive care for colorectal cancer survivors. J Gen Intern Med. 2008;23(3):254–9.
24. Ogle KS, Swanson GM, Woods N, Azzouz F. Cancer and comorbidity: redefining chronic diseases. Cancer. 2000;88(3):653–63.
25. Darby K, Davis C, Likes W, Bell J. Exploring the financial impact of breast cancer for African American medically underserved women: a qualitative study. J Health Care Poor Underserved. 2009;20(3):721–8.
26. Pezzin LE, O'Niel MB, Nattinger AB. The economic consequences of breast cancer adjuvant hormonal treatments. J Gen Intern Med. 2009;24 Suppl 2:S446–50.
27. Weaver KE, Rowland JH, Bellizzi KM, Aziz NM. Forgoing medical care because of cost: assessing disparities in healthcare access among cancer survivors living in the United States. Cancer. 2010;116(14):3493–504.
28. Donabedian A. The definition of quality and approaches to its assessment. Ann Arbor: Health Administration Press; 1980.
29. Oeffinger KC, Mertens AC, Hudson MM, Gurney JG, Casillas J, Chen H, et al. Health care of young adult survivors of childhood cancer: a report from the Childhood Cancer Survivor Study. Ann Fam Med. 2004;2(1):61–70.
30. U.S. Census Bureau. Language use and English speaking ability. 2000. Available from: http://www.census.gov/prod/2003pubs/c2kbr-29.pdf, May 31, 2010.
31. Thomas V, Richardson A, Saleem T, Baylav A, Hall A, Richards M, et al. The efficacy of bilingual health advocacy in ethnic minority patients with cancer. Nurs Stand. 2000;14(26):32–3.
32. Flores G. The impact of medical interpreter services on the quality of health care: a systematic review. Med Care Res Rev. 2005;62(3):255–99.

33. National Health Law Prgoram and Access Project. Language services action kit: Interpreter services in health care settings for people with limited English proficiency. 2004. Available from: http://www.healthlaw.org/images/stories/issues/2004.ActionKitReprint.pdf, March 14, 2011.
34. El Ansari W, Newbigging K, Roth C, Malik F. The role of advocacy and interpretation services in the delivery of quality healthcare to diverse minority communities in London, United Kingdom. Health Soc Care Community. 2009;17(6):636–46.
35. Ayanian JZ, Zaslavsky AM, Guadagnoli E, Fuchs CS, Yost KJ, Creech CM, et al. Patients' perceptions of quality of care for colorectal cancer by race, ethnicity, and language. J Clin Oncol. 2005;23(27):6576–86.
36. Wu S, Ridgely MS, Escarce JJ, Morales LS. Language access services for Latinos with limited English proficiency: lessons learned from Hablamos Juntos. J Gen Intern Med. 2007;22 Suppl 2:350–5.
37. Price-Haywood EG, Roth KG, Shelby K, Cooper LA. Cancer risk communication with low health literacy patients: a continuing medical education program. J Gen Intern Med. 2010;25 Suppl 2:S126–9.
38. Friedman DB, Corwin SJ, Dominick GM, Rose ID. African American men's understanding and perceptions about prostate cancer: why multiple dimensions of health literacy are important in cancer communication. J Community Health. 2009;34(5):449–60.
39. Beagan BL, Kumas-Tan Z. Approaches to diversity in family medicine: "I have always tried to be colour blind". Can Fam Physician. 2009;55(8):e21–8.
40. Arora NK. Importance of patient-centered care in enhancing patient well-being: a cancer survivor's perspective. Qual Life Res. 2009;18(1):1–4.
41. Epstein RM, Street RL. Patient-centered communication in cancer care: promoting healing and reducing suffering. Bethseda: National Cancer Institute, NIH Publication No. 07-62252007, 2007. Available from: http://outcomes.cancer.gov/areas/pcc/communication/pccm_flyer.pdf, March 14, 2011.
42. Davis SW, Diaz-Mendez M, Garcia MT. Barriers to seeking cancer information among Spanish-speaking cancer survivors. J Cancer Educ. 2009;24(3):167–71.
43. Ayanian JZ, Jacobsen PB. Enhancing research on cancer survivors. J Clin Oncol. 2006;24(32):5149–53.
44. Carver JR, Shapiro CL, Ng A, Jacobs L, Schwartz C, Virgo KS, et al. American Society of Clinical Oncology clinical evidence review on the ongoing care of adult cancer survivors: cardiac and pulmonary late effects. J Clin Oncol. 2007;25(25):3991–4008.
45. Schapira MM, McAuliffe TL, Nattinger AB. Underutilization of mammography in older breast cancer survivors. Med Care. 2000;38(3):281–9.
46. Earle CC, Burstein HJ, Winer EP, Weeks JC. Quality of non-breast cancer health maintenance among elderly breast cancer survivors. J Clin Oncol. 2003;21(8):1447–51.
47. Keating NL, Landrum MB, Guadagnoli E, Winer EP, Ayanian JZ. Factors related to underuse of surveillance mammography among breast cancer survivors. J Clin Oncol. 2006;24(1): 85–94.
48. Aziz NM, Rowland JH. Cancer survivorship research among ethnic minority and medically underserved groups. Oncol Nurs Forum. 2002;29(5):789–801.
49. Ries LAG, Melbert D, Krapcho M, Stinchcomb DG, Howlader N, Horner M, et al. SEER cancer statistics review: 1975-2005. National Cancer Institute. Bethesda. 2008. Available from: http://seer.cancer.gov/csr/1975_2005/, March 14, 2011.
50. Deimling GT, Sterns S, Bowman KF, Kahana B. The health of older-adult, long-term cancer survivors. Cancer Nurs. 2005;28(6):415–24.
51. Hudson MM, Mulrooney DA, Bowers DC, Sklar CA, Green DM, Donaldson SS, et al. High-risk populations identified in Childhood Cancer Survivor Study investigations: implications for risk-based surveillance. J Clin Oncol. 2009;27(14):2405–14.
52. Ganz PA, Casillas JN, Coscarelli A. Estimating the human costs of cancer survivorship in children. Ann Intern Med. 2010;152(7):465–6.

53. American Society of Clinical Oncology. ASCO cancer treatment summaries. 2009. Available from: http://www.cancer.net/patient/Survivorship/ASCO+Cancer+Treatment+Summaries, March 14, 2011.
54. Texas Children's Cancer Center and Hematology Service. Passport for Care. 2010. Available from: http://www.txccc.org/content.cfm?menu_id=128, March 14, 2011.
55. Penn Medicine's OncoLink. LIVESTRONG Care Plan. 2010. Available from: http://www.livestrongcareplan.org, March 14, 2011.
56. National Coalition for Cancer Survivorship, UCLA Cancer Survivorship Center, WellPoint Inc., Genentech. Journey Forward: Guiding survivors as they move ahead. 2010. Available from: http://www.journeyforward.org, March 14, 2011.
57. Kadan-Lottick NS, Robison LL, Gurney JG, Neglia JP, Yasui Y, Hayashi R, et al. Childhood cancer survivors' knowledge about their past diagnosis and treatment: Childhood Cancer Survivor Study. JAMA. 2002;287(14):1832–9.
58. Children's Oncology Group. Long-term follow-up guidelines for survivors of childhood, adolescent, and young adult cancers. 2008. Available from: http://www.survivorshipguidelines.org/, March 14, 2011.
59. Burg MA, Lopez ED, Dailey A, Keller ME, Prendergast B. The potential of survivorship care plans in primary care follow-up of minority breast cancer patients. J Gen Intern Med. 2009;24 Suppl 2:S467–71.
60. McInnes DK, Cleary PD, Stein KD, Ding L, Mehta CC, Ayanian JZ. Perceptions of cancer-related information among cancer survivors: a report from the American Cancer Society's Studies of Cancer Survivors. Cancer. 2008;113(6):1471–9.
61. The Lance Armstrong Foundation. What we do. 2010. Available from: http://www.livestrong.org/What-We-Do, March 14, 2011.
62. Davis C, Darby K, Likes W, Bell J. Social workers as patient navigators for breast cancer survivors: what do African-American medically underserved women think of this idea? Soc Work Health Care. 2009;48(6):561–78.
63. Casillas J, Kahn KL, Doose M, Landier W, Bhatia S, Hernandez J, et al. Transitioning childhood cancer survivors to adult-centered healthcare: insights from parents, adolescent, and young adult survivors. Psychooncology. 2010;19:982–90.
64. The Patient Protection and Affordable Care Act. Health reform for children. 2009. Available from: http://dpc.senate.gov/healthreformbill/healthbill84.pdf, March 14, 2011.
65. Monheit AC, Vistnes JP. Race/ethnicity and health insurance status: 1987 and 1996. Med Care Res Rev. 2000;57 Suppl 1:11–35.
66. Ayanian JZ, Kohler BA, Abe T, Epstein AM. The relation between health insurance coverage and clinical outcomes among women with breast cancer. N Engl J Med. 1993;329(5):326–31.
67. Bradley CJ, Given CW, Roberts C. Late stage cancers in a Medicaid-insured population. Med Care. 2003;41(6):722–8.
68. O'Malley CD, Shema SJ, Clarke LS, Clarke CA, Perkins CI. Medicaid status and stage at diagnosis of cervical cancer. Am J Public Health. 2006;96(12):2179–85.
69. Roetzheim RG, Pal N, Tennant C, Voti L, Ayanian JZ, Schwabe A, et al. Effects of health insurance and race on early detection of cancer. J Natl Cancer Inst. 1999;91(16):1409–15.

# Chapter 8
# Cancer Survivorship Plans: A Paradigm Shift in the Delivery of Quality Cancer Care

**Julia H. Rowland and Patricia A. Ganz**

## Historical Perspective

With the release in November 2005 of the Institute of Medicine Report, *From Cancer Patient to Cancer Survivor: Lost in Transition* [1], public attention was drawn to the unique, complex, and largely unmet healthcare needs of the growing population of individuals who were making, or had already made, the transition from active patient to posttreatment recovery and beyond. For many of us, this event, accompanied as these reports usually are with formal briefings and considerable media flurry, was seen as an important turning point. Just as the founding members of the National Coalition for Cancer Survivorship (NCCS) gave us new language for what it meant to be a "survivor" (http://www.canceradvocacy.org/resources/glossary.html#C), the *Lost in Transition* report firmly established a distinct place on the continuum of cancer care for research and practice addressing "survivorship." Dispensing with the outdated medical definition of a survivor that required someone to remain disease-free for a minimum of 5 years after treatment to earn this status, coalition members argued convincingly in 1986 that a person could call him- or herself a survivor from the moment of diagnosis and for the remainder of life. This, they successfully argued, was the only way to ensure that the focus of care, and cancer-related decisions, would be on achieving a full and meaningful future life, worth living, for the individual. That definition revolutionized cancer care. In a similar way, 25 years later, the *Lost in Transition* report has given us the next paradigm shift.

As with many things, the timing of the release of this document was critical to the subsequent impact it has had. Not infrequently, once released, these types of national reports languish, gathering dust on academic bookshelves. Testament to this, a number of reports declaiming the gaps in optimal quality cancer care delivery had already appeared prior to the release of *Lost in Transition* [2–4]. So, what was different now? As highlighted in the Preface to the document, three factors served to bring broad attention to and have fueled the subsequent uptake of the recommendations made

J.H. Rowland (✉)
Office of Cancer Survivorship, National Cancer Institute, Bethesda, MD, USA
e-mail: rowlandj@mail.nih.gov

M. Feuerstein and P.A. Ganz (eds.), *Health Services for Cancer Survivors*,
DOI 10.1007/978-1-4419-1348-7_8, 

within the full report. The first of these was recognition that the cancer experience does not end when treatment ends. A growing body of published studies, the pace of which accelerated dramatically with the establishment within the National Cancer Institute (NCI) in 1996 of the Office of Cancer Survivorship (OCS), shows that cancer exacts a lingering toll for most of those diagnosed and treated. Rapid advances in early detection, more effective treatment, and better supportive care mean that most individuals found to have cancer will survive their initial treatment. Today, it is estimated that for all cancers combined, 68% of those diagnosed will be alive in 5 years; among those diagnosed as children, 77% can expect to be alive in 10 years. Of the over 12 million current survivors, 14% were diagnosed 20 or more years earlier [5]. However, the majority of cancer survivors, even those considered "cured" of their disease, will live with cancer as a chronic illness.

There are few if any benign therapies. Survivors as a group are at risk for a number of serious or life-threatening conditions, from recurrence of their original disease, to second cancers [6], some related to their earlier illness and others not, to diabetes, stroke, heart disease, and osteoporosis [7, 8]. They are more likely to report higher levels of functional impairment than their peers not treated for cancer, and frequently experience worse quality of life [9]. Cancer survivors of all ages may be adversely affected by their cancer experience and cancer's impact may be felt in multiple domains: physical, psychological, social, economic, and existential. While some people experience few side effects of the disease and its treatment, some have many and still others are left permanently impaired. The result is a growing urgency in efforts to determine how best to identify those who may be at risk for adverse outcomes and to develop and deliver evidence-based interventions to prevent these conditions from occurring when possible, or ameliorating them when not.

A second factor affecting interest in survivors' care has been the rapid evolution of the field of health services research. With its emphasis on understanding the personal (employment, insurance, financial) as well as social costs (healthcare structure, delivery, and reimbursement) of health care, research, practice, and policy generated from this field has served to draw attention to the need for a better understanding and evaluation of survivors' posttreatment care needs and the most effective, efficient, and equitable way to meet these needs.

The third, and arguably most important, driver behind the rapid uptake of the IOM report's findings has been consumers themselves. The past two decades have seen a steady increase in the level of involvement by cancer survivors, and those who care for and about them, in public policy efforts to define what is meant by and promote national standards for quality cancer care. This has ranged from the establishment of local groups giving voice to the survivorship concerns of those from distinct communities (e.g., Nueva Vida, Sister's Network, Native People's Circle of Hope, The Mautner Project) to the creation of larger advocacy organizations whose missions are to highlight and galvanize research and resources to address the unique challenges faced by survivors of specific cancers (e.g., the Pancreatic Cancer Action Network, the Ovarian Cancer National Alliance, the Bladder Cancer Advocacy Network or BCAN) or all cancers (e.g., LIVE**STRONG**), to the development by cancer survivors in positions of federal leadership of legislation designed to address the quality of survivors' care (e.g., Ted Kennedy, Arlen Specter, Debbie Wasserman Schultz). Combined, these efforts ensured that once released, the *Lost in Transition* report would have a receptive constituency of supporters. But the element of the report that has thus far secured the most "traction" in promoting a sea change in the oncology world has been the focus on the development and delivery of treatment summaries and guidelines for follow-up care, which together have come to be called: survivorship care plans.

While the importance of these documents was noted in the earlier released Institute of Medicine (IOM) [10] and President's Cancer Panel [11, 12] survivorship reports, the *Lost in Transition* document carefully specified what was called for in creating these tools (see Tables 8.1 and 8.2). Importantly, the scope of follow-up care was expected to go beyond the standard and more limited purview of

**Table 8.1** Survivorship care plan: treatment summary (Reprinted with permission from *From Cancer Patient to Cancer Survivor, Lost in Transition*, 2005 by the National Academy of Sciences, Courtesy of the National Academies Press, Washington, D.C., p. 152)

| |
|---|
| Upon discharge from cancer treatment, including treatment of recurrences, every patient should be given a record of all care received and important disease characteristics. This should include at a minimum: |
| 1. Diagnostic tests performed and results |
| 2. Tumor marker characteristics (e.g., site(s), stage and grade, hormone receptor status, marker information) |
| 3. Dates of treatment initiation and completion |
| 4. Surgery chemotherapy, radiotherapy, transplant, hormonal therapy or gene, or other therapies provided, including agents used, treatment regimen, total dosage, identifying number and title of clinical trials (if any), indicators of treatment response, and toxicities experienced during treatment |
| 5. Psychosocial, nutritional, and other supportive services provided |
| 6. Full contact information on treatment institutions and key individual providers |
| 7. Identification of a key point of contact and coordinator of continuing care |

**Table 8.2** Survivorship care plan: follow-up care plan (Reprinted with permission from *From Cancer Patient to Cancer Survivor, Lost in Transition*, 2005 by the National Academy of Sciences, Courtesy of the National Academies Press, Washington, D.C., pp. 152–153)

| |
|---|
| Upon discharge from cancer treatment, every patient and his/her primary health care provider should receive a written follow-up care plan incorporating available evidence-based standards of care. This should include, at a minimum: |
| 1. The likely course of recovery from treatment toxicities, as well as the need for ongoing health maintenance/adjuvant therapy |
| 2. A description of recommended cancer screening and other periodic testing and examinations, and the schedule on which they should be performed (and who should provide them) |
| 3. Information on possible late and long-term effects of treatment and symptoms of such effects |
| 4. Information on possible signs of recurrence and second tumors |
| 5. Information on the possible effects of cancer on marital/partner relationship, sexual functioning, work, and parenting and the potential future need for psychosocial support |
| 6. Information on the potential insurance, employment, and financial consequences of cancer and, as necessary, referral to counseling, legal aid, and financial assistance |

(continued)

**Table 8.2** (continued)

| |
|---|
| 7. Specific recommendations for healthy behaviors (e.g., diet, exercise, healthy weight, sunscreen use, immunizations, smoking cessation, osteoporosis prevention). When appropriate, recommendations that first-degree relatives be informed about their increased risk and the need for cancer screening (e.g., breast cancer, colorectal cancer, prostate cancer) |
| 8. As appropriate, information on genetic counseling and testing to identify high-risk individuals who could benefit from more comprehensive cancer surveillance, chemoprevention, or risk-reducing surgery |
| 9. As appropriate, information on known effective chemoprevention strategies for secondary prevention (e.g., tamoxifen in women at high risk for breast cancer; aspirin for colorectal cancer prevention) |
| 10. Referrals to specific follow-up care providers (e.g., rehabilitation, fertility, psychology), support groups, and/or the patient's primary care provider |
| 11. A listing of cancer-related resources and information (e.g., Internet-based sources and telephone listing for major cancer support organization) |

surveillance for recurrence of disease to embrace the broader concepts of prevention, intervention, and coordination of care. It is this new vision of what constitutes survivorship generally and survivorship care more specifically that is forging the paradigm shift.

## The Need for an Integrated Approach to Drive Quality Care

After the publication of the IOM report, a number of professional organizations and groups of clinicians reviewed the recommendations and began to address those that seemed to be most pertinent to them. The number two recommendation of the *Lost in Transition* report, which states that, "Patients completing primary treatment should be provided with a comprehensive care summary and follow-up plan that is clearly and effectively explained," seemed to be directed at oncology clinicians, and thus was taken up early on by key champions within the American Society of Clinical Oncology (ASCO). A first step in this process resulted in a special workshop, sponsored by NCCS, with support from the Lance Armstrong Foundation and the National Cancer Institute, being convened in March 2006 to examine how best to proceed implementing survivorship care planning [13]. The issues addressed at this workshop are outlined in Table 8.3; many of them remain to be fully addressed. In the wake of this meeting, members of ASCO's quality of care working group were charged with developing a response to how best to format and promote the uptake of treatment summaries in the medical oncology community.

Systematic generation of a detailed treatment summary was not historically a standard part of outpatient oncology care. This may be, in part, an artifact of the evolution of cancer medicine and practice, which was largely hospital-based until the past two to three decades. The earliest and still most common treatment for cancer is surgery. Surgical operative reports have a long history and remain a mainstay of practice; these also become a standard part of a patient's medical record along

**Table 8.3** Implementing cancer survivorship care planning workshop topics of discussion (Reprinted with permission from *Implementing Cancer Survivorship Care Planning Workshop Summary*, 2007 by the National Academy of Sciences, Courtesy of the National Academies Press, Washington, D.C., p. 2)

| |
|---|
| What are the essential elements of the care plan? Will a single template work? |
| Who is responsible for creating the plan and discussing the plan with patients? |
| What are the respective roles of oncology/primary care and physicians/nurses? |
| What economic strategies could encourage implementation of care planning? |
| What barriers exist to creating the care plan? How can they be overcome? |
| What resources are currently available for completing the care plan template (survivorship guidelines, psychosocial support resources, recommendations on healthy behaviors/prevention)? |
| What is needed to adapt care plans to electronic record systems and information technologies? |
| What statewide and collaborative approaches are available for or needed to advance implementation? |
| What opportunities exist to pilot test survivorship care planning and assess its impact? |
| What is needed to evaluate and promote a research agenda for survivorship care planning? |

with the detailed pathologic findings. Similarly, radiation therapy, the prescriptions for which are carefully mapped out and charted prior to commencement of treatment, also lends itself to standardized summary formats, even if these are delivered in a nonhospital-based, stand-alone facility.

By contrast, the practice of medical oncology has been more fragmented, moving to outpatient settings with small numbers of oncology specialists working together or even as solo practitioners. Initially provided through a hospital base with access to consolidated medical record systems, chemotherapy delivery and cancer survivor follow-up care moved quickly into the outpatient setting, leading to separate charting, and limited oversight from institutional accrediting bodies such as the Joint Commission. While chemotherapy treatment in the local community setting offers substantial convenience for many patients, a significant consequence for a large proportion of patients is the loss of coordination of the patient record. Thus, to realize the goal of a comprehensive treatment summary, as well as coordination of posttreatment care between oncology and primary care physicians involved in the initial cancer diagnosis and treatment, a system to link all of these parts of the cancer care and treatment-based datasets would be necessary. The absence of such a system was painfully evident in the wake of Hurricane Katrina where cancer patients were left with missing or incomplete access to their medical records or any form of treatment plan and summary.

Toward this end, various models and platforms to facilitate such integrated documentation were reviewed and considered. As in many aspects of survivorship care, pediatric oncologists were ahead of their adult oncology colleagues in tackling this issue. Early in the new millennium, experts concerned about the long-term follow-up of childhood cancer survivors were beginning to develop tools to address this logistical challenge. At the time of the ASCO team review, one such model platform was being tested by childhood cancer survivor experts at Baylor College of Medicine and Texas Children's Cancer Center. Led by David Poplack, the group had designed a HIPAA compliant, survivor-focused web-based system intended to help childhood cancer survivors both navigate and control their own medical history in an effort to facilitate better coordination as well as standardization of their post-treatment care. Interestingly, this effort was initiated in direct response to the 2003 IOM report on childhood cancer survivorship [10]. Referred to as the Passport for Care (PFC) (http://www.txccc.org/content.cfm?menu_id=128), this platform takes advantage of the highly centralized treatment of children with cancer and the participation of most on clinical trials with standardized treatment regimens.

The simultaneous development of consensus-based surveillance guidelines by the Children's Oncology Group (COG) [14] enabled the developers of the PFC to link the treatments received by children to specific exposure-based late effects surveillance guidelines. Unique features of the PFC are that it permits the childhood cancer survivor to share his/her treatment information with other health care providers in a secure fashion, allows for regular reminders for surveillance testing and information about new findings, and also has the capacity to generate targeted and personally tailored health promotion messages. Long aware of the need for tailored follow-up care among their young and vulnerable population, the pediatric oncology community has had since the mid-1980s a number of specialized programs to meet the special needs of this population. As of June 2010, the COG web site links to 156 children's hospitals, medical centers, and institutions in the USA and Canada offering resources for addressing the long-term care needs of pediatric cancer survivors (http://www.childrensoncologygroup.org/Surveys/lateEffects/LateEffects.PublicReport.asp). This same situation is not true for adult survivors.

At the time of the release of the adult survivorship report, a prototype of the PFC platform was available, but implementation and dissemination was limited. Currently, however, efforts are underway to have all COG sites participate by entering end-of-treatment information into a specially hosted web site. Although this pioneering effort for childhood cancer survivors was appealing, it was not clear that a similar approach would be relevant for adult cancer survivors, whose care primarily occurs in the community rather than in specialized medical settings and infrequently involves enrollment in standard clinical trials.

As ASCO approached this endeavor, the thought was to develop a relatively short template to capture treatment-specific data that could be applied to a common cancer(s) for which evidence-based surveillance guidelines existed. Two diseases/settings that met these criteria (i.e., were common and had a solid evidence-base for follow-up care) were postadjuvant therapy for colon cancer and breast cancer. Because the majority of adults who are diagnosed with these diseases are older (>60 years), the use of a web-based platform did not seem appropriate. Rather, a tool that could be easily completed by the treating oncologist seemed most appropriate, with the idea being that the content of this then could either be distributed to patients and other providers through a paper or electronic medium as desired, using office-based computers and software. The linkage to the existing surveillance guidelines, for which patient versions were available, would be considered a starting place for the survivorship care plan component.

As in the pediatric setting, however, getting these treatment summaries completed was the first challenge. ASCO has serially formed working groups of clinical experts to develop each of its treatment summary templates. After a draft was agreed upon through consensus, it was pilot tested in clinical settings for feasibility and then modified [15] (http://www.asco.org/treatmentsummary). These templates are intended to facilitate provider-to-provider and provider-to-patient communication. The templates may be distributed to patients or providers as records of the care planned and received; however, they were not designed to replace detailed chart documentation, including complete patient histories or chemotherapy flow sheets. Currently available treatment plan and summary templates cover cancer treatment generally, breast cancer adjuvant treatment, colon cancer adjuvant treatment, adjuvant nonsmall cell lung cancer, limited and extensive stage small cell lung cancer, and diffuse large B-cell lymphoma. Breast cancer and colon cancer survivorship plans are also available. These templates are available in Microsoft Word documents to be filled in by hand on paper or electronically, as well as in a Microsoft Excel format. To facilitate the ready completion of these summaries, ASCO has now worked for several years with oncology-specific electronic health record vendors encouraging them to include software applications that will allow automatic preparation of these treatment summaries as part of their products. Unfortunately, the uptake of electronic records has been relatively limited and it is uncertain whether this has influenced the use of treatment summaries and care plans in oncology practice thus far.

At the same time that the first ASCO templates were being developed in 2006, collaboration was launched among several partners, including the National Coalition for Cancer Survivorship (NCCS), the UCLA Cancer Survivorship Center, Wellpoint, and Genentech, to promote a strategy that would effectively facilitate the use of treatment summaries and survivorship care plans in clinical oncology practice. As part of the collaboration, focus groups with oncology specialists, primary care providers, and patients were held, and a professional advisory board that included these same entities as well as patient advocacy organizations was established. Through this effort, it was decided that tools were needed that would help all three target groups focus on survivorship care planning, although a special emphasis was placed on encouraging oncology providers to complete treatment summaries for their patients who had recently completed therapy. The partners, who named their initiative *Journey Forward* (http://www.journeyforward.org), collectively developed a set of materials that enable cancer survivors and their doctors to work as a team after active treatment comes to an end by providing electronic tools and resources to assist providers in completing the treatment summary and survivorship care plan. In addition, there are resources for survivors and primary care providers. The key feature of *Journey Forward* is an electronic "survivorship care plan builder" that takes the content of the ASCO treatment summary templates and puts them into a user-friendly electronic format with drop-down menus and reports that are customizable. The electronic program is downloadable and thus can reside on the healthcare providers' own computer, where the data can be updated as necessary, and can serve as a component of an electronic record.

Currently, electronic templates are available on the *Journey Forward* web site (http://www.journeyforward.org) for breast and colon cancer adjuvant therapy, as well as the ASCO generic template. Technical support for navigating and populating these is also available through the web site. These materials are available free of charge and have been distributed by Wellpoint to physicians and patients in California, Colorado, and New England. The survivorship care plan component of *Journey Forward* is modest, relying on national and local resources as well as the materials from the ASCO surveillance guidelines for breast and colon cancer. The main emphasis of this effort has been on facilitating completion of the treatment summary component as a first step toward guiding and tailoring long-term follow-up care. As with any change in practice, the impact of this procedure will need to be evaluated both in terms of its overall effect on the content and quality of care delivered, as well as its influence on survivors' health outcomes. It is expected that this approach will further evolve as a result of such research.

In contrast, the LIVE**STRONG** Care Plan (http://www.livestrongcareplan.org/), which is a collaboration between the Lance Armstrong Foundation and the University of Pennsylvania's Oncolink©, focuses on providing information that relates to treatment exposures and tries to tailor a survivorship care plan to the type of cancer and treatments the patient has received. The patient or his or her provider can complete this alternate web-based tool. However, it does require having some basic information about the cancer treatments received, although detailed information about the dose of drugs or radiation is not required. A series of questions asks about symptoms and medical conditions in an attempt to tailor the information provided in the care plan. This has been a work in progress, with several evolving versions that have been modified and updated, to make the information provided more refined and targeted. Preliminary testing of this interface with survivors and healthcare providers has shown good acceptability [16]. Nevertheless, a limitation of this tool is that it resides on the Penn Medicine server and cannot be updated either by the patient or the health care provider. If a patient or provider logs in once, the information is not saved and needs to be re-entered. Further, the survivorship care plan that is produced provides links to other electronic resources outside of the care plan itself. This product is in evolution but is nevertheless a good starting point for survivors who may want more general information about potential late effects of treatment.

There are other formats for capturing and communicating treatment summaries and survivorship care plans that are being used among the various LIVE**STRONG** Survivorship Centers of Excellence Network programs [16]. This diversity reflects the need to provide documentation and care planning within the context of a variety of health care settings (e.g., free standing cancer centers as well as university-based matrix cancer centers and community sites). It is clear that there is not one way to provide these services to patients/survivors. By and large, all of these efforts draw extensively on the examples provided in the IOM report, by including key elements of the treatment history as well as the expected posttreatment complications, symptom management, and disease recurrence surveillance. In addition to these North American efforts, there are developing programs in Australia, the United Kingdom, the Netherlands, and Italy. All of these efforts are in their infancy. Most are incorporating lessons learned from the North American experience and also trying to integrate survivorship care within cancer rehabilitation services that are hospital-based and more broadly available in Canadian and European countries than in the USA.

In addition to questions around how to provide or communicate this information, the timing of provision of the treatment summary and care plan is another issue that needs further study. It is currently recommended that the treatment summary and some form of follow-up care plan should be given to the patient near the conclusion of initial treatment to facilitate the transition to less frequent follow-up and coordinated care with other providers. It is less time consuming to do a treatment summary at this point, and education around this time can be valuable for the patient whose visits to the oncologist will be less frequent. There may be subsequent time points for updates, for example, at the end of 5 years of endocrine adjuvant therapy for breast cancer. However, the details of the primary treatment will not need to be recapitulated if already described. Instead, an interval history and long-term follow-up plan can be articulated at this later date, providing specific follow-up recommendations for the primary care physician who may be able to assume all long-term care.

However, there are many millions of survivors (prevalent cases), treated in an earlier era and before the current push for documentation, who have never received a treatment summary or care plan. For these individuals, it is enormously time consuming to retrieve their original treatment records and prepare appropriate ongoing care plans. Nevertheless, this is an important need and is especially salient for the large number of childhood cancer survivors at high risk for late effects several decades later. Increasingly, long-term adult cancer survivors who have heard about efforts to coordinate posttreatment follow-up care are seeking survivorship consultations, or they may be referred by their primary care physicians who want to be certain there are no special late effects that need monitoring. Provision of survivorship consultation services is something that is currently being done at each of the LIVE**STRONG** Network sites [17]. As the demand for these types of services expands, and as primary care providers begin to expect to receive this type of information from oncology providers, we will begin to see the more universal implementation of treatment summaries and care plans; at present, we are not there yet. Nevertheless, the pressure to meet this new standard is mounting.

In an important step toward making treatment summaries and care plans a part of quality care, ASCO decided to incorporate relevant measures as part of its Quality Oncology Practice Initiative (QOPI). First opened to full ASCO membership in January 2006, QOPI was created to promote excellence in cancer care by helping oncologists create a culture of self-examination and improvement. A voluntary program, which as of June 2010 had over 590 members, QOPI provides criteria by which a physician or practice can measure his/her or its ability to meet a set of evidence-based quality indicators in caring for cancer patients seen. Data are collected using systematic chart review and information about which quality standards are being met (or not), and the information is then fed back to the practitioners as a quality improvement activity. In 2008, development and delivery to patients and their other providers of treatment summaries became an additional set of quality indicators on the QOPI core list of measures (see Table 8.4). It is expected that to the extent these metrics become more widely accepted as the desired standard for oncology practice, more clinicians will provide treatment summaries to their patients.

**Table 8.4** QOPI: core measure criteria for delivery of treatment summaries (American Society of Clinical Oncology (ASCO) Quality Oncology Practice Initiative (QOPI) standards for assessment of adherence to the development and dissemination of cancer treatment summaries; as of September 2010 there are a total of 25 items that form the core set of criteria required for completion by participating practices, including these three (http://qopi.asco.org/program))

| | |
|---|---|
| 1. | Chemotherapy treatment summary completed within 3 months of chemotherapy end |
| 2. | Chemotherapy treatment summary provided to patient within 3 months of chemotherapy end |
| 3. | Chemotherapy treatment summary provided or communicated to practitioner(s) within 3 months of chemotherapy end |

While a desirable goal in growing efforts to increase delivery of evidence-based care, there are a number of important challenges associated with implementing survivorship care plans in regular medical practice. Unlike hospital discharge summaries, which are required by facility accrediting bodies, there is no such requirement for an end-of-treatment summary after months of cancer treatment in the outpatient setting. In addition, these treatments often take place across many medical settings (hospital, radiation therapy facilities, and private oncology offices), and there is seldom an integrated medical record. Furthermore, identification or designation of the oncology team member who will take responsibility for survivorship care planning, even if someone else has done the treatment summary, is a daunting task. With so few guidelines and recommendations available, as well as limited personnel with training to deliver the content of the care plan, we are faced with considerable resistance to embrace these activities currently. Until this becomes a universal standard of care and expectation of quality oncology practice, including sufficient reimbursement and incentives, this will not become a routine part of cancer care. New efforts to identify the medical home and deliver "patient-centered care" emphasize the importance of communication and coordination of care, especially at times of transition [18].

Arguably, oncology practices might be grateful to share subsequent care of their patients with experienced primary care providers (PCPs). PCPs, who may already have a precancer relationship with the patient, can do all of the posttreatment health promotion and disease prevention and, with appropriate guidance, perform recommended cancer surveillance monitoring for these survivors, allowing oncology practitioners to see and treat more new patients, a larger source of revenue. Given the anticipated shortage in oncology providers [19], such a hand-off when possible seems desirable from both a pragmatic as well as a business model.

The studies of Grunfeld and colleagues suggest that follow-up care can be safely provided by primary care providers in the United Kingdom and Canada for early stage breast cancer patients [20, 21]. However, US breast cancer survivors seem more dubious that this will be the case, worrying that their primary care physician may not be as knowledgeable about monitoring for cancer recurrence or addressing the persistent and late occurring effects of cancer [22]. From the few studies published to date, we know that the current system of continuous follow-up care by oncology specialists alone leads to missed opportunities in necessary health promotion and disease prevention activities, and that cancer patients who have shared care visits with a primary care physician are more likely to have better quality care

[23–25]. In the USA, there has not been as much acceptance of this model as yet. As changes occur in the US health care system as a result of the 2010 national health care legislation, the extent to which oncology and primary care providers are part of the same accountable health care organizations may influence the sharing of care and implementation of survivorship care plans in this patient population [26]. Quality care means ensuring survivors do not become lost in the transition from completion of initial cancer treatment to recovery and life after cancer, with its attendant shift in focus to monitoring for potential disease recurrence, new cancers, or comorbidities, addressing functional and psychosocial challenges, promoting health, and, in some cases, negotiating end of life care. Whether this means a hand-off back to primary care, monitoring in a shared care model, or potentially enrollment in a specialty cancer survivorship clinic or program, or some combination is a key survivorship goal for the future. Regardless of who will be in charge of a survivors' posttreatment care, instigating conversations between patients and their physicians, and oncologists and the PCPs about their expectations regarding who is providing what to whom, will be a necessary component of achieving integrated care, where all parties are "on board" with the plan [27, 28].

## Reform Efforts

### *The Need for an Evidence Base*

As more clinicians and oncology practices adopt the new standard of providing cancer treatment summaries and care plans, a major challenge will be finding methods and mechanisms by which to measure the impact of this paradigm shift. Thus far, data are lacking on the benefits of care planning. A true test of the treatment summary and care plan would be its utility as a means of facilitating better quality of care outcomes. At present, this shift in practice is happening in the absence of a clear agenda for evaluation of how (or even whether) use of survivorship care plans ultimately will affect health care delivery and quality of care, and critically, cancer survivors' health-related outcomes. It is imperative that we should be considering now how we are going to tackle this issue.

Potential "metrics for success" that might be considered are outlined in Table 8.5. Reflected in this list is the promise of what survivorship care plans might hold across three levels of effect: for survivors themselves, their providers, and the healthcare systems in which care is delivered and received. It is important to note that to be of value, these outcomes are predicated on a number of underlying assumptions. First, is that treatment summaries and follow-up care plans are discussed by the physician and the patient, and that this is done in a clear and collaborative fashion, duly respecting a given patient/survivor's cultural needs. This includes efforts to ensure that the survivor "understood" what was said and the implications of this for his or her behavior and health going forward. Second, it assumes that all of

**Table 8.5** Evaluating the impact of cancer survivorship care planning

| Metrics for success | |
|---|---|
| Survivor level | Improved (perceived) patient/doctor communication |
| | Improved understanding of needed follow-up tests, their purpose and periodicity, and who will conduct these |
| | Better understanding of potential late effects of illness and what symptoms might be important to report |
| | Better adherence to recommended follow-up activities |
| | Improved ability to identify providers and resources to address persistent effects of cancer and its treatment |
| | Decreased cancer-related morbidity |
| | Improved health-related quality of life and function |
| | Improved healthy lifestyle choices |
| | Potentially, improved overall survival |
| Clinician level | Improved (perceived) doctor/patient communication |
| | Improved doctor/doctor communication |
| | Better ability to coordinate care |
| | Improved knowledge about and ultimately standardization of follow-up care behaviors |
| | Improved ability to monitor survivor's health and implement changes in care in response to new information about treatment exposures and follow-up needs |
| System level | Reduced duplication of services |
| | Improved access to information necessary to guide follow-up care; less time spent searching for this |

the kinds of information outlined in Table 8.2 are covered as part of the consultation and documented on the forms provided. Third, it assumes that a copy of this information is given to the survivor as well as provided to other healthcare professionals either designated by the survivor or known to be important to the ongoing or future medical needs of that individual (e.g., her or his primary care physician; specialist provider if this is appropriate, such as cardiologist or endocrinologist or psychiatrist; and possibly key family member or caregiver responsible for the survivors' ongoing health, and/or designated health attorney). Proponents of electronic health records reasonably argue that having this type of information readily available in an electronic database will affect the utility of these documents to influence care. It should be noted that not included in this list is the potential impact of this new model of care on family members' behavior and functioning, although this could certainly be considered and corresponding metrics developed.

While a decrease in duplication of services (e.g., visits to multiple providers – the cancer surgeon, radiation oncologist, and medical oncologist – for receipt of cancer follow-up care) and unnecessary screening procedures (e.g., routine chest x-rays, bone scans, or biomarker assays among breast cancer survivors) would be expected to reduce the cost of survivorship care, no other economic assumptions are made in this evaluation model, although they too could be included. To date, it remains unknown what the cost/benefit ratio will be of this modification to existing practice. Because the shift being made is toward adoption of a combined chronic care and prevention model, the upfront economic costs are expected to be high, with the hope of reducing long-term costs of care for conditions that could have been prevented or caught early or simply better and more efficiently managed. It is clear that at present, it is costly in terms of both time and personnel to capture cancer treatment summary information and use this to generate a tailored cancer survivorship care plan. It is also expensive for a clinician to take the time to talk through this information with a survivor. How this should best be done (e.g., in person, by phone, using the Internet, augmented by different formats for conveying the information such as paper, DVD, audiotape, on a flash drive phone), by whom, and when after treatment ends are questions that remain to be studied. Finally, without measuring what may be changed by this process, we will be unable to determine the true impact of what is beginning to look like an important paradigm shift.

## *Delivery and Access*

A second set of evaluation criteria are needed to assess the best way (most efficient, effective, equitable, and patient-centered) to deliver long-term survivorship care. To date, while clinical experience may suggest these are particularly useful, especially for complex cases, cancer survivorship clinics and specialty follow-up programs have yet to prove that they are better than "usual care" (admittedly hard to define for survivors) in improving survivors' outcomes; specifically, data are lacking to show they reduce cancer-related morbidity and mortality. Even if these do prove to be highly effective, the sheer number of cancer survivors, and their geographic dispersion, precludes the possibility that each of these individuals can be seen in a specialty clinic. At the same time, there are millions who probably do not need such intensive or highly specialized care (e.g., most of those with early stage colorectal, breast, or prostate cancer). The question then becomes who should receive intensive follow-up in a survivorship clinic or with specially trained personnel, who can be returned quickly to the primary care setting, and who may need some intermediate type of surveillance in a shared-care model? Can we develop and test (using the metrics in Table 8.5) the impact of different models of care delivery, including those leveraging telemedicine and mobile health technologies?

An additional subset of studies is needed to determine how best to care for our oldest survivors, those 65 and older. It is estimated that by 2050 the number of men and women aged 65 and older diagnosed with cancer will double, assuming incident rates remain the same and do not increase [29]. Currently, there are approximately seven million survivors in this older age group [5]. To date, survivorship research has largely ignored this population in studies conducted despite the fact that they represent the largest constituent group (60%) of those alive today with a cancer history [30]. The National Cancer Policy Forum held hearings in November 2006 covering topics in elderly cancer survivors such as: (1) the implications of the aging of our society on oncology practice; (2) the consequent demands on delivery capacity and training; (3) the special rehabilitation needs of this population of survivors; (4) challenges to quality cancer care of a shaky Medicare system, and (5) the reality of cancer becoming a chronic illness for many older adults in particular, and the resulting impact of this for informal caregivers (many of whom are family members; most of whom are women) [31]. Much of the work currently underway to advance survivorship care planning is still focused largely on younger groups of survivors, not our older, more vulnerable aging population of survivors. This will have to change if we are to positively impact the future for these individuals and rein in the cost of cancer care in the USA and globally.

## Advocacy

Propelling collectively the diverse efforts in this area, and a reason why the survivorship care planning initiative will continue to have strong momentum going forward, are a number of more recent confluent events. The first of these includes the release of the IOM report, *Cancer Care for the Whole Patient: Meeting Psychosocial Health Needs* [32]. This document, with its call for the monitoring of systems to address the human side of cancer, complements well the requirement that care plans evaluate and provide quidance for managing the chronic effects of cancer for those transitioning to recovery. Many of these persistent effects encompass or are compounded by social and emotional issues (e.g., concern about employment and financial status, problems with interpersonal relationships, depression, fear of recurrence, stigma, social isolation), beyond just the physical sequelae. Since Spring 2008, ASCO has also begun to incorporate standards for such care in their QOPI indicators (see Table 8.6).

At the same time, the US has turned its attention to healthcare reform. With the number of cancer survivors expected to continue to grow into the foreseeable future, finding ways to reduce the cost of this illness to these individuals and the larger public will necessarily be an area of high interest. The clinical research community, in response to these pressures, is reviving interest in rehabilitation programs for survivors. A standard in many European nations and north of the US border in Canada, cancer rehabilitation programs largely disappeared across the US over the last three decades. With broader recognition that cancer for most will be a chronic health condition, interest in delivering interventions that promote recovery and encourage self-management of health is rapidly kindling.

**Table 8.6** QOPI core indicators for measurement of emotional well-being (American Society of Clinical Oncology (ASCO) Quality Oncology Practice Initiative (QOPI) standards for assessment of adherence to the development and dissemination of cancer treatment summaries; as of September 2010 there are a total of 25 items that form the core set of criteria required for completion by participating practices, including these two (http://qopi.asco.org/program))

| |
|---|
| 1. Patient emotional well-being assessed by the second office visit |
| 2. Action taken to address problems with emotional well-being by the second office visit |

Three final trends in healthcare will contribute to the success of survivorship care planning. These include: new attention to the identification of a "medical home" for each individual, growing emphasis placed by the senior leadership at the National Institutes of Health on realizing the vision of "personalized medicine" [33], and finally, deeper understanding of the key role that good patient–physician communication will necessarily play if we are to achieve both of these goals [34]. As proposed, the survivorship care plan can help achieve all three of these goals.

## Summary

As the population of both pediatric and adult survivors continues to grow and age clinicians and researchers will be challenged to find ways to reduce the burden of long-term survivorship on these individuals, their families, and society. New approaches to posttreatment rehabilitation, health-promotion and disease prevention, and broader dissemination of these to diverse communities will be required to successfully meet this challenge. In the wake of the release of the IOM report, *From Cancer Patient to Cancer Survivor: Lost in Transition*, a major shift has occurred in how cancer survivors are viewed on the one hand, and how they are cared for as they transition to posttreatment recovery and beyond on the other. One example is the introduction of the use of treatment summaries and survivorship care plans for patients making the transition to recovery. This new initiative has the potential to change how oncology and primary care clinicians are practicing and how patients themselves navigate and manage their posttreatment health. Multiple hurdles remain in realizing the goal of delivering these forms to all those completing their primary cancer care. While this shift has the potential to alter many long-term outcomes, efforts are urgently needed to study this process, measure its true impact, and as needed, course correct for the future.

## References

1. Hewitt M, Greenfield S, Stovall Ellen, editors. From cancer patient to cancer survivor: lost in transition. Washington, DC: Institute of Medicine, National Academies Press; 2005.
2. Hewitt M, Simone JV, editors. Ensuring quality cancer care. Washington, DC: Institute of Medicine, National Academies Press; 1999.
3. Crossing the quality chasm: a new health system for the 21st century. Institute of Medicine, National Academies Press: Washington, DC; 2001.
4. Foley KM, Gelband H, editors. Improving palliative care for cancer. Washington, DC: Institute of Medicine, National Academies Press; 2001.
5. Altekruse SF, Kosary CL, Krapcho M, Neyman N, Aminou R, Waldron W, Ruhl J, Howlader N, Tatalovich Z, Cho H, Mariotto A, Eisner MP, Lewis DR, Cronin K, Chen HS, Feuer EJ, Stinchcomb DG, Edwards BK, editors. SEER Cancer Statistics Review, 1975–2007, National

Cancer Institute. Bethesda, MD, http://seer.cancer.gov/csr/1975_2007/, based on Nov 2009 SEER data submission, posted to the SEER web site, 2010.
6. Mariotto AB, Rowland JH, Ries LAF, Scoppa S, Feuer EJ. Multiple cancer prevalence: a growing challenge in long-term survivorship. Cancer Epidemiol Biomark Prev. 2007;116(3):566–71.
7. Ganz PA. Late effects of cancer and its treatment. Semin Oncol Nurs. 2001;17(4):241–8.
8. Ganz PA, editor. Cancer survivorship: today and tomorrow. New York: Springer; 2007.
9. Hewitt M, Rowland JH, Yancik R. Cancer survivors in the United States: age, health, and disability. J Gerontol Med Sci. 2003;58(1):82–91.
10. Hewitt M, Weiner SL, Simone JV, editors. Childhood cancer survivorship: improving care and quality of life. Washington, DC: Institute of Medicine, National Academies Press; 2003.
11. President's Cancer Panel Report 2003/2004. Living beyond cancer: finding a new balance. National Cancer Institute: Bethesda MD; 2004.
12. President's Cancer Panel Report 2005/2006. Assessing progress, advancing change. National Cancer Institute: Bethesda, MD; 2006.
13. Implementing Cancer Survivorship Care Planning: Workshop Summary. Washington, DC: National Academies Press; 2007.
14. Landier W, editor. Establishing and enhancing services for childhood cancer survivors: Long-term follow-up program resource guide. Children's oncology group nursing discipline, Clinical Practice Subcommittee/Survivorship in collaboration with the Late Effects Committee, 2007 (http://www.survivorshipguidelines.org/).
15. ASCO's library of treatment plans and summaries expands. J Oncol Pract 2008; 4(1):31–6.
16. Hill-Kayser CE, Vachani C, Hampshire M, Jacobs LA, Metz JM. An Internet tool for creation of cancer survivorship care plans for survivors and health care providers: design, implementation, use and user satisfaction. J Med Internet Res. 2009;11(3):e39.
17. Shapiro C, McCabe M, Syrjala K, Friedman D, Jacobs L, Ganz P, et al. The LIVESTRONG Survivorship Center of Excellence Network. J Cancer Surviv. 2009;3:4–11.
18. Bechtel C, Ness DL. If you build it, will they come? Designing truly patient-centered health care. Health Aff. 2010;29:914–20.
19. Erickson C, Salsberg E, Forte G, Bruinooge S, Goldstein M. Future supply and demand for oncologists: challenges to assuring access to oncology services. J Oncol Pract. 2007;3(2):79–86.
20. Grunfeld E, Mant D, Yudkin P, Adewuyi-Dalton R, Cole D, Stewart J, et al. Routine follow up of breast cancer in primary care: randomised trial [see comments]. BMJ. 1996;313:665–9.
21. Grunfeld E, Levine MN, Julian JA, Coyle D, Szechtman B, Mirsky D, et al. Randomized trial of long-term follow-up for early-stage breast cancer: a comparison of family physician versus specialist care. J Clin Oncol. 2006;24:848–55.
22. Mao JJ, Bowman MA, Stricker CT, DeMichele A, Jacobs L, Chan D, et al. Delivery of survivorship care by primary care physicians: the perspective of breast cancer patients. J Clin Oncol. 2009;27:933–8.
23. Earle CC, Burstein JH, Winer EP, Weeks JC. Quality of non-breast cancer health maintenance among elderly breast cancer survivors. J Clin Oncol. 2003;21:1447–51.
24. Earle CC, Neville BA. Underuse of necessary care among elderly colorectal cancer survivors. Cancer. 2004;101:1712–9.
25. Nathan PC, Greenberg ML, Ness KK, Hudson MM, Mertens AC, Mahoney MC, et al. Medical care in the long-term survivors of childhood cancer: a report from the Childhood Cancer Survivor Study. J Clin Oncol. 2008;26:4401–9.
26. Lin J, Donehower RC. Make quality cancer survivorship care possible in the era of workforce shortage. J Oncol Pract. 2010;6(1):52–3.
27. Cheung WY, Neville BA, Cameron DB, Cook EF, Earle CC. Comparison of patient and physician expectations for cancer survivorship care. J Clin Oncol. 2009;27:2489–95.
28. Grunfield E, Earle CC. The interface between primary and oncology specialty care: treatment through survivorship. J Natl Cancer Inst Mongr. 2010;40:25–30.
29. Edwards BK, Howe HL, Ries LAG, Thun MJ, Rosenberg HM, Yancik R, et al. Annual report to the nation on the status of cancer, 1973–1999, featuring implications of age and aging on U.S. cancer burden. Cancer. 2002;94(10):2766–92.

30. Bellizzi KM, Rowland JH. Role of comorbidity, symptoms and age in the health of older survivors following treatment for cancer. Aging Health. 2007;3(5):625–35.
31. Cancer in elderly people: workshop proceedings. Washington, DC: Institute of Medicine, National Academies Press; 2007.
32. Adler NE, Page AEK, editors. Cancer care for the whole patient: meeting psychosocial health needs. Washington, DC: Institute of Medicine, National Academies Press; 2008.
33. Hamburg MA, Collins FS. The path to personalized medicine. N Engl J Med. 2010;363(4): 301–4.
34. Epstein RM, Street RL, Jr. Patient-centered communication in Cancer care: Promoting Healing and Reducing Suffering. National Cancer Institute, NIH Publication No. 07-6225. Bethesda, MD; 2007.

# Part III
# Optimizing Care Across Clinical Settings

# Chapter 9
# Optimizing Health: Primary Care

**Kevin C. Oeffinger and Larissa Nekhlyudov**

## Introduction

There are over 11 million cancer survivors in the United States, and this number is expected to grow [1]. Survivors are also living longer and whereas most of the cancer survivors are early in their phase of survivorship, about half have survived for at least 10 years. The rates of cancer survivors among those aged 65 and older has grown, and the number of elderly cancer survivors is projected to be quite significant over the next few decades. As such, a growing population of cancer survivors will have cancer and noncancer-related concerns and comorbidities which will require long-term follow-up and management. The medical needs of cancer survivors include cancer-related care, such as surveillance for recurrences, follow-up for complications of treatment, and other cancer screening. Cancer survivors also have noncancer-related health care needs, including disease prevention and chronic disease management. Further, cancer survivors face an array of psychosocial issues which require ongoing monitoring and evaluation, including quality of life, financial burdens of cancer and noncancer illness, and implications of cancer and cancer survivorship on their family. Each of the components of cancer survivorship requires coordination of care between primary care providers, cancer specialists, nursing, and others who may be involved.

Primary care providers are involved in caring for cancer survivors; their role is likely to expand in the upcoming years as the number of survivors grows, comorbidities increase, and the availability of oncologists becomes insufficient to provide survivorship care [2]. This chapter addresses the current state of knowledge about the role for primary care providers in the caring for cancer survivors and ways in which this care may be optimized.

K.C. Oeffinger (✉)
Memorial Sloan-Kettering Cancer Center, New York, USA
e-mail: oeffingk@mskcc.org

M. Feuerstein and P.A. Ganz (eds.), *Health Services for Cancer Survivors*,
DOI 10.1007/978-1-4419-1348-7_9, © Springer Science+Business Media, LLC 2011

## Risk-Based Survivorship Health Care

The authors of the Institute of Medicine (IOM) report, *From Cancer Patient to Cancer Survivor: Lost in Transition*, recommend lifelong health care for all cancer survivors [1]. This recommendation is based on the observation that cancer survivors often develop a health problem as a direct or indirect consequence of the cancer or the cancer therapy. One approach to survivorship care is based on individualized risk assessment. These problems may occur during therapy and persist as a chronic disease, such as bleomycin-induced lung injury in a male treated for testicular cancer [3]. In contrast, some health problems, such as late-onset anthracycline-induced cardiomyopathy, may not become clinically manifested until many years or even decades after the cancer therapy [4]. Collectively, these persistent and late occurring chronic diseases are generally referred to as late effects. The development and progression of a late effect of the therapy may be influenced by other noncancer comorbidities and preexisting conditions. For example, a woman treated for Hodgkin lymphoma at the age of 40 years with mediastinal irradiation has a substantially elevated risk of coronary artery disease. Traditional cardiovascular risk factors, such as dyslipidemia or tobacco use, further increase this risk [5]. Similarly, a woman with newly diagnosed breast cancer and with preexisting heart disease has an increased risk of acute and late-onset anthracycline cardiotoxicity [6]. Recognizing that the risk and severity of many late effects can be reduced with preventive strategies or early detection, a systematic plan for lifelong screening, surveillance, and prevention that incorporates risks based on the previous cancer, cancer therapy, genetic predispositions, lifestyle behaviors, and comorbid health conditions should be developed for all survivors. Content, intensity, and frequency of health care vary from survivor to survivor. Survivors treated with less intense or tissue damaging therapies are unlikely to experience a late effect and consequently have less health care needs other than surveillance for a recurrence of the primary cancer. However, those treated with radiation, intensive chemotherapy, and organ altering surgery (e.g., left lung lobectomy) generally need more attentive monitoring and surveillance.

Psychological difficulties arising from the cancer experience may not correlate with the risk of late effects, necessitating periodic screening for depression, anxiety, and somatization for all cancer survivors [1, 7]. In addition, some survivors benefit from special services, including outcome-specific multidisciplinary programs (e.g., lymphedema program, cognitive rehabilitation) and more generalized services (e.g., physical, occupational, and speech therapy; career counseling; peer support programs; genetic testing and counseling) [8–10].

## Current State of Cancer Survivorship Care

While many specialized cancer survivorship programs have emerged [11], most cancer survivors, including childhood cancer survivors, receive care in community primary care settings alone or in combination with oncology care [12–18].

Many cancer survivors are not receiving the health care that they need, including surveillance for recurrences [19–22], management of comorbid conditions [23, 24], and screening for late effects and subsequent cancers [17, 25, 26]. Many cancer survivors, including those at highest risk, are altogether lost in the system and are not followed [13–17, 26], while others receive more aggressive and possibly duplicative care [27].

The documented discrepancies in cancer survivorship care have resulted in further research addressing whether under-utilization of recommended health services is affected by the type of provider the cancer survivor sees following cancer treatment. Using SEER Medicare data to evaluate patterns of care for cancer survivors, Snyder et al. [13] found that in year 1 following diagnosis, approximately 40% of colorectal cancer survivors saw their primary care provider and oncologist, over 40% saw their primary care provider only, and less than 10% saw their oncologist only. About 10% saw neither provider. Over the following 5 years, fewer survivors saw oncologists and more saw their primary care providers alone. In assessing utilization of services, the authors found that survivors mostly seeing oncology specialists were more likely to receive cancer-related services, such as surveillance and screening; those who were mostly seeing primary care providers were more likely to have noncancer-related services, such as vaccinations, cholesterol screening, and evaluation for osteoporosis. Similar patterns of care and utilization of cancer and noncancer-related services were observed among breast cancer survivors [14]. Interestingly, when survivors were cared for by oncology specialists and primary care providers, more of cancer and noncancer-related services were received. While it is not surprising that oncology-based care is focused on cancer-related areas and primary care–based care is focused on prevention, this study demonstrates the need for elucidating the goals for cancer surveillance and screening as patients transition from the oncologist to primary care settings. The study findings may also lead to the conclusion that a shared care approach to cancer survivorship care is optimal; while that may be true, however, it is important to note that while shared care is a potential solution, it does present questions about when shared care may be potentially duplicative, unnecessary and potentially present a significant burden to the patients, the health care system, and society. In a recent study, Pollack et al. [12] analyzed the SEER data and found that in years 6–12 after cancer diagnosis, patients had 8–9 clinical visits per year with their primary care providers, cancer specialists, nononcology specialists, and other providers.

Few studies have directly assessed the differences in outcomes when survivorship care is provided by primary care providers compared with oncology specialists. Grunfeld et al. [28] conducted a randomized controlled trial in Canada where 968 women with early-stage breast cancer who had completed adjuvant chemotherapy and/or radiation therapy, were disease free, and were between 9 and 15 months after diagnosis were allocated to follow-up in the cancer center (usual care) or with their own family physician. The family physicians received a one-page guideline with surveillance recommendations, including intervals for physical examinations and mammography. For women on tamoxifen, they were advised to inquire about vaginal bleeding and to perform a pelvic examination annually. The family physicians were advised to refer patients back to the cancer center if a recurrence or new primary breast cancer developed. Patients were followed for up to 5 years. The study found no differences in the rates recurrences, deaths or recurrence-related serious clinical events among the women in the two groups. There were also no statistically significant differences in self-reported health-related quality of life. In an interesting study, Blaauwbroek and her Dutch colleagues invited a random sample of 123 adult survivors of childhood cancer to participate in piloting a shared care model that transitioned survivors from the oncologist to the primary care physician (Dutch family doctor) [29]. Almost all family doctors invited to participate enrolled in the study (98%), 85% returned all forms (including test findings), and only 3% were dissatisfied with the shared-care program. Possibly as a result of the information provided by the oncologists to the family doctors, only 7% of patients felt the family doctors did not know what they were expected to do. Additionally, the oncology team educated the adult survivors on their health risks and the need for longitudinal care and facilitated the visit to the family doctor. Few of the survivors (11%) were dissatisfied with the survivor-focused care they received from the family doctors. Furthermore, the study population was representative of adult survivors of pediatric cancer; this was not a simple low-risk group, as shown by the fact that 40% of the cohort had a moderate-to-severe chronic sequelae and 70% had multiple health conditions. While important lessons may be learned from these two studies, due to differences in the health care system, the findings may not be reproducible to the United States. It is essential that studies testing outcomes of different models of care are conducted and in different health care systems.

## Care of the Cancer Survivor by the Primary Care Physician

It is important for the primary care physician to be involved in the care of most if not all cancer survivors. Notably, primary care physicians generally have expertise in chronic disease management and working with subspecialists in a shared care model [30–33]. The cornerstone of shared care is personal communication and a periodic two-way transfer of information between the specialist and the primary care physician. To facilitate survivor care, it is ideal when the primary care physician follows the patient through the diagnosis and cancer therapy. This can sometimes be difficult with the number of appointments and type of health care needed for the cancer patient; however, for many patients primary care providers continue to play an important role in their care. A recent survey of 1,694 primary care providers who were identified by colorectal and lung cancer patients as filling one or more key roles in their care, over 90% of providers reported participating in their patients' general medical care, managing comorbid conditions, symptom control, and referring to hospice care [34]. During cancer therapy, receipt of a summary of the planned cancer therapy from the oncologist, as recommended in the IOM report [1], along with periodic updates can facilitate the maintenance of the bond between the patient and the primary care physician. Then upon completion of the cancer therapy, it is important for the oncologist (or the cancer

SUMMARY OF CANCER TREATMENT
**Date of preparation:** 7/8/2009

| | | | |
|---|---|---|---|
| **Name:** Jane Doe | | **Date of Birth: 1/1/1987** | |
| **Cancer Diagnoses:**<br>1. Hodgkin Lymphoma, Stage IIIB (nodular sclerosing)<br>2. Myelodysplasia/treatment-related AML | | | |
| Treatment center: Memorial Sloan-Kettering Cancer Center<br>Date of diagnosis: 7/2001; age at diagnosis: 14 ½ years old<br>Date of diagnosis of MDS: 12/2002<br>Date of diagnosis of AML: 6/2003<br>Date of completion of therapy: 8/21/03 | | | |
| **Radiation Therapy** | | | |
| **Start** | **Stop** | **Field** | **Dose (cGy)** |
| 2/18/02 | 3/5/02 | Modified mantle (bilateral neck; mediastinium; right axilla) | 2100 |
| 3/6/02 | 3/21/02 | Para-aortic nodes | 2100 |

| **Chemotherapy:** (Hodgkin: BEACOPP 8/2001-1/2002) (BMT protocol 01-055) | |
|---|---|
| **Drug Name** | **Dose (units or mg/m$^2$)** |
| Doxorubicin | 272 mg/m$^2$ |
| Bleomycin | 78 IU/m$^2$ |
| Cyclophosphamide | 14 grams |
| Prednisone | |
| Procarbazine | |
| Vincristine | |
| Etoposide | 2400 mg/m$^2$ |
| **MDS** | |
| Cytarabine | |
| L-Asparaginase | |
| **Mismatched unrelated allogeneic T-cell depleted peripheral stem cell transplant:** 8/21/2003<br>**Cytoreduction:** Busulfan, Melphalan, Fludarabine. | |
| **Potential Late Effects** | **Screening Recommendations**** |
| • Heart problems<br>• Lung problems<br>• Osteoporosis<br>• Thyroid problems<br>• Fertility problems<br>• Bladder problems<br>• Dental problems<br>• Secondary malignancies | • Annual labs to include: CBC, comp profile, TSH, urinalysis, lipid profile, insulin, CRP, Vit 25-OH.<br>• Echocardiogram/EKG every 1-2 years<br>• Pulmonary Function Test every 1-3 years<br>• Bone density study (DXA) baseline and as clinically indicated<br>• Breast MRI and mammogram yearly starting at age 25<br>• Colonoscopy every 5 yrs starting at age 35 |

**Screening recommendations adapted from the CureSearch Children's Oncology Group Long-Term Follow-Up Guidelines
http://www.survivorshipguidelines.org

**For any questions, please contact:**
Kevin Oeffinger, MD
Adult Long-Term Follow-Up Program
Memorial Sloan-Kettering Cancer Center
1275 York Avenue, NY, NY 10065
646-888-4730

**Fig. 9.1** Summary of cancer treatment and recommended screening

center staff) to prepare a cancer treatment summary that includes a concise description of the cancer diagnosis, therapy, key potential late effects, and recommendations for follow-up care. Figure 9.1 provides an example of the cancer treatment summary used at Memorial Sloan-Kettering Cancer Center. A more in-depth discussion about cancer care summaries is presented in a separate chapter of this book.

Survivors at low risk of late effects (e.g., those with Stage 1 breast or colorectal cancer or Stage 1 Wilms tumor) and without persistent toxicity of therapy should be transitioned with a cancer treatment summary (including recommendations for surveillance for recurrence) to the primary care physician soon after completion of therapy. The oncologist and the primary care physician should determine and clearly communicate who is responsible for surveillance for recurrence. For this group of survivors, it is essential that the oncologist provides both the patient and the primary care physician contact information to facilitate prompt evaluation for any suspected recurrence or serious problem potentially related to the cancer. In general, it is important to avoid "over medicalizing" this group of survivors with the ordering of unnecessary tests while addressing the physical and psychosocial problems that may have arisen as a result of the cancer.

Most survivors with a moderate risk of late effects or moderate persistent toxicity of therapy (e.g., breast cancer survivors treated with anthracycline-based adjuvant chemotherapy, testicular cancer survivors treated with platinum-based chemotherapy, or childhood acute lymphoblastic leukemia survivors) can be transitioned back to the primary care physician about 2–5 years after completion of therapy, depending upon their risk of recurrence (Figure 9.2, Panel A). This group of patients will require more regular communication between the oncologist and the primary care physician. In particular, the cancer treatment summary should include specific recommendations for surveillance for late effects or other key care needs. Because the understanding about late effects is an evolving process, it is important for the oncologist (or the cancer team) to periodically update the primary care physician with any new recommendations. Similarly, as demonstrated in the Dutch study [29], the primary care physician should send back results of surveillance testing or any other new cancer-related developments to the cancer center. As with the low risk population, clear delineation of responsibilities and contact information is essential. While both short- and long-term communication strategies present a challenge, particularly as patients, clinicians, and health care systems are not static, use of electronic reminders, registries, and personal health records have the potential to enhance this process.

Survivors at high risk of serious late effects (e.g., Hodgkin lymphoma survivors treated with mantle or mediastinal irradiation) or with moderate-to-severe multiorgan disease (e.g., allogeneic hematopoietic stem cell transplant recipients) require close monitoring. If this cannot be provided through the practice of the primary care physician, then continued follow-up care at the cancer center or by the oncologist is warranted (Figure 9.2, Panel B). However, even in this setting, it is important for the survivor to maintain contact with their primary care physician for the management of noncancer-related health problems.

In the last few years, several comprehensive cancer centers have developed specialized survivorship programs for moderate-to-high risk survivors [35]. Several models are being studied. One model used by several centers incorporates a one-time consultative survivorship visit in which a cancer treatment summary and care plan is prepared and discussed with the cancer survivor. In another model, survivors

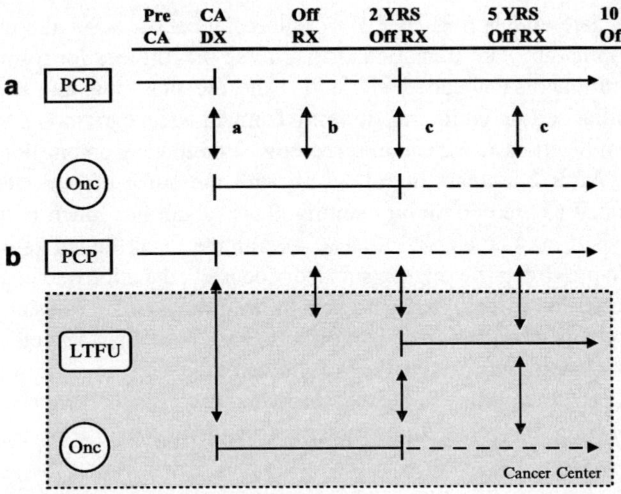


Panel (A) community-based follow-up care of cancer survivors at low or moderate risk of late effects;
Panel (B) cancer center-based follow-up care of high risk cancer survivors.

Abbreviations: CA, cancer; DX, diagnosis; Off RX, completion of cancer therapy; PCP, primary care physician; Onc, oncologist; LTFU, Long-term follow-up program

Solid line connotes primary responsibility; dashed line connotes secondary responsibility.

**Roles and Responsibilities**

***Oncologist:***

- Cancer therapy
- Keep primary care physician informed
- Guidance in long-term survivorship care
- Transition of patient to primary care physician at appropriate time
- Availability for questions, consults, referrals

***Primary care physician:***

- Ensure physical and emotional health needs of the survivor are addressed
- Assume responsibility for aspects of care of the chronic disease that are feasible in the primary care setting
- Refer for problems and/or periodic evaluations
- Consult in areas of uncertainty

**Communication Points**

a. Cancer diagnosis, stage and/or TNM classification, planned therapeutic approach, brief overview of chemotherapy, radiation therapy, and/or surgery
b. *Survivorship Care Plan* : summary of cancer and cancer therapy, a list of potential late effects, up-to-date recommendations for recurrence and late effects, contact information
c. Continued update with changes in surveillance recommendations and new information regarding potential late effects.

*Adapted with permission from the *Journal of Clinical Oncology* 24:5117–24, 2006

**Fig. 9.2** Care of cancer surviors stratified by risk of late effects (Oeffinger and McCabe, Models for Delivering Survivorship Care, J Clin Oncol. Reprinted with permission. © 2008 American Society of Clinical Oncology. All rights reserved) at moderate risk for late effects (e.g., breast or colorectal cancer survivors treated with adjuvant chemotherapy) are transitioned to a nurse practitioner for follow-up care. The nurse practitioner is embedded within the cancer team setting, thus keeping the patient in a familiar setting while transitioning from an acute care model to one promoting long-term health issues through screening, surveillance, counseling, and targeted education. After 2–5 years of follow-up with the nurse practitioner, the survivor is transitioned to the community setting. This model has much potential for cancer centers, as it may be a cost-effective alternative to continued care with the oncologist while providing the intense survivor-focused education and counseling for a short time period prior to transitioning to the primary care physician. In another model, survivors at high risk of late effects (e.g., bone marrow transplant recipients, Hodgkin lymphoma survivors) are followed long-term by a multidisciplinary team with special expertise in cancer survivors. Overall, the proportion of cancer survivors followed in such settings remains small [17].

## Are Primary Care Physicians Interested in Following Cancer Survivors and Are They Capable of Doing This?

Numerous studies have shown that primary care providers alone, or together with an oncologist and/or another provider, already care for most cancer survivors [13–18, 28, 36]. Only about half reported being comfortable in having responsibility for surveillance of cancer recurrences [37]. A recent study surveyed 330 primary care providers (response rate, 52%) in Canada found 50–55% were willing to assume exclusive responsibility for the follow-up of breast, prostate, and colorectal cancer survivors within 2 years following completion of treatment, and 42% were willing to accept exclusive care of patients with lymphoma [38]. In the Northern Netherlands, 358 primary care physicians participated in a postgraduate course on late effects in pediatric cancer survivors [39]. After the course, they were asked to complete a ten-item questionnaire on motivation to participate in the regular follow-up of adult survivors of childhood cancer. Of the responders (response rate, 65%), almost all (97%) were willing to participate in a shared care model for follow-up and 64% felt that it was their responsibility to be in charge of childhood cancer survivors. The main requirements for participation were the availability of guidelines (64%), sufficient information about the patient's medical history (37%), and short communication lines (45%). The main barriers to participate were workload (16%), lack of knowledge (15%), and lack of communication (13%). In the United States, a survey by Cheung et al. [40] found that most of the 255 primary care providers (response rate, 66%) were willing to be responsible, either solely or in collaboration with the oncologist, for all domains of cancer survivorship care, including monitoring for cancer recurrence, screening for other cancers, management of other medical conditions, and disease prevention. Primary care–based follow-up would be facilitated with the availability of patient-specific letters from the specialist, printed guidelines, and, if needed, expedited means of referring the patient back to the specialist [38].

However, despite their interest and willingness to assume the care for cancer survivors, primary care providers have also expressed concerns about the time and training involved in providing survivorship care plans and communication problems with oncologists [41]. About half of the 227 primary care providers (response rate, 76%) surveyed in one study found that they were not prepared to evaluate and manage long-term effects of cancer; however, only 14% reported that late effects should be mainly managed by oncologists [42]. Lack of formal training was mostly cited by these primary care providers as a barrier in providing cancer survivorship care. A survey of 54 general practitioners in the United Kingdom found that the most commonly cited barriers to providing survivorship care reported were budgetary restrictions, demands on time, and lack of expertise [43].

Oncologists have also been surveyed about their views of having primary care providers engaged in caring for cancer survivors. One survey of 123 oncologists (response rate, 30%) found that while they expected to provide follow-up for cancer recurrence and screening for other cancers, they did not expect to be involved in general preventive care or treatment of other medical problems [40]. The previously cited study in the United Kingdom found that of the 421 oncology providers who were also surveyed, approximately 60% reported that follow-up of cancer survivors in primary care follow-up would increase their availability for acute cancer care. About 80% felt that primary care providers lacked expertise about cancer survivorship and 60% perceived that primary care providers have too many other priorities. Further, the majority felt that primary care–based care would result in loss of outcomes data about late effects of treatment. Interestingly, over 60% felt that primary care–based follow-up would increase patient anxiety [43]. In a recent survey of pediatric oncologists in the United States (response rate, 57%), Henderson et al. reported that many pediatric oncologists are increasingly uncomfortable with caring for survivors as they age and have suboptimal knowledge regarding the current surveillance recommendations for second malignant neoplasms and late effects [44].

Cancer survivors' attitudes toward receiving survivorship care from primary care providers have been mixed. Cancer treatment presents a unique time for bonding between patients and their oncologists following successful cancer treatment, survivors and their oncologists often do not wish to part [45]. This bond often complicates the potential "hand off" of patients to the primary care provider settings. Further, survivors' confidence in their primary care providers' ability to care for them is often lacking. Mao et al. [46] found that while most of the 300 breast cancer survivors (response rate, 81%) with stage I–III cancer were confident in their primary care providers' ability to provide general care, psychosocial support, and health promotion skills, only half reported that their primary care providers were knowledgeable about cancer follow-up, late effects of treatment, and treating symptoms related to cancer or its treatment. Only 28% felt that their oncologist and primary care provider communicated well. A recent United Kingdom survey of 255 young adult cancer survivors aged 18–45 (response rate 66%), including breast cancer ($n=71$), hematologic cancers ($n = 102$), and testicular cancer ($n = 82$), similarly found that hospital-based oncology care was preferable to general practitioner-based care [47]. While these studies offer important insights into patient preferences, it is important to note that the participants were receiving care at major cancer centers and therefore, the results may not be generalizable to the majority of cancer survivors followed in community-based settings.

## What Tools Do Primary Care Providers Need to Provide Cancer Survivorship Care?

In order to promote quality cancer survivorship care by primary care providers, further research needs to take place in order to monitor cancer survivors for late effects of treatment. This should lead to the development of risk stratification tools that may be used to identify survivors who are at a high risk for complications related to cancer and/or its treatment. Such an approach has been developed for childhood cancer survivors treated in the United Kingdom by Wallace and colleagues [48]. High-risk survivors may be most appropriate for shared care or mostly oncology-based care. Survivors found to be at moderate or lower risk for recurrences and/or complications, may be safely cared for mostly in primary care settings, with intermittent consultation in oncology. For patients who do transition to primary care, it is critical that primary care providers in community settings have direct access to cancer survivorship experts who can continue to offer guidance [38] or to local generalists who may develop expertise in cancer survivorship [11]. Primary care providers need to work together with oncology specialists to improve transitions of care, evaluate care models, and develop comprehensive care summaries that include the relevant elements needed for primary care practice. Primary care providers may not need detailed information about the course of treatment and radiation doses, but do need recommendations about the (1) modalities to be used for cancer recurrence surveillance, including the periodicity of surveillance and duration; (2) types of risk-based cancer screening needed; (3) surveillance for and management of treatment-related morbidities, including potential interactions between cancer and noncancer medications and/or treatments; (4) prevention and behavioral risk-modifying strategies such as diet or exercise that may be of specific benefit for the cancer survivor; (5) genetic risk of prior cancer on the patient, his/her family members and children; (6) resources that may be available for survivors to assist with long-term financial and psychosocial concerns; and as previously addressed (7) coordination of care if needed, with whom, and when (Table 9.1) [49].

The effectiveness of summaries by patients and primary care providers and their effects on outcomes of care, including quality and costs, need to be evaluated. Both short- and long-term communication strategies between specialists and primary care providers have to be refined and tested. Finally, primary care providers need to be educated about cancer survivorship care. This may be achieved though formal training and continuing medical education programs, journal supplements, medical textbooks, and Internet resources. Primary care providers who may not be aware

**Table 9.1** Basic information needed by primary care providers in caring for cancer survivors*

- Modalities to be used for cancer recurrence surveillance, including the periodicity of surveillance and duration
- Types of risk-based cancer screening needed
- Surveillance for and management of treatment-related morbidities, including potential interactions between cancer and non-cancer medications and/or treatments
- Prevention and behavioral risk-modifying strategies such as diet or exercise that may be of specific benefit for the cancer survivor
- Genetic risk of prior cancer on the patient, his/her family members and children
- Resources that may be available for survivors to assist with long-term financial and psychosocial concerns
- Coordination of care if needed, with whom, and when

*This information may be included in care planning summaries as well as educational programs aimed at enhancing primary care providers knowledge about cancer survivorship care.

**Table 9.2** Cancer survivorship resources available for primary care providers

Institute of Medicine Reports, also available at http://www.iom.edu

Hewitt M, Weiner SL, Simone JV (editors). *Childhood Cancer Survivorship: Improving Care and Quality of Life*. Washington, DC, The National Academies Press, 2003

Hewitt M, Greenfield S, Stovall E (editors). *From Cancer Patient to Cancer Survivor – Lost in Transition*. Washington, DC, The National Academies Press, 2006

Hewitt M, Ganz PA (editors). *Implementing Cancer Survivorship Care Planning – Workshop Summary*. Washington, DC, The National Academies Press, 2007

Other reports

Centers for Disease Control and Prevention and the Lance Armstrong Foundation: A National Action Plan for Cancer Survivorship: Advancing Public Health Strategies. Atlanta, GA, Centers for Disease Control and Prevention, 2004. http://www.cdc.gov/cancer/survivorship/pdf/plan.pdf

Chapter books

Ganz P (editor). *Cancer Survivorship: Today and Tomorrow*. New York, Springer, 2007

Feuerstein M (editor). *Handbook of Cancer Survivorship*. New York, Springer, 2007

Miller K (editor). *Medical and Psychosocial Care of the Cancer Survivor*. Jones and Bartlett Publishers, Sudbury, MA, 2010

Wallace WHB, Green DM (editors). *Late Effects of Childhood Cancer*. Arnold Press, London, UK, 2004

Journal special editions or supplements

*Journal of Clinical Oncology,* November 2006

*Cancer,* June 2008

*American Academy of Family Physicians* Monograms, Home Study: Care of Cancer Survivors 352:11–44, 2008

*Journal of Clinical Oncology,* May 2009 – Childhood Cancer Survivors Study

*Cancer,* September 2009

*Journal of General Internal Medicine,* November 2009

*Primary Care: Clinics in Office Practice,* December 2009

(continued)

**Table 9.2** (continued)

| |
|---|
| Internet resources |
| National Cancer Institute Office of Cancer Survivorship, http://dccps.nci.nih.gov/ocs/ |
| National Comprehensive Cancer Network Guidelines in Oncology, http://www.nccn.org |
| Guidelines for Follow up of Childhood Cancer Survivors. Children's Oncology Group, http://www.survivorshipguidelines.org |
| LIVESTRONG Foundation, http://www.livestrong.org |
| National Coalition for Cancer Survivorship, http://www.canceradvocacy.org |
| Internet resources – cancer survivorship links available through search engine |
| American Cancer Society, http://www.cancer.org |
| Centers for Disease Control and Prevention, http://www.cdc.gov |
| American Academy of Family Physicians, http://www.aafp.org |
| American Society of Clinical Oncology, http://www. asco.org |
| Children's Oncology Group, http://www.childrensoncologygroup.org |
| Online educational programs |
| UpToDate – new cancer survivorship chapters pending 2011 |
| American Society of Clinical Oncology – cancer survivorship modules in development |
| LIVESTRONG Survivorship Centers of Excellence |
| Abramson Cancer Center, University of Pennsylvania |
| Dana-Farber Cancer Institute |
| Fred Hutchinson Cancer Research Center |
| Memorial Sloan-Kettering Cancer Center Survivorship Program |
| The Ohio State University Comprehensive Cancer Center |
| UCLA's Jonsson Comprehensive Cancer Center |
| University of Colorado Cancer Center |
| University of North Carolina at Chapel Hill, Lineberger Comprehensive Cancer Center |

of guidelines developed by specialized organizations, such as the Children's Oncology Group, American Society of Clinical Oncology, or the National Comprehensive Cancer Network, should be provided with information about available guidelines and readily access them at the clinical point of contact. Table 9.2 provides a list of resources available to primary care providers who are interested in learning more about cancer survivorship care. As general internists gain expertise in cancer survivorship, they may serve as local experts in both academic and community-based settings. Lastly, medical education efforts need to provide students and/or residents with specific knowledge and skills needed to care for cancer survivors. Few curricula currently exist [50]; these should be tested and refined to meet the needs of the learners and the patients whom they serve. Cancer survivors can play an important role in educating clinicians and those in training.

## Future Directions

Several studies are in process in the United States, Canada, Europe, Asia, Australia, and New Zealand assessing the content and usability of cancer treatment summaries and testing methods to transition cancer survivors from the oncologist to the primary care physician. Further research is needed to better understand the long-term risks following cancer therapy and the harms and benefits associated with surveillance for late effects. Opportunities for enhancing knowledge and skills in cancer survivorship have to be developed in medical school, residency and fellowship curricula, as well as in continuing medical education programs. Although primary care providers currently care for a large population of cancer survivors, as the oncology force begins to lag behind the growing demand [2], the need for primary care provider care may also surpass the currently available workforce [51]. These issues are also critical as we move forward in cancer survivorship care.

## References

1. Hewitt M, Greenfield S, Stovall E. From cancer patient to cancer survivor: lost in transition. Washington, DC: The National Academies Press; 2006.
2. Erikson C, Salsberg E, Forte G, Bruinooge S, Goldstein M. Future supply and demand for oncologists, challenges to assuring access to oncology services. J Oncol Pract. 2007;3:79–86.
3. Sleijfer S. Bleomycin-induced pneumonitis. Chest. 2001;120:617–24.
4. Jensen BV. Cardiotoxic consequences of anthracycline-containing therapy in patients with breast cancer. Semin Oncol. 2006;33:S15–21.
5. Aleman BM, van den Belt-Dusebout AW, De Bruin ML, et al. Late cardiotoxicity after treatment for Hodgkin lymphoma. Blood. 2007;109:1878–86.
6. Doyle JJ, Neugut AI, Jacobson JS, et al. Chemotherapy and cardiotoxicity in older breast cancer patients: a population-based study. J Clin Oncol. 2005;23:8597–605.
7. Ganz PA. Psychological and social aspects of breast cancer. Oncology (Williston Park). 2008;22:642–6, 650; discussion 650, 653.
8. Tesauro GM, Rowland JH, Lustig C. Survivorship resources for post-treatment cancer survivors. Cancer Pract. 2002;10:277–83.
9. Matthews BA, Baker F, Spillers RL. Oncology professionals and patient requests for cancer support services. Support Care Cancer. 2004;12:731–8.
10. van Weert E, Hoekstra-Weebers J, Grol B, et al. A multidimensional cancer rehabilitation program for cancer survivors: effectiveness on health-related quality of life. J Psychosom Res. 2005;58:485–96.
11. Hong S, Nekhlyudov L, Didwania A, et al. Cancer survivorship care: exploring the role of the general internist. J Gen Intern Med. 2009;24 Suppl 2:S495–500.
12. Pollack LA, Adamache W, Ryerson AB, et al. Care of long-term cancer survivors: physicians seen by Medicare enrollees surviving longer than 5 years. Cancer. 2009;115:5284–95.
13. Snyder CF, Earle CC, Herbert RJ, et al. Preventive care for colorectal cancer survivors: a 5-year longitudinal study. J Clin Oncol. 2008;26:1073–9.
14. Snyder CF, Earle CC, Herbert RJ, et al. Trends in follow-up and preventive care for colorectal cancer survivors. J Gen Intern Med. 2008;23:254–9.
15. Snyder CF, Frick KD, Peairs KS, et al. Comparing care for breast cancer survivors to non-cancer controls: a five-year longitudinal study. J Gen Intern Med. 2009;24:469–74.
16. Snyder CF, Frick KD, Kantsiper ME, et al. Prevention, screening, and surveillance care for breast cancer survivors compared with controls: changes from 1998 to 2002. J Clin Oncol. 2009;27:1054–61.
17. Nathan PC, Greenberg ML, Ness KK, et al. Medical care in long-term survivors of childhood cancer: a report from the childhood cancer survivor study. J Clin Oncol. 2008;26:4401–9.
18. Oeffinger KC, Mertens AC, Hudson MM, et al. Health care of young adult survivors of childhood cancer: a report from the Childhood Cancer Survivor Study. Ann Fam Med. 2004;2:61–70.
19. Doubeni CA, Field TS, Ulcickas Yood M, et al. Patterns and predictors of mammography utilization among breast cancer survivors. Cancer. 2006;106:2482–8.

20. Geller BM, Kerlikowske K, Carney PA, et al. Mammography surveillance following breast cancer. Breast Cancer Res Treat. 2003;81:107–15.
21. Keating NL, Landrum MB, Guadagnoli E, et al. Factors related to underuse of surveillance mammography among breast cancer survivors. J Clin Oncol. 2006;24:85–94.
22. Lash TL, Silliman RA. Medical surveillance after breast cancer diagnosis. Med Care. 2001; 39:945–55.
23. Earle CC, Burstein HJ, Winer EP, et al. Quality of non-breast cancer health maintenance among elderly breast cancer survivors. J Clin Oncol. 2003;21:1447–51.
24. Earle CC, Neville BA. Under use of necessary care among cancer survivors. Cancer. 2004;101:1712–9.
25. Hudson SV, Hahn KA, Ohman-Strickland P, et al. Breast, colorectal and prostate cancer screening for cancer survivors and non-cancer patients in community practices. J Gen Intern Med. 2009;24 Suppl 2:S487–90.
26. Nathan PC, Ford JS, Henderson TO, et al. Health behaviors, medical care, and interventions to promote healthy living in the Childhood Cancer Survivor Study cohort. J Clin Oncol. 2009;27:2363–73.
27. Keating NL, Landrum MB, Guadagnoli E, et al. Surveillance testing among survivors of early-stage breast cancer. J Clin Oncol. 2007;25:1074–81.
28. Grunfeld E, Levine MN, Julian JA, et al. Randomized trial of long-term follow-up for early-stage breast cancer: a comparison of family physician versus specialist care. J Clin Oncol. 2006;24:848–55.
29. Blaauwbroek R, Tuinier W, Meyboom-de Jong B, et al. Shared care by paediatric oncologists and family doctors for long-term follow-up of adult childhood cancer survivors: a pilot study. Lancet Oncol. 2008;9:232–8.
30. Ciardullo AV, Daghio MM, Brunetti M, et al. Changes in long-term glycemic control and performance indicators in a cohort of type 2 diabetic patients cared for by general practitioners: findings from the "Modena Diabetes Project". Nutr Metab Cardiovasc Dis. 2003;13:372–6.
31. Holm T, Lassen JF, Husted SE, et al. A randomized controlled trial of shared care versus routine care for patients receiving oral anticoagulant therapy. J Intern Med. 2002;252:322–31.
32. Jones C, Roderick P, Harris S, et al. An evaluation of a shared primary and secondary care nephrology service for managing patients with moderate to advanced CKD. Am J Kidney Dis. 2006;47:103–14.
33. Renders CM, Valk GD, de Sonnaville JJ, et al. Quality of care for patients with Type 2 diabetes mellitus – a long-term comparison of two quality improvement programmes in the Netherlands. Diabet Med. 2003;20:846–52.
34. Klabunde CN, Ambs A, Keating NL, et al. The role of primary care physicians in cancer care. J Gen Intern Med. 2009;24:1029–36.
35. Shapiro CL, McCabe MS, Syrjala KL, et al. The LIVESTRONG Survivorship Center of Excellence Network. J Cancer Surviv. 2009;3:4–11.
36. Grunfeld E, Mant D, Vessey MP, et al. Specialist and general practice views on routine follow-up of breast cancer patients in general practice. Fam Pract. 1995;12:60–5.
37. Nissen MJ, Beran MS, Lee MW, et al. Views of primary care providers on follow-up care of cancer patients. Fam Med. 2007;39:477–82.
38. Del Giudice ME, Grunfeld E, Harvey BJ, et al. Primary care physicians' views of routine follow-up care of cancer survivors. J Clin Oncol. 2009;27:3338–45.
39. Blaauwbroek R, Zwart N, Bouma M, et al. The willingness of general practitioners to be involved in the follow-up of adult survivors of childhood cancer. J Cancer Surviv. 2007;1:292–7.
40. Cheung WY, Neville BA, Cameron DB, et al. Comparisons of patient and physician expectations for cancer survivorship care. J Clin Oncol. 2009;27:2489–95.
41. Kantsiper M, McDonald EL, Geller G, et al. Transitioning to breast cancer survivorship: perspectives of patients, cancer specialists, and primary care providers. J Gen Intern Med. 2009;24 Suppl 2:S459–66.

42. Bober SL, Recklitis CJ, Campbell EG, et al. Caring for cancer survivors: a survey of primary care physicians. Cancer. 2009;115:4409–18.
43. Greenfield DM, Absolom K, Eiser C, et al. Follow-up care for cancer survivors: the views of clinicians. Br J Cancer. 2009;101:568–74.
44. Henderson TO, Hlubocky FJ, Wroblewski KE, et al. Physician preferences and knowledge gaps regarding the care of childhood cancer survivors: a mailed survey of pediatric oncologists. J Clin Oncol. 2010;28:878–83.
45. Mariscotti J. A delicate dance: negotiating the doctor-patient relationship during cancer treatment. Oncologist. 2008;13:1205–6.
46. Mao JJ, Bowman MA, Stricker CT, et al. Delivery of survivorship care by primary care physicians: the perspective of breast cancer patients. J Clin Oncol. 2009;27:933–8.
47. Absolom K, Eiser C, Michel G, et al. Follow-up care for cancer survivors: views of the younger adult. Br J Cancer. 2009;101:561–7.
48. Wallace WH, Blacklay A, Eiser C, et al. Developing strategies for long term follow up of survivors of childhood cancer. BMJ. 2001;323:271–4.
49. Nekhlyudov L. "Doc, should I see you or my oncologist?": a primary care perspective on opportunities and challenges in providing comprehensive care for cancer survivors. J Clin Oncol. 2009;27:2424–6.
50. Potter J, Johnston K. Keeping up with survivors: education across the spectrum of cancer. J Gen Intern Med. 2009;24 Suppl 2:S501–2.
51. Hauer KE, Durning SJ, Kernan WN, et al. Factors associated with medical students' career choices regarding internal medicine. JAMA. 2008;300:1154–64.

# Chapter 10
# Optimizing Health: Oncology Care

Linda A. Jacobs, Jun J. Mao, K. Scott Baker, and Patricia A. Ganz

## Introduction

Since more than 40% of people born today in the United States will be diagnosed with cancer at some point in their lives [1], it is critical that the increasing number of cancer survivors receive optimal care. This is a complicated issue and this chapter will attempt to identify and discuss components of care that should ultimately result in cancer survivors receiving the services essential to maintaining health, decreasing risk for disease recurrence and new cancers, and improving overall quality of life.

The Institute of Medicine (IOM) report in 2006, "From Cancer Patient to Cancer Survivor: Lost in Transition" [2], identified cancer survivorship as a distinct phase of care and reported that this phase has been neglected in the areas of advocacy, education, clinical practice, and research. They outlined four essential, broad, and very general components of patient-centered survivorship care (Table 10.1) and made ten, also broad and general, recommendations for improving the care that is delivered (Table 10.2) [2].

These components of care and recommendations for improving care have provided a frame of reference for identifying areas of needed research and raising questions regarding the how, when, where, and by whom survivorship care should be provided. In this phase of care, the focus turns to monitoring for disease recurrence as well as to surveillance for and management of long-term and late effects that occur as a result of cancer and its treatment and to routine health promotion and prevention of disease. The IOM report identified the need for surveillance guidelines that will better inform the identification and treatment of physical and psychosocial late effects of cancer, as well as the monitoring for disease recurrence. The report also identified the need to overcome health care system challenges, provide access to adequate and affordable health insurance, and to coordinate care among specialists and primary care providers. Although an important call to action,

L.A. Jacobs (✉)
Abramson Cancer Center, University of Pennsylvania, Philadelphia, PA, USA
e-mail: linda.jacobs@uphs.upenn.edu

M. Feuerstein and P.A. Ganz (eds.), *Health Services for Cancer Survivors*,
DOI 10.1007/978-1-4419-1348-7_10, © Springer Science+Business Media, LLC 2011 

**Table 10.1** Essential components of survivorship care (Republished from Hewitt et al. [2]. Copyright National Academies Press. With kind permission)

| |
|---|
| Prevention of recurrent and new cancers, and other late effects |
| Surveillance for cancer spread, recurrence, or second cancers; assessment of medical and psychosocial late effects |
| Intervention for consequences of cancer and its treatment |
| Coordination between specialists and primary care providers to ensure that all of the survivor's health needs are met |

**Table 10.2** IOM recommendations for survivorship care (Republished from Hewitt et al. [2]. Copyright National Academies Press. With kind permission)

| |
|---|
| Raise awareness of cancer survivorship |
| Provide a care plan for survivors |
| Develop clinical practice guidelines for cancer survivors |
| Define quality health care for cancer survivors |
| Overcome health care system challenges |
| Address survivorship as a public health concern |
| Provide survivorship education and training of health care professionals |
| Address employment concerns of cancer survivors of all ages |
| Improve access to adequate and affordable health insurance |
| Invest in research |

the IOM report does not offer an algorithm to guide practitioners through the maze of possible treatments, potential late effects of these treatments, surveillance options, and schedules for follow-up care for cancer survivors. There has been considerable research in recent years examining a wide array of adult cancer survivorship issues; however, despite these efforts, there continues to be a lack of evidence based on sound research to guide decisions regarding follow-up care, which translates into little clarity regarding what constitutes optimal care. This presents a major challenge for cancer survivors who are seeking care and advice to maintain an optimal state of health broadly defined.

Historically, the majority of cancer survivors have been followed in busy oncology practices where surveillance for disease recurrence is the focus of follow-up visits. Cancer survivors are generally followed within the practice setting where they were treated by the team who delivered that care, and in most cases there is little or no discussion of symptoms or problems patients are experiencing posttreatment. Patients hesitate to report and burden their oncology team with seemingly trivial problems and complaints that they may perceive as non-oncology issues or clearly have been told that these issues should be evaluated by their primary care provider (PCP), GYN, or another specialist. In addition, symptoms and medical issues that arise in this population may be viewed by patients and providers as simply expected comorbidities of aging. This is often an explanation provided to younger and middle-aged adults.

Cancer survivorship care requires a thoughtful, organized approach to addressing the recommendations made by the IOM and other groups. However, the current numbers of survivors who require follow-up care pose significant and immediate challenges to the medical community as this population continues to grow exponentially.

The IOM also examined the oncology workforce in the recent "Ensuring Quality Cancer Care through the Oncology Workforce: Sustaining Care in the 21st Century" workshop and publication [3] and noted that the aging and retiring of health care providers in oncology and primary care, as well as the increasing number of cancer survivors, will create a significant crisis in the coming years. In addition, long-term follow-up care needs of survivors combined with the increasing focus on health promotion and disease prevention, diet, exercise, and general well-being will further tax the resources of available oncology practitioners and place new and significant demands on PCPs who do not feel adequately prepared to care for cancer survivors [3–8]. As the numbers of survivors increase and the traditional oncology workforce diminishes, primary and specialty care practices will be caring for more long-term cancer survivors and they must be prepared to do so.

The role of the PCP in cancer survivorship care is evolving, and the communication between the oncology team and primary care must include critical diagnosis and treatment information, as well as a care plan for the PCP to organize an appropriate follow-up plan for care. Templates for organizing treatment data and creating a written survivor care plan at the end of treatment have been developed by a number of sources. These plans are based on a combination of the best available clinical information, evidence-based standards, and in some cases, institutional practices [9]. Care plans are only as good as their content, and there is considerable debate among oncology providers as to who should be responsible for developing a personalized plan for posttreatment care and what should be considered and included when developing that plan. The IOM suggested the elements to be included in a care plan; however, the lack of research makes it impossible to determine, with any certainty or consensus, what really should be included.

This chapter will explore the current state of and what constitutes optimal oncology follow-up care for cancer survivors, and how effective communication and collaborations with PCP can contribute to cancer survivors receiving optimal care.

## Guidelines for Care as Outlined by the IOM

In charting recommendations for posttreatment survivorship care, the 2006 IOM report [2] noted the paucity of clinical practice guidelines on this topic. Due to the diversity of cancer sites, variations in treatment exposures even within common tumors (e.g., breast, colon, prostate), the introduction of new treatments and exposures, and lack of systematic follow-up data linking exposures to outcomes, it is difficult for professional and government organizations to adopt authoritative guidelines with specific recommendations for which providers should be held accountable. As a result, many existing guidelines are based on consensus or "best guess" and may risk either over or under-utilization of tests/procedures for monitoring of risk for recurrence or late effects of cancer treatment.

In this chapter, we review current strategies for optimizing the health of survivors in the posttreatment setting that are based on best practices outlined by evolving survivorship programs around the country at a number of comprehensive cancer centers. Good quality care in the posttreatment follow-up period should be aimed at facilitating the recovery of the patient from the acute effects of cancer and its treatment, as well as guiding survivors regarding the care they need as they move into a future that is clouded by uncertainty about the effects of past treatments. This should include evidence of coordinated health care between oncology specialists and primary care providers, with an emphasis on addressing the physical, emotional, informational, and social needs of the person who has just completed cancer therapy (and/or may still require ongoing maintenance therapy, e.g., endocrine therapy for breast cancer). The transition from patient on active treatment to post-treatment survivor requires considerable adjustments, including a decrease in frequency of contact with members of the cancer treatment team (can be good and bad at the same time), a decrease in toxicity from therapies that are often noxious and burdensome, an increase in anxiety and uncertainty about the future, as well as an expectation that everything should be back to "normal" within a reasonable time frame. All of these adjustments occur over the weeks to months to years after active treatment ends. While energy and interest in nonmedical activities may be returning, persistence of the physical and psychological scars of active treatment remain for some individuals. Patients who knew exactly what the drill was during active treatment are now faced with a whole host of questions about what they should do to maintain their health, prevent a recurrence, and ensure that they will recover from the acute effects of treatment. Few cancer survivors appreciate that there is limited knowledge about the late effects of cancer treatment as well as who may be at risk. In addition, many are unaware of what may reduce their risk for persistence or exacerbation of long-term problems that developed during treatment.

Although there is ongoing research to provide systematic documentation of the late effects of cancer treatment [10–12], research is far more advanced in pediatric oncology than in the field of adult oncology. Since many of these individuals are now alive 30–40 years after treatment exposures, and since most children have been treated on clinical trials, it is easier to catalog the frequency of specific organ toxicities, employment, emotional, cognitive, interpersonal, and educational limitations, as well as secondary health problems in this small population of cancer survivors. As a result, the pediatric oncology community has developed specific programs to address survivorship care (specialized clinics within treatment centers) [13] and exposure-related guidelines (http://www.childrensoncologygroup.org/disc/le/). Since the vast majority of cancer survivors are adults at diagnosis, these follow-up approaches may have limited relevance to how care should be organized for adult cancer survivors in the posttreatment period. However, the growing number of these survivors and the constraints in the oncology workforce [14] indicate that strategies to deliver adult cancer survivorship care that goes beyond the traditional oncology treatment setting must be established.

Many adults diagnosed with cancer have a PCP or will access one at the time of symptoms and cancer diagnosis. Often this health care provider has had a long-term relationship with the patient and may have ordered the screening or diagnostic test(s) that led to the cancer diagnosis. With other chronic conditions that co-occur with the cancer, the PCP should be and often is an important member of the cancer treatment team. Unfortunately, in many cancer treatment settings, the person diagnosed with cancer is swept into a complex and fragmented cancer care system that is dominated by multiple specialists (surgery, medical oncology, radiation oncology) who may or may not practice within an integrated delivery system. In many cases, limited communication occurs between cancer specialists and the PCP during the course of treatment, as well as after completion of treatment, which can be 1–2 years later, when patients resume follow-up with the PCP. The patient is often the primary source of information regarding the cancer treatment they received as well as any related problems that they experienced, and this often unclear picture coupled with the PCP's limited knowledge of cancer care can leave the PCP unsure of how to best serve the ongoing needs of the posttreatment cancer survivor.

As adult cancer survivors age and require ongoing care by a PCP for common health problems associated with aging, the IOM report as well as a related symposium [2, 15] strongly advocate for a shared care model of posttreatment care. The shared care model requires that complex specialty care such as the diagnosis, management, and ongoing care of a patient with cancer be shared with the PCP through regular communication (written and verbal), and among oncology care providers and PCPs.

## Oncology Follow-up Care

As noted, oncology follow-up care should include surveillance for recurrent disease, discussion with and education of the survivor regarding their risk for long-term and late effects of cancer treatment, and participation in routine age appropriate cancer screening (Table 10.3), health screening, risk assessment, and health promotion and disease prevention activities (Table 10.4).

## Long-Term and Late Effects of Cancer Therapy: Risk-Adapted Care for Survivors

Long-term side effects of cancer treatments are considered to be those concerns that develop during active treatment and may then persist for months or years. These effects must be considered and understood by providers of oncology follow-up care. Examples of long-term effects include peripheral neuropathies, weakness, pain, fatigue, cognitive impairments, and sexual difficulties. Late effects of treatment, on the other hand, are considered to be those conditions that are not present

**Table 10.3** Recommended by the American Cancer Society [16–20]

*American Cancer Society Guidelines for the early detection of cancer*

The American Cancer Society recommends these screening guidelines for most adults

*Breast cancer*

- Yearly mammograms are recommended starting at age 40 and continuing for as long as a woman is in good health
- Clinical breast exam (CBE) about every 3 years for women in their twenties and thirties and every year for women 40 and over
- Women should know how their breasts normally look and feel and report any breast change promptly to their health care provider. Breast self-exam (BSE) is an option for women starting in their 20s

The American Cancer Society recommends that some women – because of their family history, a genetic tendency, or certain other factors – be screened with MRI in addition to mammograms. (the number of women who fall into this category is small: less than 2% of all the women in the United States.) Talk with your doctor about your history and whether you should have additional tests at an earlier age. For more information, call the American Cancer Society and ask for our document, *Breast Cancer: Early Detection*

*Colorectal cancer and polyps*

Beginning at age 50, both men and women should follow one of these testing schedules:

*Tests that find polyps and cancer*

- Flexible sigmoidoscopy every 5 years,[a] or
- Colonoscopy every 10 years, or
- Double-contrast barium enema every 5 years,[a] or
- CT colonography (virtual colonoscopy) every 5 years[a]

*Tests that primarily find cancer*

- Yearly fecal occult blood test (gFOBT),[b] or
- Yearly fecal immunochemical test (FIT) every year,[b] or
- Stool DNA test (sDNA), interval uncertain[b]

The tests that are designed to find both early cancer and polyps are preferred if these tests are available to you and you are willing to have one of these more invasive tests. Talk to your doctor about which test is best for you

The American Cancer Society recommends that some people be screened using a different schedule because of their personal history or family history. Talk with your doctor about your history and what colorectal cancer screening schedule is best for you. For more information on colorectal cancer screening, please call the American Cancer Society and ask for our document, *Colorectal Cancer: Early Detection*

*Cervical cancer*

- All women should begin cervical cancer screening about 3 years after they begin having vaginal intercourse, but no later than 21 years old. Screening should be done every year with the regular Pap test or every 2 years using the newer liquid-based Pap test
- Beginning at age 30, women who have had three normal Pap test results in a row may get screened every 2–3 years. Women older than 30 may also get screened every 3 years with either the conventional or liquid-based Pap test, plus the human papilloma virus (HPV) test
- Women 70 years of age or older who have had three or more normal Pap tests in a row and no abnormal Pap test results in the last 10 years may choose to stop having Pap tests
- Women who have had a total hysterectomy (removal of the uterus and cervix) may also choose to stop having Pap tests, unless the surgery was done as a treatment for cervical cancer or precancer. Women who have had a hysterectomy without removal of the cervix should continue to have Pap tests

(continued)

**Table 10.3** (continued)

Some women – because of their history – may need to have a different screening schedule for cervical cancer. Please see our document, *Cervical Cancer: Early Detection* for more information

*Endometrial (uterine) cancer*

The American Cancer Society recommends that at the time of menopause, all women should be informed about the risks and symptoms of endometrial cancer. Women should report any unexpected bleeding or spotting to their doctors

Some women – because of their history – may need to consider having a yearly endometrial biopsy. Please talk with your doctor about your history

*Prostate cancer*

The American Cancer Society recommends that men make an informed decision with their doctor about whether to be tested for prostate cancer. Research has not yet proven that the potential benefits of testing outweigh the harms of testing and treatment. The American Cancer Society believes that men should not be tested without learning about what we know and do not know about the risks and possible benefits of testing and treatment

Starting at age 50, talk to your doctor about the pros and cons of testing so you can decide if testing is the right choice for you. If you are African American or have a father or brother who had prostate cancer before age 65, you should have this talk with your doctor starting at age 45. If you decide to be tested, you should have the PSA blood test with or without a rectal exam. How often you are tested will depend on your PSA level. For more information, please see our document, *Prostate Cancer: Early Detection*

*Cancer-related check-up*

For people aged 20 or older having periodic health exams, a cancer-related check-up should include health counseling and, depending on a person's age and gender, exams for cancers of the thyroid, oral cavity, skin, lymph nodes, testes, and ovaries, as well as for some nonmalignant (noncancerous) diseases

*Take control of your health and reduce your cancer risk*

- Stay away from tobacco
- Stay at a healthy weight
- Get moving with regular physical activity
- Eat healthy with plenty of fruits and vegetables
- Limit how much alcohol you drink (if you drink at all)
- Protect your skin
- Know yourself, your family history, and your risks
- Have regular check-ups and cancer screening tests
- For information on how to reduce your cancer risk and other questions about cancer, please call us anytime, day or night, at 1-800-227-2345 or visit us online at http://www.cancer.org

[a] If the test is positive, a colonoscopy should be done

[b] The multiple stool take-home test should be used. One test done by the doctor in the office is not adequate for testing. A colonoscopy should be done if the test is positive

or identified during or shortly after treatment and rather develop later as a consequence of treatment. These can be impairments or dysfunction of organs or organ systems or can be related to psychological impairments or distress. In order to determine a patient's risk for the development of these potential problems one must first examine what their significant treatment exposures were including exposure to radiation therapy (including total dose and site), which chemotherapeutic agents

**Table 10.4** Recommendations by the American Academy of Family Physicians [21] (Copyright 2010 AAFP)

| |
|---|
| Example of items to consider: health screening, risk assessment, health promotion and disease prevention |
| Tests to check your general health or the health of certain parts of your body |
| Regular measurements of weight, cholesterol levels, and blood pressure |
| Advice about diet, exercise, tobacco, alcohol and drug use, stress and accident prevention |
| Immunizations ("shots") for both children and adults |
| Special tests at certain times in your life, such as during pregnancy and after age 50 |
| Do not use any form of tobacco |
| Eat a healthy diet |
| Practice safe sex |
| Exercise regularly |
| Drink alcohol in moderation, if at all |
| Do not use illegal drugs |
| Use seat belts (and car seats for children) when riding in a car or truck |
| See your doctor regularly for preventive care |

were utilized (including total cumulative doses for some), and what types of surgical procedures were performed (identifying any vital structures that were removed or altered).

However, as shown in Fig. 10.1, individual risks of late effects from the various treatment modalities are modified by several other intrinsic and extrinsic factors that must also be taken into account including the patients age at treatment, gender, other pre-existing medical conditions already present at the time of diagnosis, social concerns (support systems, financial issues, etc.), and lifestyle factors such as smoking, alcohol use, dietary habits, etc. Another consideration for which there is little information currently available is the contribution that underlying genetic factors have in the variability that exists between individuals who when exposed to identical therapies may experience very disparate acute or long-term toxicities. As discussed elsewhere in this book, an individual treatment summary of all cancer therapies received, including acute toxicities and co-morbid conditions, is the first step towards defining what will be necessary for optimal long-term follow-up care of the cancer survivor. It is important to note that survivors may also have significant psychosocial needs and concerns, and for some patients these can be of more urgent importance than concerns they may have related to their physical health. There is a need to consider both. Therefore, an assessment of survivors concerns related to relationships, return to work or school, financial difficulties, and persistent levels of distress, anxiety, depression, or fear of recurrence should be evaluated.

## *Surveillance: Recurrence and Second Cancers*

One of the major recommendations from the 2006 IOM report [2] was that survivors be provided with services for the prevention, surveillance, and detection of new and

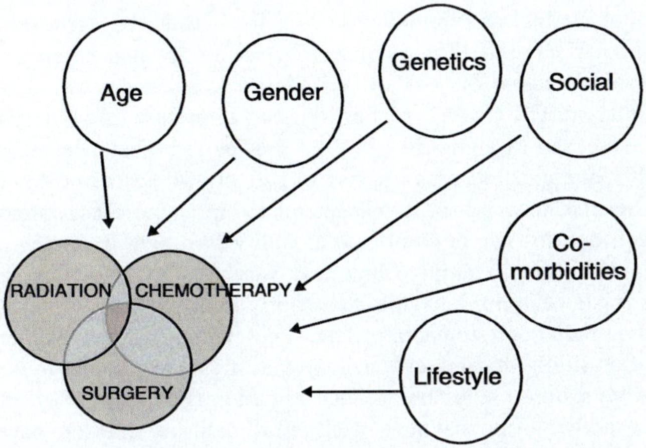


**Fig. 10.1** Factors to be considered in risk of late effects of therapy

recurrent cancers. Surveillance methodologies including radiographic scans, lab tests such as tumor markers, clinical exams, and symptom assessment are quite variable depending on the particular diagnosis and sometimes controversial regarding recommended screening and frequency of that screening. Evidence-based screening recommendations for recurrence exist for some cancers (such as colon, breast, and lung), have been developed by the American Society of Clinical Oncology, and can be found on their web site (http://www.asco.org). At this time, formal recommendations do not exist for many cancers and are frequently formulated on an individual basis. Patients should be informed of the "best recommendations available at this time" regarding screening for cancer recurrence and should be provided with a schedule for the frequency and duration of this screening when they complete their therapy. While it is appropriate for this surveillance to occur in the oncology practice setting during the highest risk period for recurrence, consideration should also be given, and a plan established, for when this screening can be managed by a PCP.

Despite successful treatment of their primary cancer, survivors face a life-long higher risk of developing new malignancies. The etiology of these second cancers is not entirely known but in some cases has been linked to treatment exposures including certain chemotherapy agents, ionizing radiation, as well as prolonged immune suppression and infection. It is also likely that in some patients, there may exist an underlying genetic susceptibility including gene–environment and gene–gene interactions that impact risks from numerous issues related to treatment exposure and possibly the risk of developing cancer itself [22]. One must remember that lifestyle factors such as tobacco smoking and alcohol intake are risk factors for the development of cancer in the general population including cancer survivors. The issue of secondary malignant neoplasms (SMN) is significant and it has been estimated cancer survivors have a 14% higher risk of developing a new malignancy by 25 years since diagnosis of their first cancer compared to the general population [23]. Much of the published data on SMN in adult cancer survivors have recently been summarized [24] and are highlighted briefly here.

Survivors of Hodgkin's lymphoma have a significant risk of developing solid tumors, particularly breast [25] and lung [26] in a dose dependant manner after radiation exposure where the risk of secondary breast cancer was 3.2-fold (95% confidence interval [CI] 1.4–8.2) higher for a radiation dose of 4 Gy or more to the breast, and increased to eightfold (95% CI 2.6–26.4) higher when the dose was more than 40 Gy compared with the risk in patients who received lower doses of radiation. This risk may be somewhat attenuated after more contemporary treatment protocols and the use of combined modality treatment including involved or limited field radiation therapy techniques. Survivors of testicular cancer have higher risks for developing leukemia and solid tumors related to the use of para-aortic or pelvic radiation (stomach, pancreas, colorectal, kidney, bladder) or mediastinal radiation (lung, thyroid, esophagus) with higher risks seen in patients who were treated with both chemotherapy and radiation (RR 2.9) [27]. Breast cancer survivors are another group that have been well studied and shown to have increased risk for SMN including sarcomas, lung, and/or esophageal cancers in women treated with radiation [28, 29]. Women are at a slightly increased risk for acute myeloid leukemia after regional radiotherapy alone (relative risk, 2.4), alkylating agent chemotherapy alone (relative risk, 10.0, although at higher dose than typically utilized today), and especially after combined radiation and chemotherapy (relative risk, 17.4) [30]. In addition, a twofold higher risk of endometrial cancer has been described in women who have been treated with tamoxifen [31]. There are many other examples where elevated risks for subsequent malignancies in survivors exist, with the most common treatment exposure risk being radiation therapy [24]. Differences in age at exposure, radiation dose, and length of follow-up impact this risk, such that in general, younger age at exposure, higher dose, and longer length of follow-up all lead to a higher incidence of SMNs.

The issue of SMN in survivors of childhood cancer is also of significant concern. In adult survivors of childhood leukemia, the cumulative incidence of SMN at 25 years is 5.2% overall and 6.2% in irradiated patients vs. 3.1% in nonirradiated [32]. Eighty-one percent of the SMN that were reported occurred in irradiated patients and 53% of those were in the central nervous system, highlighting this unique risk in childhood leukemia patients. In a large study of childhood cancer survivors, the highest nonrelapse cause of late mortality was from subsequent malignancies (SMR = 19.4), and the most significant treatment-related associations were present for exposure to radiation, alkylating agents, and epipodophyllotoxins [33].

There are a greater number of studies that have examined the risk of SMN in patients after hematopoietic cell transplantation (HCT), and data from single institutional analyses have shown that the cumulative incidence for the development of any posttransplant malignancy was 6.9% at 20 years post HCT and the cumulative incidence for invasive solid cancers was 3.8% [34]. In a large study published recently examining the development of new solid tumors in over 28,000 recipients of allogeneic HCT, it was found that overall, survivors after transplant developed new solid cancers at twice the rate that was expected based on general population rates [35]. This risk increased to threefold for patients who were followed for 15 years or more.

Guidelines developed by the Children's Oncology Group are available for survivors of childhood cancers that detail the screening recommendations for SMN based on treatment exposures, particularly radiation therapy (http://www.survivorshipguidelines.org). There are no published guidelines for screening adult cancer survivors for SMN; therefore, patients should be informed of the potential risk for developing an SMN based upon their treatment exposures, and this information should be conveyed to their PCP. In the absence of guidelines, survivors should be strongly encouraged to comply with age appropriate screening and early detection strategies (e.g., breast and testicular self-exams, mammography, pap smears, colonoscopy, PSA, DREs, etc.) and avoidance of any additional exposures that impact the risk of cancer (such as sunburns, smoking, and excessive alcohol use).

## Coordination of Oncology Follow-up Care

The question of where cancer survivors should receive their follow-up care is complex and complicated by several factors including the type of cancer, likelihood of recurrence, and socio-demographic factors related to proximity and access to health care services (hospital-based services, cancer center or oncologist office, primary care, etc.). Other considerations include the psychosocial impact involved when transitioning patients from frequent cancer focused health care visits to less frequent follow-up visits or transferring care to a survivorship clinic and/or to primary care. There are also psychosocial implications for survivors who are followed indefinitely by their oncologists where the focus of follow-up visits is typically upon surveillance for recurrence of the primary cancer.

It is certainly appropriate that survivors should have routine follow-up with their medical and/or radiation oncologist during the period of highest risk for disease recurrence to assure the coordination of appropriate surveillance. Survivors should also be evaluated for health and psychosocial concerns related to the long-term and late effects of treatment. It is rare that the issues facing survivors are adequately addressed in the context of clinical evaluations focused on surveillance for recurrence and should include a comprehensive evaluation of the survivors overall health care needs. There are several clinical models of care that have been utilized in programs that are providing survivorship focused care and evaluations for their patients (discussed in more detail elsewhere in this book), and these can easily be adapted to the unique circumstances of care settings. In most of these models, the clinical services are provided by mid-level providers such as nurse practitioners, physician's assistants, either in conjunction with, or with the oversight of, a physician.

One model of care provides survivorship services within the context of the primary oncology practice where active treatment was received. After the completion of therapy and early recurrence surveillance, the focus shifts and includes survivorship-related issues. Other models involve the development of survivorship clinics that function either as a consultative-based service with limited routine follow-up or as disease-specific survivorship clinics that focus on long-term wellness of survivors and provide ongoing long-term follow-up. The ultimate goal for these models is to transition patients, if appropriate, back to the community and primary care. Finally, some programs have established multidisciplinary survivorship clinics that are staffed by a multidisciplinary team that may consist of a variety of professionals (oncology, endocrinology, neuropsychology, nutrition, rehabilitation medicine, physical/occupational therapy), where each provider evaluates the survivor for potential issues focused on their area of expertise. This clinic model is less common and more frequently utilized in pediatric oncology programs where the risks for certain complications (such as endocrine sequelae and growth abnormalities) are frequent, and where screening the majority of the patients being evaluated is justified. This model has also been established in some disease-specific survivorship clinics such as clinics for brain tumor or head and neck cancer patients where specialized care for treatment-related sequelae and long-term complications are required.

It is important in any of these models of care that a local referral network of subspecialists be established who have a specific interest in the unique complications that cancer survivors can develop so that appropriate evaluation and intervention can occur without unnecessary delay. As discussed in the next section, it is important that survivors have a PCP since the risk for heart disease, hypertension, hyperlipidemia, osteopenia, and other chronic health conditions is still present (and in some cases increased) for cancer survivors. The development of a treatment summary and survivor care plan can provide a road map for this transition to primary care with assurances that appropriate cancer-related treatment risks are monitored on a long-term basis.

## The Role of the PCP in Survivorship Care

Although a significant number of cancer survivors continue to receive cancer follow-up care from oncologists and are not followed routinely by their PCPs after a diagnosis of cancer, there are also a number of survivors who continue to receive care from PCPs for non-oncology-related comorbidities [36]. The complexity of the health issues faced by survivors requires coordinated and patient-centered care. Additionally, the myriad of health issues combined with the experience of surviving cancer requires a shift in the paradigm from disease-focus during acute cancer treatment to wellness-centered comprehensive care during the survivorship phase of care. Furthermore, as survivorship care focuses on restoring health and preventing recurrence, the care model needs to be personalized, preventative, and participatory. Active involvement of PCPs in survivorship care is essential in order to provide quality, optimal care for cancer survivors [37].

### *Transition from Oncology to Primary Care*

In order for PCPs to actively participate in survivorship care, a seamless transition from oncology to primary care must occur. Studies often cite lack of clear communication as a major limiting factor in this transition. Patients build strong relationships with their oncology team through the course of the intense treatment regimen and may feel that the oncologist has become their primary health care provider. Transitioning back to a PCP is difficult for many survivors because they often see their oncologist as someone who saved their life and thus trust them with the management of their care thenceforth. The transition may also be difficult for oncologists and the oncology team because they may see survivors as their success stories and the emotional bond shared with some patients can be significant.

The transition of care needs to be negotiated among the providers to create an individualized patient-centered plan and health care providers should actively engage patients in the shared decision making to formulate a survivorship care plan [38]. In this plan, the providers should communicate the expected frequency of follow-up visits with each specific provider over the next several years with a clear designation as to the role each provider will have (e.g., screening for cancer recurrence and other cancers, preventative health measures, and ongoing comorbidity management). The survivorship care plan may be an important tool to enhance the communication between oncology and PCPs. In many cases, this document could replace the consultation note sent to PCPs and may decrease the chance of redundancy in the care provided. The survivorship care plan needs to be brief and clear, explicitly outlining the screening tests PCPs should perform and in what intervals they should be ordered for the specific survivor [39]. Oncologists should also explicitly communicate to PCPs the extent to which they will continue to participate in the survivor's care.

In some cases, it may work best for PCPs and oncologist to share the survivorship care and one way to do this is for survivors to rotate visits between providers. For example, a patient may choose to see their oncologist every other or even every 5 years rather than yearly and maintain their PCP as their main health care provider. Some institutions are establishing clinical programs for cancer survivors that are staffed by nurse practitioners who focus clinical visits on educating survivors regarding the late effects of treatment that they may be at risk for developing, individual surveillance schedules to monitor for disease recurrence, management of symptoms and problems they report that are related to the treatment they received, as well as on general health promotion and disease prevention.

## Electronic Medical Record to Enhance Communication

The development of survivorship care plans is challenging and requires time and resources, two commodities that are hard to come by for busy oncology practices in the current health care environment. There are numerous electronic vehicles to gather and organize patient data. Some institutions utilize electronic tablets that have patient questionnaires that are completed prior to clinical visits and have the capacity to transfer that information directly into the patient's electronic medical record (EMR). The EMR is a helpful tool for organizing and communicating patient-related

**Table 10.5** The EMR in survivorship care

| |
|---|
| Facilitate interspecialty communication |
| Create automatic survivorship care plans |
| Improve adherence to guidelines by using the preventative health reminder system |
| Generate patient education and resource lists for patients to access |

information among providers. Patient records can be viewed by the multidisciplinary practices within an institution, allowing quick and easy access to up-to-date treatment information, problems encountered, plans formulated, and outcomes for medical and psychosocial issues reported by cancer survivors, or detected and/or treated by various providers. The EMR allows PCPs to have a more concise, clear, and accurate understanding of the entire picture surrounding the cancer experience for each patient. It also requires less time for a PCP to review and plan the appropriate care for a cancer survivor, making the experience more positive for PCPS and survivors. In some cases, visit notes can be routed directly from the PCP to the oncology team, increasing confidence among oncologists that their patients are receiving optimal follow-up care. At this time, however, although institutions may use the same EMR system, communication among providers and access to a patient's confidential medical information can only occur within a single institution.

The EMR is in its infancy in oncology care, however, with collaboration among clinicians, researchers, and health technology specialists; it has the potential to decrease workload, further improve accuracy of health information, enhance clinical care, and possibly save money (Table 10.5).

## Creating a Primary Care–Based Patient-Centered Medical Home for Cancer Survivors

With the advancement in health information technology, creating a financially sustainable model of primary care–based survivorship care is a reasonable goal. In recent years, several leading primary care organizations, such as the American Academy of Family Physicians (AAFP), American College of Physicians, American Academy of Pediatrics, and the American Osteopathic Association, have advocated and piloted test models of a "patient-centered medical home" [40]. In chronic disease management, this model includes continuity, coordination, and integration of care as well as improved quality and safety for each patient [41].

Quality measures, patient experience, health information technology, and practice organization are the four domains that must be considered if a patient-centered medical home is being established in a practice. These domains have numerous items outlined in a checklist that guides clinicians when developing medical home centered practices [41]. Figure 10.2 depicts a model of a Patient-Centered Medical Home (PCMH). This model, described by the AAFP, provides a diagram of the four domains with Family Medicine/the PCP as the foundation of this model home. For more information on this topic, see http://www.aafp.org/pcmh.

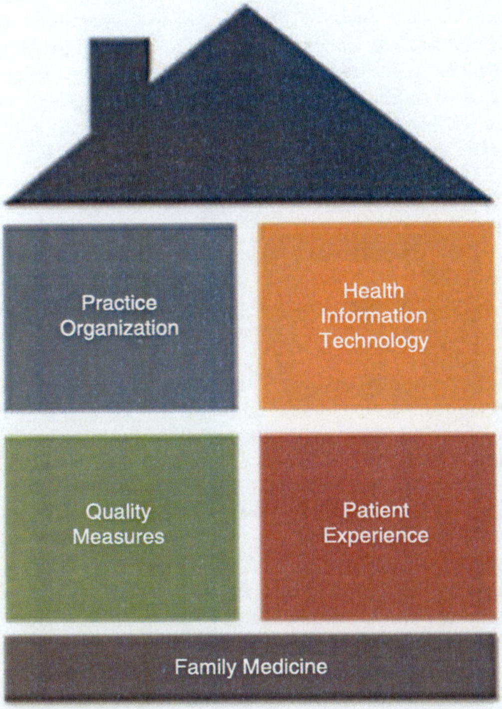


**Fig. 10.2** Model of a patient-centered medical home (PCMH) (Copyright 2010, permission granted AAFP)

The medical home model holds great potential for the delivery of survivorship care. In this model, the primary care practice is home for cancer survivors and the PCP coordinates care by communicating and consulting with oncologists, other specialists, and care providers and facilitating referrals as needed, allowing patients to feel confident that all of their providers continue to be involved in their care. Having a PCP who has an enduring relationship with the patient and is knowledgeable regarding survivorship care and general medical care can help to assure optimal survivorship care.

Ongoing research examining the delivery and outcome of survivorship care by primary care, oncology, and specialty care providers is critical in order to determine the best model of care for all cancer survivors [7].

## References

1. Travis LB, Yahalom J. Preface. Hematol Oncol Clin N Am. 2008;22(2):xi–xii.
2. Hewitt M, Greenfield S, Stovall E, editors. From cancer patient to cancer survivor: lost in transition. Washington, DC: National Academies Press; 2006.
3. Patlak M, Levit L. Ensuring quality cancer care through the oncology workforce. Institute of Medicine, National Cancer Policy Forum. Washington, DC: The National Academies Press; 2009.

4. Hewitt M, Bamundo A, Day R, Harvey C. Perspectives on post-treatment cancer care: qualitative research with survivors, nurses, and physicians. J Clin Oncol. 2007;25(16):2270–3.
5. Nissen M, Beran M, Lee M, Mehta SR, Pine DA, Swenson KK. Views of primary care providers on follow-up care of cancer patients. Fam Med. 2007;39(7):477–82.
6. Earle CC, Burstein HJ, Winer EP, Weeks JC. Quality of non-breast cancer health maintenance among elderly breast cancer survivors. J Clin Oncol. 2003;21(8):1447–51.
7. Mao JJ, Bowman MA, Stricker CT, DeMichele A, Jacobs L, Chan D, et al. Delivery of survivorship care by primary care physicians: the perspective of breast cancer patients. J Clin Oncol. 2009;27(6):933–8.
8. Starfield B, Fryer Jr GE. The primary care physician workforce: ethical and policy implications. Ann Fam Med. 2007;5(6):486–91.
9. Jacobs LA, Palmer SC, Schwartz LA, DeMichele A, Mao JJ, Carver J, et al. Adult cancer survivorship: evolution, research, and planning care. CA Cancer J Clin. 2009;59(6):391–410.
10. Ganz PA, Hussey MA, Moinpour CM, Unger JM, Hutchins LF, Dakhil SR, et al. Late cardiac effects of adjuvant chemotherapy in breast cancer survivors treated on Southwest Oncology Group Protocol S8897. J Clin Oncol. 2008;26(8):1223–30.
11. Janov A, Anderson J, Cella DF, Zukerman E, Kornblith AB, Holland JC, et al. Pregnancy outcome in survivors of advanced Hodgkins disease. Cancer. 1992;70(3):492.
12. Fossa S. Long-term sequelae after cancer therapy – survivorship after treatment for testicular cancer. Acta Oncol. 2004;43(2):134–41.
13. Aziz NM, Oeffinger KC, Brooks S, Turoff AJ. Comprehensive long-term follow-up programs for pediatric cancer survivors. Cancer. 2006;107(4):841–8.
14. Erikson C, Salsberg E, Forte G, Bruinooge BA, Goldstein M. Future supply and demand for oncologists: challenges to assuring access to oncology services. J Oncol Pract. 2007;3(2):79–84.
15. Hewitt M, Ganz PA. From cancer patient to cancer survivors – lost in transition: an American Society of Clinical Oncology and Institute of Medicine Symposium. Washington, DC: National Academies Press; 2006.
16. American Cancer Society. Cancer facts and figures 2010. Atlanta, GA: American Cancer Society; 2010.
17. Levin B, Lieberman DA, McFarland B, Smith RA, Brooks D, Andrews KS, et al. Screening and surveillance for the early detection of colorectal cancer and adenomatous polyps, 2008: a joint guideline from the American Cancer Society, the US Multi-Society Task Force on Colorectal Cancer, and the American College of Radiology. CA Cancer J Clin. 2008;58(3):130–60.
18. Saslow D, Boetes C, Burke W, Harms S, Leach MO, Lehman CD, et al. American Cancer Society guidelines for breast screening with MRI as an adjunct to mammography. CA Cancer J Clin. 2007;57:75–89.
19. Smith RA, Cokkinides V, Eyre HJ. American Cancer Society guidelines for the early detection of cancer, 2006. CA Cancer J Clin. 2006;56:11–25.
20. Smith RA, Cokkinides V, Brawley OW. Cancer screening in the United States, 2008: a review of current American Cancer Society guidelines and cancer screening issues. CA Cancer J Clin. 2008;58:161–79.
21. American Academy of Family Physicians. http://www.aafp.org/online/en/home/aboutus/theaafp/about/permissions.html.
22. Travis LB, Rabkin CS, Brown LM, Allan JM, Alter BP, Ambrosone CB, et al. Cancer survivorship – genetic susceptibility and second primary cancers: research strategies and recommendations. J Natl Cancer Inst. 2006;98(1):15–25.
23. Fraumeni JF, Curtis RE, Edwards BK, Tucker MA. Chapter 1, Introduction. In: Curtis RE, Freedman DM, Ron E, Ries LAG, Hacker DG, Edwards BK, Tucker MA, Fraumeni Jr JF, editors. New Malignancies Among Cancer Survivors: SEER Cancer Registries, 1973–2000. Bethesda, MD: National Cancer Institute NIH Publ. No. 05-5302; 2006.
24. Ng AK, Travis LB. Second primary cancers: an overview. Hematol Oncol Clin North Am. 2008;22(2):271–89.

25. Travis LB, Hill DA, Dores GM, Gospodarowicz M, van Leeuwen FE, Holowaty E, et al. Breast cancer following radiotherapy and chemotherapy among young women with Hodgkin disease. JAMA. 2003;290(4):465–75.
26. Travis LB, Gospodarowicz M, Curtis RE, Clarke A, Andersson M, Glimelius B, et al. Lung cancer following chemotherapy and radiotherapy for Hodgkin's disease. J Natl Cancer Inst. 2002;94(3):182–92.
27. Travis LB, Fossa SD, Schonfeld SJ, McMaster ML, Lynch CF, Storm H, et al. Second cancers among 40,576 testicular cancer patients: focus on long-term survivors. J Natl Cancer Inst. 2005;97(18):1354–65.
28. Roychoudhuri R, Evans H, Robinson D, Moller H. Radiation-induced malignancies following radiotherapy for breast cancer. Br J Cancer. 2004;91(5):868–72.
29. Neugut AI, Robinson E, Lee WC, Murray T, Karwoski K, Kutcher GJ. Lung cancer after radiation therapy for breast cancer. Cancer. 1993;71(10):3054–7.
30. Curtis RE, Boice Jr JD, Stovall M, Bernstein L, Greenberg RS, Flannery JT, et al. Risk of leukemia after chemotherapy and radiation treatment for breast cancer. N Engl J Med. 1992;326(26):1745–51.
31. Fisher B, Costantino JP, Redmond CK, Fisher ER, Wickerham DL, Cronin WM. Endometrial cancer in tamoxifen-treated breast cancer patients: findings from the National Surgical Adjuvant Breast and Bowel Project (NSABP) B-14. J Natl Cancer Inst. 1994;86(7):527–37.
32. Mody R, Li S, Dover DC, Sallan S, Leisenring W, Oeffinger KC, et al. Twenty-five-year follow-up among survivors of childhood acute lymphoblastic leukemia: a report from the Childhood Cancer Survivor Study. Blood. 2008;111(12):5515–23.
33. Mertens AC, Yasui Y, Neglia JP, Potter JD, Nesbit ME, Ruccione K, et al. Late mortality experience in five-year survivors of childhood and adolescent cancer: the Childhood Cancer Survivor Study. J Clin Oncol. 2001;19(13):3163–72.
34. Baker KS, DeFor TE, Burns LJ, Ramsay NK, Neglia JP, Robison LL. New malignancies after blood or marrow stem-cell transplantation in children and adults: incidence and risk factors. J Clin Oncol. 2003;21(7):1352–8.
35. Rizzo JD, Curtis RE, Socie G, Sobocinski KA, Gilbert E, Landgren O, et al. Solid cancers after allogeneic hematopoietic cell transplantation. Blood. 2009;113(5):1175–83.
36. Snyder CF, Earle CC, Herbert RJ, Neville BA, Blackford AL, Frick KD. Preventive care for colorectal cancer survivors: a 5-year longitudinal study. J Clin Oncol. 2008;26(7):1073–9.
37. Grunfeld E. Primary care physicians and oncologists are players on the same team. J Clin Oncol. 2008;26(14):2246–7.
38. Ganz PA, Hahn EE. Implementing a survivorship care plan for patients with breast cancer. J Clin Oncol. 2008;26(5):759–67.
39. Nekhlyudov L. "Doc, should I see you or my oncologist?": a primary care perspective on opportunities and challenges in providing comprehensive care for cancer survivors. J Clin Oncol. 2009;27(15):2424–6.
40. Rittenhouse DR, Shortell SM. The patient-centered medical home: will it stand the test of health reform? JAMA. 2009;301(19):2038–40.
41. Kellerman R, Kirk L. Principles of the patient-centered medical home. Am Fam Physician. 2007;76(6):774–5.

# Chapter 11
# Optimizing Survivorship Care: Academic and Community Clinic Models

**Mary S. McCabe, Scott K. Baker, Caroline Huffman, and Ken Miller**

## Introduction

Due to advances in early detection and treatment, more individuals than ever are surviving cancer. Dissemination of these new, effective interventions into clinical practice has transformed cancer into largely a chronic condition, rather than an acute disease. Cancer survivors are living longer, and with one-third of the American population experiencing a cancer diagnosis in their lifetime, the need for focused attention on the long-term needs of cancer survivors is critical [1].

The Institute of Medicine (IOM) and many other national health advisory bodies worldwide recognize the range of medical, functional, and psychosocial issues faced by individuals who have completed cancer treatment and view survivorship as a distinct phase of cancer care. Although there are several variations defining when the phase of cancer survivorship begins, including the moment of diagnosis, completion of acute therapy, and living five years beyond diagnosis, the IOM definition of cancer survivorship as the "phase of care that follows primary treatment" is the one being used for the purpose of outlining the need for specialized follow-up services [2].

As the number of cancer survivors in the USA approaches 12 million, and the challenges grow in magnitude and complexity, there will be increasing need for new models of survivorship care and research [3]. Because extended cancer survival is a relatively new denouement, the development of effective models of care lags behind the need. There are several reasons: knowledge about survivorship care is limited; there is a lack of evidence-based interventions; survivorship care tends to be fragmented and not complementary to primary treatment and care; and there is a lack of meaningful collaboration among the stakeholders in addressing survivorship issues, including survivors, their family members, caregivers, social service providers, health care professionals, and researchers [4, 5].

M.S. McCabe (✉)
Memorial Sloan-Kettering Cancer Center, Weill Medical College,
Cornell University, New York, NY, USA
e-mail: mccabem@mskcc.org

M. Feuerstein and P.A. Ganz (eds.), *Health Services for Cancer Survivors*,
DOI 10.1007/978-1-4419-1348-7_11, 

In 2006, the IOM's report, *From Cancer Patient to Cancer Survivor: Lost in Transition*, cited specialized survivorship clinics as a promising model for delivering survivorship care [1]. Survivorship clinics provide a coordinated approach to follow-up care, enabling issues related to an individual's cancer treatment to be diagnosed and managed in one location. These clinics also provide a comprehensive follow-up program for posttreatment cancer survivors that include education and counseling. This specialized care can reduce the risk of misdiagnosis, limit unnecessary tests and procedures, and increase productivity of survivors. At the same time, these survivorship clinics conduct research on the late effects of cancer treatment.

Delivering care to cancer survivors presents many challenges to health care providers and the health care delivery system [6–9]. One of the most daunting challenges is the complexity of survivorship care delivery dictated by the diversity of patients, diagnoses, treatments, and potential sequelae. Health care professionals often lack awareness of treatment-related risks and the potential interactions of these risks with common comorbid conditions, such as obesity, diabetes, cardiovascular disease, anxiety, and depression [3, 10–12].

Despite the fact that there is currently no consensus regarding the best strategy for providing survivorship care to the rapidly growing survivorship population, new models are being developed to meet the needs of a variety of institutions and patient populations [13, 14]. These innovative care models for cancer survivors are currently being implemented and evaluated at a growing number of cancer centers and community hospitals across the country as survivorship care is increasingly seen as an integral and important phase of the cancer care continuum. Regardless of the model or system of survivorship care delivery, well-coordinated, effective, and comprehensive survivorship services are required in order for cancer survivors to have the best chance for achieving their optimal level of health following cancer treatment (Fig. 11.1).

## Models of Survivorship Care

With the expected doubling of the number of cancer survivors over the next decade, there is an increasing need for providing health care services specifically for cancer survivors [15]. The usual practice where survivors continue to be followed indefinitely by the oncologist is no longer feasible, nor is that practice necessarily in the best interest of the survivor [8]. It has become increasingly apparent that the needs of survivors are unique and that their health care needs extend far beyond surveillance for recurrence of their underlying malignancy (Table 11.1). Services provided to survivors should include prevention and/or early detection of possible long-term complications, providing education regarding their specific diagnosis, the treatments that they have received, and the potential long-term complications associated with that treatment [16, 17]. If problems are detected, they should be provided access to referrals with specialists who are familiar with complications that may result from exposure to cancer treatments. Survivors should also have a regular assessment of their psychosocial needs, including needs of affected family members and consideration of issues related to school, work, financial, and insurance

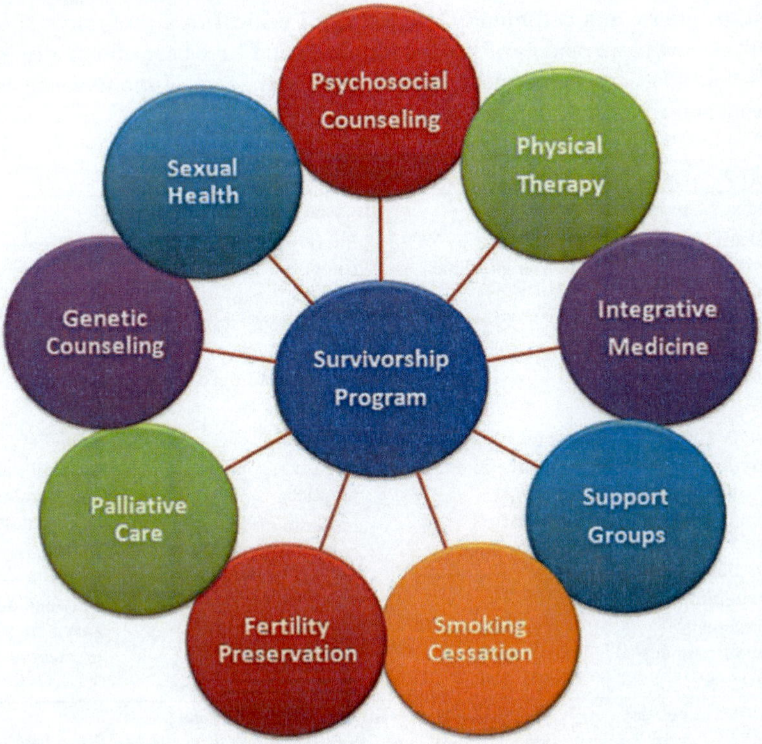


**Fig. 11.1** Comprehensive survivorship services

**Table 11.1** Essential components of survivorship care [2]

| |
|---|
| • Surveillance for recurrence |
| • Screening for new cancers |
| • Identification of and interventions for consequences of cancer and its treatment |
| • Health promotion strategies |
| • Coordinator between oncology specialties and primary care providers |

issues [18]. Another important aspect of survivorship care should be to ensure that survivors have an established "primary care home" and provider, and that survivors are provided with healthy lifestyle and wellness recommendation to incorporate into their daily life [19, 20]. Finally, survivors should be equipped with resources to allow them to navigate the complex health care system and to advocate on behalf of their own health care needs.

How these goals are best met, however, needs to be carefully evaluated and many factors taken into consideration when services for survivors are being developed. The two lessons that most established survivorship programs have learned are that (1) a *one-size fits all* approach rarely works and (2) that simply *opening a survivorship clinic* does not necessarily mean that patients will come. There are many obstacles and barriers that exist and thus careful consideration of institutional, patient, provider, and community needs are all critical to a program's success. We will review basic models of survivorship care that have been commonly implemented and that have been successful, pointing out some of the advantages and disadvantages of each (Table 11.2).

**Table 11.2** Clinical models for survivorship care

| **Multidisciplinary** | | **Disease/treatment specific** | |
|---|---|---|---|
| • Patients seen/evaluated by different providers in the context of a single clinic visit<br>• Oncology, endocrinology, neuropsychology, neurology, social work, nutrition, etc. | | • Survivorship clinic for specific disease category (breast)<br>• Stem cell transplant patients frequently seen in separate clinic from general oncology<br>• Can be developed for psychosocial services only | |
| *Advantages* | *Challenges* | *Advantages* | *Challenges* |
| • Easy for patients<br>• Comprehensive<br>• Good model for complex patient (brain tumors)<br>• Common pediatric model | • Resource intense<br>• Difficult to coordinate<br>• Not everyone needs all services | • Focused scope of practice<br>• Easier to make consensus guidelines for follow-up<br>• Good model for complex patients (brain tumors, HCT)<br>• Good way to start out | • Inequality ("everything is for breast cancer survivors …")<br>• May exclude survivors with greatest needs |
| **Consultative service** | | **Integrated care model** | |
| • One time consult visit to cover general survivorship issues and distribute treatment summary/care plan, frequently NP staffed<br>• Some may see annual returns<br>• Referral to subspecialist, PT, nutrition, psych, etc.<br>• Establish primary care home for survivor | | • Survivorship visit in the context of same oncology clinic<br>• Survivorship NP<br>• Frequently ongoing yearly visits | |
| *Advantages* | *Challenges* | *Advantages* | *Challenges* |
| • Serves unrestricted survivor population, outside referrals<br>• Provides core service, treatment summary/care plan<br>• Reinforces need for primary care follow-up and transition out of cancer clinic setting | • Difficult to be "expert" in long-term follow-up issues for all diseases<br>• Difficult to have consensus guidelines for follow-up for all<br>• Buy in from multiple different oncologist for patient referral difficult | • Easy transition for patients<br>• Access to treatment history<br>• Works well for surveillance of recurrent/new cancer as well as for late effects<br>• Improved referral rates for survivorship visit | • May restrict to certain diseases<br>• Patients may be reluctant for transition to primary care<br>• Requires busy clinical practice to justify |

## Clinic Models

### *Multidisciplinary Clinics*

In this type of clinical setting, a survivor will be seen by more than one clinician during a single clinic visit. This may include a provider (physician and/or nurse practitioner) with expertise in long-term follow-up care, as well as one or more additional subspecialists such as endocrinology, cardiology, neurology, neuropsychology, social work, nutrition, and others. These clinics are typically cancer center or hospital-based and are advantageous for patients with very complex long-term follow-up needs such as brain tumor survivors or for patients who have received hematopoietic cell transplants (HCT). This model has been much more commonly employed in a pediatric survivorship setting where annual and ongoing long-term follow-up by different specialists may frequently be required. The disadvantages of this model are that it is very resource intense requiring an ongoing time commitment by different providers and clinic staff. These clinics are also very difficult to coordinate and not every patient may need to be seen by all providers. It is also not a model that will lend itself to serving a large population of survivors.

### *Disease- or Treatment-Specific Clinics*

These models are useful for settings where there is a sufficient population of survivors of one particular type of cancer (breast or prostate cancer, for example) or for survivors who have all received a similar kind of treatment, such as HCT. In a model such as this, the survivor can receive very individualized follow-up care and detailed disease-specific recommendations. From a provider standpoint, this model allows for a focused scope of practice where it will be easier to develop and maintain consensus follow-up guidelines and perhaps easier to provide a more detailed evaluation of potential risk factors for late effects. Similar to the multidisciplinary model, this also is a good model for patients with complex medical needs and is frequently utilized for centers that perform HCT as the needs of those survivors are more complex, including issues related to chronic graft vs. host disease. This disease-centered approach is also useful for institutions that are initiating a survivorship program since it allows them to develop high-quality services for one or two diagnoses to begin with and then to expand to other diseases in an incremental fashion. This model is also advantageous for any program that has a research component and where there is a desire to focus on a particular type of cancer. The disadvantages of this model is that it establishes inequality within an institution by providing a highly desired service for only a subset of survivors, most commonly for breast cancer survivors since they comprise the largest number of survivors overall. This model may also then exclude survivors who actually have the greatest needs and fewest internal or external resources.

## *Consultative Clinics*

This model is common and relatively easy to establish. Survivors are typically seen in a clinical setting that is separate from where they received their primary oncology care and these clinics are commonly staffed by nurse practitioners or physician assistants. Survivors are seen for a one time consult visit to cover general survivorship issues and to distribute a treatment summary and survivorship care plan, although some may offer annual return visits also. For individual issues that are identified, survivors are referred to medical subspecialists, physical therapy, nutrition counseling, or for psychological/psychiatric services. Another important component of this model is that a primary care home for the survivor be established and that the treatment summary and survivorship care plan be sent to that provider. An advantage of this model is that it typically serves an unrestricted survivor population (no limitations based on type of cancer) and can accommodate patients who did not necessarily receive treatment in the same institution in which the clinic is located. These clinics provide core survivorship services, including the generation of a treatment summary and care plan, and reinforce the need for primary care follow-up and transition out of cancer clinic setting. Some challenges that arise are that it is difficult for providers to be "expert" in long-term follow-up issues for all diseases and it is an arduous task to develop consensus guidelines for follow-up for such a wide variety of diseases and treatments. For patients who have received treatment in a different institution, access to and obtaining required medical records can be a significant task in order to generate a treatment summary. In addition, buy-in from multiple different oncologists/oncology clinics for patient referrals can be challenging.

## *Integrated Clinics*

In this clinical model, survivorship visits occur in the context of same oncology clinic where the primary cancer treatment was provided (Fig. 11.2). Again in this model, the survivorship visit is commonly performed by a nurse practitioner or physician assistant. Patients are frequently seen for ongoing yearly visits and may also still be receiving surveillance for recurrence of their primary disease. The advantage of this model is that there is an easy transition for patients from "oncology follow-up" to "survivorship follow-up." This model also provides easy access to the patient's complete treatment history, making the completion of a treatment summary an easier task. The integrated model works well for diseases where surveillance of recurrent cancer is long term and can be incorporated into the surveillance for late effects as well. Finally, this model improves referral rates for survivorship visits as it typically becomes part of the standard practice in that clinic. The disadvantages of this model are that it requires more resources to establish unless the services are going to be restricted to a certain diagnosis or to a particular clinic. Since patients remain in the same clinic they received their treatment from, they may be more reluctant to transition to primary care. This model also requires busy clinical practice to justify a separate provider(s) dedicated to survivorship follow-up.

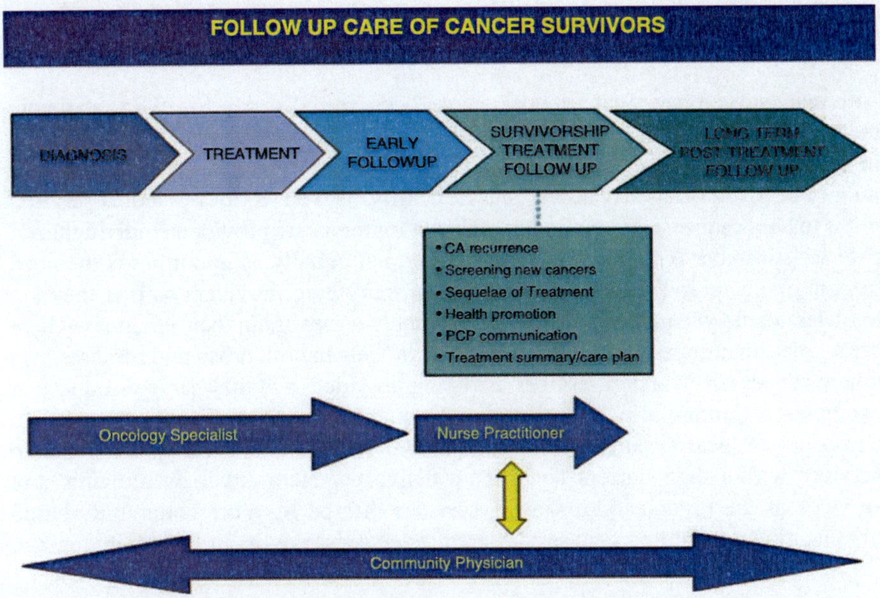


**Fig. 11.2** Integrated care by nurse practitioners (With the permission of the Survivorship Program at Memorial Sloan-Kettering Cancer Center)

## Provider Models

In addition to how the survivorship care models are physically structured, as discussed above, there are different models of who is providing the care in each setting. The vast majority of successful survivorship programs have been established with clinical visits being provided by a nurse practitioner rather than a physician. The reasons for this are varied but include economic realities, time limitations, need to see newly diagnosed patients, focus on wellness and rehabilitation, and the lack of desire/time to deal with psychosocial concerns on the part of oncologists. Obviously clinics primarily staffed by nurse practitioners have collaborating physicians who provide backup and consultation as needed. In many clinics that are staffed by physicians, there frequently are nurse practitioners who are working in conjunction with the physician during those visits. Another issue related to providers is their background training. Most commonly, the physicians and nurse practitioners have oncology training, but it is becoming more common for survivorship programs to include a physician with primary care (family medicine, internal medicine, combined medicine-pediatrics) training which is an ideal situation for clinics where longitudinal follow-up of survivors is desired or in the pediatric setting where transition from pediatric-based care to adult care also needs to take place.

## Unique Community Models

Although survivorship care models have been initially developed in academic medical centers, the basic elements of this type of care are essential for survivors in a community setting as well. In addition, cancer survivorship care in the community needs to offer easy access and flexibility, as well as offer practical services if it is to help cancer survivors and be efficient for their care providers. Individualized care for survivors is important in this setting, but equally as important is the need to communicate and collaborate with the primary care providers so that they are knowledgeable when caring for the many cancer survivors in their practices. There are a growing number of unique community models in both urban and rural settings where cancer survivorship services are being provided, and they serve as important examples for community organizations, hospitals, and private practices to assess and adapt to local circumstances. Each model focuses on providing survivorship services within their current health care delivery system either by utilizing core services of the organization, sharing services offered by other community-based organizations, or adding new services requested by survivors in their community.

### *Private Practice Model of Survivorship Care*

In a large community practice in a rural state, the oncologists have developed formal survivorship services utilizing dedicated staff. Upon completion of treatment, patients have a onetime consult visit with a nurse practitioner who reviews with the patient their cancer diagnosis and treatment history, as well as a patient-specific follow-up plan that has been developed in collaboration with the oncologist. This visit also serves as an opportunity for patients to "debrief" about their treatment experience and prepares them for the transition to surveillance-focused care. The patient, primary care physician, and oncologist all receive a copy of the Survivorship treatment summary and care plan [16, 21]. This survivorship consult was initially provided only to breast cancer survivors, but has now been expanded to all survivors who have completed treatment. Beginning with one disease group allowed for a focused beginning and for feedback from an interested group of patients who were eager to have the services.

### *Primary Care Model of Survivorship Services*

A large multi-specialty medical group serving an extensive suburban area has developed formal survivorship services that are provided by a set of internists who have an interest and expertise in survivorship follow-up care. Cancer survivors are preferentially referred to this select group of internists (both by oncologists in the group and outside oncologists) and ongoing care is provided to these survivors as they are incorporated into their practices.

This arrangement provides an opportunity for the survivor to have their cancer-related problems addressed by one provider along with other medical problems that may impact late and long-term treatment sequelae. A treatment summary and care plan is requested from the oncologist and this document serves as the template for future care and referrals. The "survivorship internists" utilize the many resources of the multi-specialty group, such as counseling, physical therapy, and integrative medicine, and are able to provide a focus on wellness, all in the same convenient location.

## *Community Health Center*

A well-established community health center in an urban area developed a unique survivorship program that includes unique offerings, such as evening hours, and utilizes its strong navigator program to identify cancer survivors within the clinic population, explain the program, and enthusiastically support and facilitate patient participation. The survivorship clinic itself is staffed by primary care physicians and benefits from having a nurse and social worker who are bilingual and bicultural. Equally important are two case managers who work to facilitate the patients care based on the treatment summary and care plan that are developed by the internists. Some patients coming to the health center have never had follow-up after their cancer treatment or general cancer screening, and the case managers have been very successful in making sure these services are obtained. Another major emphasis of this survivorship program is patient education about "healthy cancer survivorship." During the survivorship visit the patients dietary, exercise, and health-related behaviors are assessed and discussed and recommendations or referrals are made. Mental health screening is also a priority and patients are referred to appropriate services either within the clinic or in the nearby community.

Building on the ongoing education programs already in existence, the community health center also hosts monthly "listening and learning" sessions for survivors and each month a different topic such as nutrition, exercise, body image, or sexuality is discussed. These group sessions are very successful and promote healthy camaraderie between survivors who learn that they share common concerns.

## *Community Hospital-Based Resource Center*

Many community-based hospitals serve one or more oncology practices and a dedicated "survivorship clinic" may not be feasible in either the hospital setting or within the practices despite the desire to provide such services. This is the case at a hospital in a remote rural area where the hospital staff are also constrained by the large geographic region that they serve. To best meet the needs of their population, they have established a Survivorship and Wellness Program that is based on an education/resource center model that also relies significantly on the involvement of patient navigators. They provide educational resources, including a Survivorship and Wellness Resource Library, workshops and other survivorship-oriented presentations to survivors, as well as to community oncologists and other health care providers. This approach is unique for a community-based center in that the focus of their activities is not only on the survivor, but also on health care providers, so that they may continually gain more education regarding the unique health care needs of cancer survivors. Other activities include survivor support groups, a Healing Arts Program, and a survivorship-focused rehabilitation program within their physical/occupational therapy department. They have also partnered with a regional health club to provide a community-based exercise and nutrition program specific for cancer survivors.

### *Public Hospital Survivorship Clinic*

One large, urban public hospital with a busy and successful cancer program combines survivorship care with internal medicine services into one clinic staffed by two internists (one is bilingual) with the goal of providing comprehensive long-term medical and psychosocial services to a multiethnic, low-income population of adult cancer survivors. This model was developed because of a desire to keep patients in the medical care system after cancer treatment in order to manage their many, medical comorbidities while at the same time addressing their posttreatment medical and psychosocial needs. These patients have few resources to travel back and forth between oncology providers and primary care, so a system of providing a wide range of health care services in one setting is not only efficient, but necessary. Because of the international patient community, translation services are essential, as are skills in working with a culturally diverse population. Since the hospital has limited resources to meet the psychosocial needs of this survivor population, outside community groups that have ongoing programs such as counseling and nutrition programs are invited to offer these services at the hospital. These collaborations have been very successful since the community organizations are eager to have access to an expanded population of patients and the hospital can offer needed services not financially possible.

## Considerations for Getting Started

> The beginning is the most important part of the work
>
> Plato: *The Republic*

Any significant change proposed or considered by an organization, especially by elements of the health care system, requires a careful, logical assessment even before a plan can be developed and implemented. In particular, when deciding how to implement survivorship care and services, whether in an academic institution or in a community outpatient facility, there are first-order questions to ask that will have important impact on the extent, pace, and direction of any proposed change. The answers to these questions will lead to a plan that fits into the overall institutional mission and can be supported by both leadership and staff. Spending time on this organizational assessment – getting as much good information as possible – will be critical in assuring success.

## *Asking the First-Order Questions*

Most Survivorship Programs will be implemented in already existing institutions and practices, so where does one begin?

*Why* – Understanding why a clinical survivorship program would be valued in an organization establishes a rationale for what eventually becomes a plan and leads logically into the development of a set of goals.

*For Whom* – Here it becomes important to define the terms "survivor" and "survivorship." Any and all plans for services, staffing, and budget will be derived from these decisions. In this chapter, we are focusing on the third phase of a patient's care following diagnosis and treatment. The plans for a survivorship clinic that will include individuals with many different diagnoses (consultative) will be very different from one that focuses on the multidisciplinary needs of one population, such as breast cancer survivors. Whatever the decision, the important thing is to understand and keep the focus on the intended population.

*With Whom* – Engaging the organizational leadership at the very beginning is essential. It matters that those who have the ultimate responsibility for making the decisions in the facility are in support of any plans, especially those that will require change and use of resources. In addition, since the needs of survivors are frequently multidisciplinary, the backing of well-respected individuals across disciplines is critical in getting plans off the ground, supporting growth, and working as a team to assure sustainability.

*What* – An essential part of planning a clinical survivorship program is to begin with a thorough assessment of the strengths and weaknesses of an institution's existing services, combined with a critical assessment of what gaps in these services exist. One needs as thorough and complete an assessment as possible of the current environment to understand how best to plan and proceed. For example, the organization may have a very strong oncology product line where new survivorship clinical services would be a natural fit. However, there may be critical gaps in the availability of certain subspecialties requiring referrals to the community.

*When* – There is no ideal time frame for a planning process, but rather, what matters more is whether certain objectives are accomplished during the planning process. Requirements before you begin include securing the needed “buy-in” from leadership and staff, acquiring an understanding of the culture of change in your facility, and developing an outline of short- and long-term goals including a listing of the resources needed to achieve those goals. Even then, a stepwise roll out (beginning with one disease group) may be the most prudent and effective way of getting a clinical program started.

## Utilize Guidance in Developing the Plan

Although the Survivorship movement is relatively new in terms of being a dedicated period of care with a set of defined services, there are a number of national reports upon which to draw. Each has a unique focus and valuable information that can be applied locally. The best known and most referred to publication is the 2006 Institute of Medicine Report (IOM), *From Cancer Patient to Cancer Survivor: Lost in Transition* that is referred to earlier in the chapter. The reason for its prominence as a resource document is that it is the most comprehensively referenced assessment of survivor needs and challenges. In addition to this IOM report, there are other valuable resources. The 2004 *President's Cancer Panel Report* presents a list of recommendations for the care of cancer survivors across the life span and identifies areas of needed research [22]. This valuable information serves as a national needs assessment since it was developed through town hall meetings conducted across the country with survivors and their families. *The National Action Plan for Cancer Survivorship* published in 2004 is just as the title suggests [23]. This action plan, developed by the Lance Armstrong Foundation and the Centers for Disease Control and Prevention (CDC), supplies us with a strategic framework that is useful when connecting plans for a local survivorship program to a national strategy. It includes a call for the establishment of clinical practice guidelines and metrics for all survivorship services as a means of assuring continued quality improvement and being able to evaluate impact over time. Most recently in 2007, the IOM has produced another relevant report entitled, *Cancer Care for the Whole Patient* [24]. This publication focuses on the psychosocial needs of the patient and challenges us to address these needs by building clinical capacity to ensure resource availability.

## Know Who You Are and What Can Be Achieved

From the very beginning, it is critically important to understand the institutional culture and align survivorship planning efforts with the long-range plans and strategic direction of the institution since the attention of leadership and allocation of monetary resources will be devoted to fulfilling these plans. Still, the clinic is not assured of success unless one is realistic about the inevitability of competing priorities. This reality may mean doing more with less in the beginning, or it may be that funds and support will be easier to obtain. In either case, moving in the same direction as the overall institution will give the clinical program visibility and a solid base from which to grow. For example, because of the predicted shortage of medical oncologists, some organizations may be very amenable to considering survivorship clinics that utilize nurse practitioners to provide long-term follow-up care, thus freeing up physicians to see new patients. Another goal may be to improve relations with the community and referral of survivors to community programs, such as smoking cessation or integrative medicine services may be beneficial in that effort.

## *Assembling the Team*

In addition to reaching high up in the organization for support, it is also important to identify champions early on in the planning phase. These individuals will likely be strong clinicians who are early adapters of institutional change or they may be staff who head up services, such as cardiology, psychiatry, and physical rehabilitation that would be an integral part of the services provided to survivors. They, in turn, may be eager to have their services better utilized. Even more broadly, it is important to spend time getting buy-in from staff throughout the institution, hospital, or practice setting. It is also important to include patients in the planning process. The program is, after all, for survivors and they can often be an influential voice with administrators. As the initial clinic planning begins, thought needs to be given to the development of a management team with a focus on how to include individuals with both expertise and influence. Having these individuals serve as a steering committee to guide development will fulfill multiple objectives: provide direction, keep projects alive and going, and maintain interest in the effort over time.

## *Pilot Programs Provide Opportunity*

Since all health care facilities are increasingly focused on the economics of service delivery, it may be a wise approach to pilot the initial survivorship clinic in a stepwise approach to both demonstrate the value of the effort and to assure administrative leadership that unsuccessful programs will not continue without review. Piloting a clinic will provide opportunity and flexibility. It will allow you to begin wherever you can as a proof of principle, and then to revise as needed using an adaptive design model. An important guide when initiating pilots during the beginning stages of program development is to be willing to make mistakes and to stop doing what is not working, revise, and try again. Pilot projects allow us to do these things and recover.

## *Cultural Change*

Institutional change is hard and can be attributed to multiple factors that are useful to be aware of. There are some who are protecting turf in an institution, others who fear failure if things change, there may also be inertia and an unwillingness to learn. To counter the inevitable resistance, regardless of the source, the support of leadership and key decision makers, as previously suggested in the chapter, is essential. An ongoing communication strategy about what is planned and how things are going is also important. To have the facts always out front in a transparent way, with the strategic goals broken out into segments, makes any new program less onerous and threatening. Change can be hard, but over time, change can be made with the support of most. There will always be some who resist, and one must be willing and able to move forward without them.

## *Program Metrics*

The demand for evaluation is made throughout all quarters of heath care, and survivorship is no exception. Yet, currently little guidance exists for how to evaluate survivorship clinics. With limited practice guidelines (whether evidence- or consensus-based), it is difficult to apply process measures that are worthy surrogates for outcomes of medical and psychosocial importance to survivors and their health care providers, but this should not dissuade us from simple, meaningful evaluation. Since survivorship clinics are so new, the evaluation of the feasibility of various models along with satisfaction with services and financial sustainability are practical and meaningful evaluations that should be undertaken and to date have not been adequately conducted.

## *Community Lessons Learned*

Although academic medical centers have been the early adopters of survivorship programs since they often have the financial and manpower resources to do so, we are now seeing a steady growth in the development of community survivorship programs as well. This is a critically important advance since the majority of cancer survivors receive their treatment and care in the community and only with the addition of these types of services close to where survivors live will we see a real change in the quality of posttreatment care and ultimately in health outcomes for this population. Some community-specific recommendations for establishing successful services include:

1. Having practice or clinic leadership who are committed to providing this care is essential.
2. These programs benefit from strong patient navigation, including identifying patients, facilitating participation, and then following up on the care plan recommendations.
3. The staffing for a community-based program must reflect the individual needs of the community including cultural and linguistic competency.

4. Learning about late and long-term health problems may not be enough to spark a patient's interest or commitment. The personal relationship with the navigator, nurse, or primary care physician is often more crucial.
5. Many health centers have excellent ancillary care services, including social work and nutrition counseling. Community survivorship care can facilitate patients receiving these needed services in their own community, regardless of where they received their cancer treatment.
6. Cancer survivorship education can occur one-on-one or in a group setting.
7. Education programs for health care providers are an excellent way to increase their interest and expertise in cancer survivorship.

## Future Directions

Since the publication of the IOM report, much has been accomplished to improve the care and health outcomes of cancer survivors. Models of care are being developed, implemented, and evaluated with the goal of meeting patient need within the constraints of institutional and national resources. At this juncture, the key to sustained progress in the evolution and maturation of care models will require continued momentum across a comprehensive set of related activities: (1) a greater international acknowledgment of the necessity of care for the posttreatment patient; (2) greater allocation of resources for research, especially studies focused on the etiology of long-term and late effects and interventions to prevent and reduce them; (3) formal assessments of care delivery models with an emphasis on novel provider arrangements and health outcomes of importance; (4) public and professional education about the medical, psychosocial, and economic issues that survivors face; and (5) formal training programs for health care providers to provide this survivorship care in both the pediatric and adult care settings. The long-term success of clinical survivorship programs depends on the development of sustainable, efficient models that provide improved health and quality of life to survivors across varied health care setting and systems.

## References

1. Travis LB, Yahalom J. Preface. Hematol Oncol Clin North Am. 2008;22(2):xi–xii.
2. Hewitt M, Greenfield S, Stoval E, editors. From cancer patient to cancer survivor: lost in transition. Washington, DC: National Academies Press; 2006.
3. Rowland JH. Cancer survivorship: rethinking the cancer control continuum. Semin Oncol Nurs. 2008;24(3):145–52.
4. Carver JR, Shapiro CL, Ng A, Jacobs L, Schwartz C, Virgo KS, et al. American society of clinical oncology clinical evidence review on the ongoing care of adult cancer survivors: cardiac and pulmonary effects. J Clin Oncol. 2007;25(25):2991–4008.
5. Nissen M, Beran M, Lee M, Menta SR, Pine DA, Swenson KK. Views of primary care providers on follow-up care of cancer patients. Fam Med. 2007;39(7):477–82.

6. Hewitt ME, Bamundo A, Day R, Harvey C. Perspectives on post-treatment cancer care: qualitative research with survivors, nurses and physicians. J Clin Oncol. 2007;25(16):2270–3.
7. Earle CC, Burstein HJ, Winer EP, Weeks JC. Quality of non-breast cancer health maintenance among elderly breast cancer survivors. J Clin Oncol. 2003;21(8):1447–51.
8. Erickson C, Slasberg E, Forte G, Bruinooge BA, Goldstein M. Future supply and demand for oncologists: challenges to assuring access to oncology services. J Oncol Pract. 2007;3(2):79–84.
9. Earle C, Neville B. Underuse of necessary care among cancer survivors. Cancer. 2004;101(8):1712–9.
10. Rowland JH, Hewitt M, Ganz PA. Cancer survivorship: a new challenge in delivering quality cancer care. J Clin Oncol. 2006;24(32):5101–4.
11. Stanton A. Psychological concerns and interventions for cancer survivors. J Clin Oncol. 2006;24(32):5132–7.
12. Mao JJ, Bowman MA, Stricker CT, DeMichele A, Jacobs L, Chan D, et al. Delivery of survivorship care by primary care physicians: the perspective of breast cancer patients. J Clin Oncol. 2009;27(6):933–8.
13. Oeffinger KC, McCabe MS. Models for delivering survivorship care. J Clin Oncol. 2006;24(32):5117–24.
14. McCabe MS, Jacobs L. Survivorship care: models and programs. Semin Oncol Nurs. 2008;24(3):202–7.
15. Warren JL, Mariotto AB, Meekins A, Topor M, Brown ML. Current and future utilization of services from medical oncologists. J Clin Oncol. 2008;26(19):3242–7.
16. Earle CC. Failing to plan is planning to fail: improving the quality of care with survivorship care plans. J Clin Oncol. 2006;24(32):5112–6.
17. Findley P, Sambamoorthi U. Preventive health services and lifestyle practices in cancer survivors: a population health investigation. J Cancer Surviv. 2009;3(1):43–58.
18. Bellizzi KM, Rowland JH, Jeffrey DD, McNeel T. Health behaviors of cancer survivors: examining opportunities for cancer control intervention. J Clin Oncol. 2005;23(34):8884–93.
19. Grunfeld E. Primary care physicians and oncologists are players on the same team. J Clin Oncol. 2008;26(14):2246–7.
20. Nekhlyudov L. "Doc, should I see you or my oncologist?" A primary care perspective on opportunities and challenges in providing comprehensive care for cancer survivors. J Clin Oncol. 2009;27(15):2424–6.
21. Ganz PA, Casillas J, Hahn EE. Ensuring quality care for cancer survivors: implementing the survivorship care plan. Semin Oncol Nurs. 2008;24(3):208–17.
22. President's Cancer Panel. Living beyond cancer: finding a new balance. Bethesda: National Cancer Institute; 2004.
23. A national action plan for cancer survivorship: advancing public health strategies. Atlanta: Centers for Disease Control and Prevention; 2004.
24. Adler NE, Page AE, editors. Cancer care for the whole patient. Washington, DC: National Academies Press; 2007.

# Chapter 12
# The Final Phase of Cancer Survivorship: End-of-Life Care

**Betty Ferrell, Carla Munévar, and Virginia Sun**

## Description of the Current Situation

In the past decade, significant attention has been given to two seemingly unrelated areas of quality care in oncology – cancer survivorship and end-of-life care. It is of note that the Institute of Medicine (IOM) held consensus meetings and issued major reports in each of these areas [1, 2]. While at first glance the issues of cancer survivorship and end-of-life care may appear as unrelated concerns, these issues are in fact highly related.

While there have been important advances in cancer diagnosis, treatment, and survivorship, recent data published by the American Society of Clinical Oncology [3] in their report "Clinical Cancer Advances 2009" illustrate the continuing reality of poor prognosis for many cancers. Table 12.1 illustrates 5-year survival rates from 1975 to 2004 for those cancers which have less than a 50% survival. It is of note that for many cancers, there has been very limited change in survival. A pivotal statistic is that in 2009, over 570,000 people in the USA died of cancer [4].

The focus on cure and long-term survivorship over the past few decades has in many ways added to the long-standing history of avoiding issues of mortality in cancer. Major media attention has been given to cancer survivorship and prominent media personalities diagnosed with cancer often portray only the most positive of outcomes. From the time of initial diagnosis, a singular focus on survivorship often ultimately leads to deficiencies in care for those who will die from their disease.

This chapter is intended to fill an often missing piece in the overall picture of cancer survivorship – the final phase. We begin with a discussion of the key deficiencies in end-of-life care and an exploration of how these may be even more pronounced for those who have experienced a period of survivorship. The chapter also includes a review of key literature to describe studies examining the experience of end-of-life care when survivors face cancer recurrence or progression of disease.

---

B. Ferrell (✉)
Division of Nursing Research and Education, Department of Population Sciences, City of Hope, Duarte, CA, USA
e-mail: bferrell@coh.org

M. Feuerstein and P.A. Ganz (eds.), *Health Services for Cancer Survivors*,
DOI 10.1007/978-1-4419-1348-7_12, © Springer Science+Business Media, LLC 2011

**Table 12.1** 5-year survival rates, 1975–2004 (select cancers) [3]

| Cancer type | 1975–1977 | 1984–1986 | 1996–2004 |
|---|---|---|---|
| Leukemia (%) | 35 | 42 | 51 |
| Ovary (%) | 37 | 40 | 46 |
| Brain (%) | 24 | 29 | 35 |
| Multiple myeloma (%) | 26 | 29 | 35 |
| Stomach (%) | 16 | 18 | 25 |
| Esophagus (%) | 5 | 10 | 17 |
| Lung (%) | 13 | 13 | 16 |
| Liver (%) | 4 | 6 | 11 |
| Pancreas (%) | 2 | 3 | 5 |

We have included in this chapter a series of case illustrations in order to best describe unique aspects of survivorship and end-of-life care. Just as the term "survivorship" encompasses a broad diversity of people living with cancer, the discussion of end-of-life care in survivorship also includes widely divergent scenarios illustrated through these cases. The chapter also presents potential solutions to this key aspect of oncology practice. As with other major areas of quality care, improved end-of-life care in cancer survivorship will require additional research as well as changes in health policy, practice, and reimbursement. While a paradigm that recognizes end-of-life care as the final phase of survivorship may be a major shift in thinking for many professionals, ultimately such a perspective will attribute significantly to quality cancer care.

The following case illustrates the complexity and challenges of impacting oncology care:

Mr. James was diagnosed in 1989 with lymphoma at age 25 while a graduate student in mathematics. He underwent an aggressive course of chemotherapy and radiation and experienced complete remission of his disease. From the time of his initial diagnosis, Mr. James was recognized by his family and health-care team as a "fighter," extremely optimistic, and a strong advocate for cancer survivorship. Mr. James married and had three children and a successful career in an engineering firm. He also continued to volunteer in his community at the Wellness Community and local American Cancer Society as a visitor for newly diagnosed patients and he was a sought after speaker for panels on survivorship. He always shared his commitment to a healthy lifestyle and adherence to annual health monitoring. The oncology program often referred to him as their "poster child," a model of health, successful treatment, and long-term survivorship.

After 18 years of disease-free survival, Mr. James' lymphoma recurred. Both he and his family were shocked and voiced great distress at his recurrence after such a long period of survivorship and especially since he had "done everything right." Mr. James' cancer was advanced at the time of recurrence and did not respond to treatment but he persisted in treatment options including clinical trials. His disease continued to advance and he also experienced numerous treatment complications as well as significant symptom concerns. After 12 months of various treatments, Mr. James' oncologist introduced the option of forgoing treatment and considering hospice care, this suggestion prompted by several repeat hospitalizations for poorly controlled symptoms. Mr. James declined hospice, insisting that he wanted to continue to fight his disease. His insurance company was also a factor in this decision, since admission to hospice would mean that any disease-focused care would no longer be approved.

Three months later, he unfortunately developed sepsis and died in the oncology unit with tremendous distress for Mr. James, his family, and the oncology staff.

The case of Mr. James is indicative of the many factors influencing optimum end-of-life care. Patient, family, professional, and system factors often combine to preclude the desired outcome of a death which is supported by good symptom management, consultation with palliative care professionals, timely referral to hospice, and psychosocial and spiritual care essential in terminal illness.

Table 12.2 summarizes key characteristics cited in palliative care literature as essential to quality care. The table lists the eight domains of quality palliative care as defined by the national guidelines in the field, the National Consensus Project for Quality Palliative Care [5]. The table then applies these domains to the unique needs of cancer survivorship.

**Table 12.2** National Consensus Project for quality palliative care domains of care applied to needs of cancer survivors [5]

| Domain | Application to end-of-life care for cancer survivors |
|---|---|
| Structure and processes of care | System and structures are needed to assess the needs of survivors who experience advancing disease or recurrence. Coordination of oncology care and palliative care is needed to insure transition to optimum end-of-life care. |
| Physical aspects of care | Cancer survivors may face complex symptom concerns including symptoms of advanced disease, treatment-related, and delayed effects of treatment symptoms. |
| Psychological and psychiatric aspects of care | Cancer survivors facing end of life may experience extreme distress associated with the shock of recurrence and destroyed hope for long-term survivorship. |
| Social aspects of care | The impact of cancer recurrence on families causes extreme family distress. Family members of survivors may require support in the transition from survivorship to grieving the death of the patient. |
| Spiritual, religious and existential aspects of care | Survivors may face existential suffering related to disease recurrence, feelings of religious abandonment and they may search for meaning in life now altered by impending death. |
| Cultural aspects of care | Cultural beliefs regarding cancer, survivorship, and death influence end-of-life care. |
| Care of the imminently dying | Cancer survivors need transition to hospice or palliative care for expert management of symptoms and psychosocial needs which emerge in the final months of life. |
| Ethical and legal aspects of care | Cancer survivors need support in making difficult choices regarding forgoing further treatment and completion of advance directives. |

## Research That Help Us Understand the Problem

Cancer survivorship, through the years, has been defined in numerous ways. Some of the definitions describe survivorship beginning at the completion of initial treatment [1]. Another definition has described survivorship as the period beginning 5 years beyond diagnosis and yet another describes it as a point in time after diagnosis or initial treatment [1]. The most common and accepted definition is that a person is considered a survivor from the moment of diagnosis [6].

With improved treatment, early detection, better supportive care, and the growth of the elderly population, end of life care after survivorship has been added to the map of the cancer care trajectory (Fig. 12.1). Since the National Coalition for Cancer Survivorship's introduction of the term "survivorship" to cancer care [7], not only has there been an evolution and refinement of the definition but it has also opened new opportunities for research. Much has begun but there are still areas yet to be explored. Much has been studied about the treatment effects, follow-up care, economic sequelae, health disparities, and family and caregiver issues, but little has been focused on end-of-life care of those "surviving" patients. As the number of survivors continue to grow there are accompanying challenges for providing an excellent continuum of care. Greater demand is being placed on the health-care system to provide necessary systems to transition patients from cancer survivors to palliative care. This system would need to provide not only for their medical needs as cancer survivors but more importantly their needs related to their psychosocial well-being. It is of no surprise then, that according to a poll taken by the Lance Armstrong Foundation [8], nearly half of those responding indicated that the American health-care system failed to meet their nonmedical needs [8].

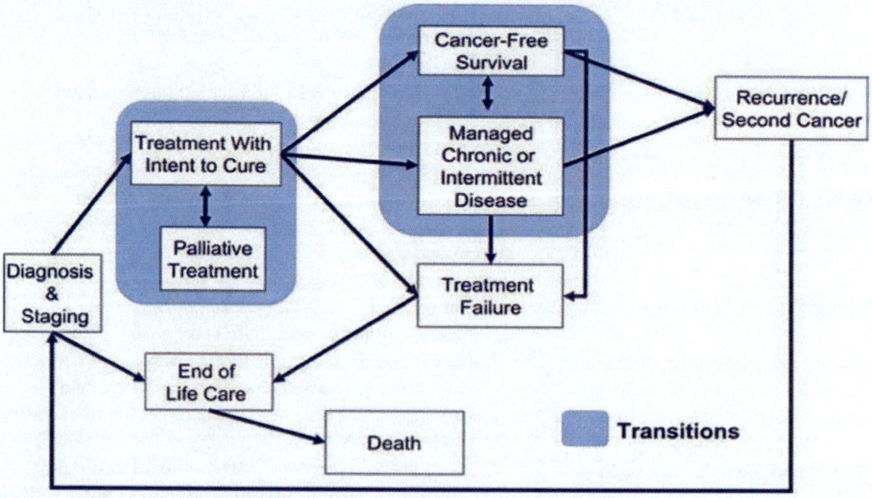


**Fig. 12.1** Cancer care trajectory (Adapted with permission from Hewitt et al. [1])

As contradictory as it may sound, end-of-life concerns are very real to those who have been able to initially survive cancer but are now faced with recurrence or late-stage disease. This area of survivorship care, as important as it is, needs to be explored further. In our review of the literature, limited research directly addressed this topic and available literature was primarily on the topics of continued care, transition, and cancer recurrence. More has to be done if health-care providers are to address the needs of this growing population.

The lack of attention to palliative care needs in survivors is particularly frustrating given that approximately 1.2 million individuals are diagnosed with cancer recurrence each year [9]. That is, one out of six cancer survivors will be diagnosed with a recurrent cancer [10]. Of those 1.2 million, more than one-half will progress rapidly and die of their disease [11]. These are sobering statistics, perhaps not familiar to the patients with the recurrent disease but nonetheless the thought and reality of dying are very eminent and real to them. In a study to further investigate the psychosocial meaning of recurrent cancer, Mahon [12] notes that issues of death and dying became a very central issue when discussing recurrence. Death and dying begins to play a more active role in their thinking and they no longer see cancer as having a cure but most likely their future cause of death. Participants in the study expressed a decrease in their belief and hope of remission in spite of receiving reassurance from their physician and those with an initial cancer diagnosis made at an early age (younger than 50 years of age) had fear that due to the recurrence, they would be more likely to experience a premature death [12]. It seems that perhaps a new perspective and deeper understanding is gained by those who have successfully finished their first treatment for cancer and are now faced with the same challenge only this time more aware of the reality of death.

The current literature supports the notion that recurrence is experienced differently than when the disease was newly diagnosed [12]. According to subjects in a study exploring the psychological meaning of recurrence [12], their feelings about being diagnosed with cancer again has given them a keener awareness of the diagnosis. Subjects stated that they were "numbed" during the initial diagnosis and treatment, but now, after recurrence, realize how horrible the reality of cancer really was [12]. A better understanding of the difficulty in treating the cancer was also better understood. One woman with a recurrent lymphoma described it: "[I]t's not just the dying thing. It's just that you realize that there are things you have no control over and that's hard to swallow. I realize now that the cancer will probably never go away. I mean I might get another remission and as far as everyone can tell it might go away, but it will always be there. It makes you feel very vulnerable because you know it could come back at any time without any warning. I know that now and I'll never forget it. I didn't feel as vulnerable the first time [12]." Since thoughts of death and dying are more prominent in recurrent cancer, the transition must also therefore differ from when the patient was initially diagnosed with their first cancer. Patients suffering from a recurrence no longer see treatment as a fight against cancer but perhaps seek to find a more peaceful way to coexist with their cancer [12]. As one woman stated, "this time I'm getting chemo, but I don't think of it as an active war. I mean I'm not giving up or anything, it's more like something I have to do [12]."

This new attitude lays the platform in which the patients will be beginning their new journey in transitioning from cancer-free to cancer patient.

The patient's ability to cope with the recurrence will greatly impact the transition and quality of life the patient will have. For health professionals, cancer has many aspects and it varies greatly from symptoms, treatment, and prognosis. For the patient, all cancers are perceived the same; therefore the patient's way to cope with a recurrent cancer is influenced greatly by their previous coping ability or their experience with other cancer survivors and how they have been able to cope [12]. Patients who had previously had a recurrence of cancer said that they were not surprised by the new diagnosis of recurrence because it had already happened to them before. These patients were more optimistic and hopeful that remission could be achieved once again [12]. In contrast, patients who had a negative experience with recurrent cancer in the family or with friends tended to be more pessimistic and generally felt that their prognosis was poor. Cancer was no longer perceived as a curable disease but rather a disease that "gets you a little at a time [12]." This coping mechanism, described by Lazarus and Folkman [13], illustrates how patients may draw on previous experiences to develop coping abilities required to deal with their current situation.

Some studies have shown that emotional and psychosocial distress experienced with recurrence has been the same or less distressing than when they were given their first cancer diagnosis [14]. This was attributed to their familiarity with the disease and treatment and with the support group that was developed during their first diagnosis. Yet others have shown that past experiences of living with cancer and undergoing treatment may also contribute to the high levels of distress during recurrence [14, 15]. Studies reveal that patients are acutely aware of the high probability of recurrent disease following initial treatment, and fears of future diagnostic tests and a general fear of recurrence are common [16–19]. This awareness, however, does not seem to diminish the negative impact that news of a recurrence brings [20]. In a study conducted among patients undergoing initial treatment, survey results revealed that over half of the women involved in the study had four or more significant concerns related to their illness experience [21]. The concerns were evaluated at first interview and at the 6-month interview. A sample of women diagnosed with a gynecological cancer demonstrated the main concerns to be their current illness, the future, and treatment-related issues [21]. At the 6-month interview, the concerns were very similar to the first but with more emphasis on physical symptoms and being unable to continue with their daily activities [21]. Psychological responses to cancer recurrence have been described in the literature as including depressive symptoms, loss of hope for recovery [22], anxiety, fears of death, and difficulties with functional decline [12, 23, 24]. At this difficult time during recurrence, patients are faced with the reality that standard treatment, which was supposed to provide the best chance for a cure, has failed [20, 25].

Perhaps the transition from remission to cancer patient could be best understood by the "Making Sense of Living Under the Shadow of Death" model described by Sarenmalm [15]. Data were collected from 40 in-depth interviews with 20 women diagnosed with recurrent breast cancer. The core category illustrated the process of "making sense of living under the shadow of death," and was based on the women's experiences of adjusting to living with persistent life-threatening illness [15]. Meaning of their recurrence was created in the context of a threat to life. A new view to life was required in coming to terms with the recurrence. Personal growth and transformation was sought through rediscovering changes in attitude and relationships and important life values. The core category encompassed three subcategories: (a) confronting, involving shifting expectations and shifting awareness; (b) struggling/easing distress, entailing losing/fearing, letting go/being reassured; and (c) transcending, involving reevaluating, repatterning relationships, and creating wellness [15]. The first step to be taken to begin this process was confronting the new diagnosis and coming to terms with it. This required a shifting of expectations from cure to palliation and from quantity of life to quality of life [15]. It was observed that a dialectical movement brought the women in the study into suffering the experience of distressful losses and fears, and then moving on to the healing process of easing the distress by letting go of the losses and being reassured [15]. This thought process enabled them to develop meaning and transcendence to their current situation. Sarenmalm described this model to be an "ongoing and interactive process, nonlinear and nonsequential … An overlapping, emerging, fading, and reemerging movement between categories [15]." Ultimately, as individuals manage and adapt to the myriad of changes precipitated by the disease and its treatment, adjustment to cancer will be an ongoing personal transition [26]. Brennan explains that the degree of adjustment depends on the appraisal of and coping response to the huge diversity of experience faced by people living with cancer [26]. Transitions have been described as a process that involves the changes in identity, role and relationship, abilities, and behaviors as patients begin to internalize and come to terms with their new diagnosis [27–30].

The experience lived through the end of the survivorship journey may not be a new experience but rather an exacerbation of the previous encountered emotions and physical distresses already experienced [31]. As more and more patients reach the end of their cancer trajectory, it is crucial for more research to develop and investigate areas of end-of-life care among those survivors that are now succumbing to their cancer or the chronic effects of their cancer treatment. Cancer survivorship research has been defined as those services which "seek to identify, examine and prevent and control adverse cancer related and treatment related outcomes (such as pain, lymphedema, sexual dysfunction, second cancers, functional impairment and poor quality of life) – provide a knowledge base regarding optimal follow up care and surveillance of cancer survivors – optimize health after cancer treatment [32]." Currently, Feuerstein's Biopsychosocial Model of Cancer Survivorship is the only model that incorporates end-of-life care to the definition of cancer survivorship [33]. The definition that is most accepted now is one that encompasses all areas of the cancer trajectory, from diagnosis to death. Perhaps expanding this definition of survivorship research to encompass end of life will underscore the importance of end-of-life care for cancer survivors.

## Cases

In order to illustrate the diversity of needs in cancer survivors who now face the end of life, the following cases are presented.

### *Prolonged Survival Followed by Recurrence and End of Life*

Beth G was a cancer survivor first diagnosed with lymphoma while a college student. She underwent chemotherapy and radiation and did very well with no evidence of further disease. Beth resumed her usual activities and was able to complete her college degree, obtain masters in accounting, and launch a successful accounting firm. Beth was a strong advocate for other cancer survivors and was an active volunteer at the cancer center where she was treated. She had also become very focused on an aggressive exercise program and maintained a healthy diet and was very diligent in routine follow-up medical care. Beth was initially hesitant to form any serious relationship but at age 40 she was married. Unfortunately, at age 42 Beth experienced a recurrence of her lymphoma with extensive metastasis and despite an intensive course of chemotherapy her disease did not respond to treatment.

Beth and her husband have been informed that her disease has progressed and that her prognosis is poor. Both Beth and her husband are shocked to hear this news, both questioning the accuracy of the latest scans. Both described the unfairness of the cancer recurrence when she has tried so hard to be healthy.

### *Poor Prognosis Cancer/Advanced at Time of Diagnosis but Still Seeking Treatment*

Max W was a 55-year-old plumber who had experienced GI symptoms over several months prior to being diagnosed with pancreatic cancer. He avoided seeking health care as he was busy with a demanding job, three teenagers, and caring for his wife who was disabled from lupus. Although Max was informed at diagnosis that his tumor was advanced and prognosis poor, Max insisted that he would be a survivor. He was quick to remind everyone that he had much to live for and would be a fighter.

Max underwent extensive chemotherapy including participation in clinical trials. He struggled to maintain his home and work responsibilities and generally coped by trying to deny his illness. At his most recent office visit, the oncologist and nurse attempted to discuss with Max the completion of an advance directive and that he should also consider transition to hospice care as he now has extensive metastasis. Max refused, still insisting that he was confident the treatment would work and he would “beat” the cancer.

## *End-of-Life Care for Survivors with no Evidence of Disease but Fatal Toxicities*

Emma H was a 52-year-old woman diagnosed with breast cancer. She underwent surgery, chemotherapy, and radiation and recovered from the initial treatment with some problems of persistent fatigue and depression. After 2 years of disease-free status, Emma developed delayed toxicities including pulmonary and cardiac failure. Her follow-up breast cancer surveillance continued to confirm no evidence of recurrent disease, but despite aggressive attention to her cardiopulmonary problems, she developed progressive heart failure.

Emma's depression worsened as she confronted the reality that she had survived cancer yet was now disabled from the toxicities of treatment. Emma voiced regret at having received such aggressive treatments. She has told her family that she is considering seeking alternative treatment in Mexico as she feels that traditional treatments have failed her and she is desperate for continued survival.

## *The Existential/Spiritual Crisis of End of Life*

Jonathan R was a college athlete whose renal cell cancer was diagnosed during an x-ray he received following a sports injury. Jonathan was aware that he was fortunate that his cancer was diagnosed so early and that his excellent prognosis would not have been possible had his cancer been diagnosed at a later stage, far more common in renal cell cancer.

Over the next 20 years, Jonathan struggled to find meaning in his life as a cancer survivor. He gave up his earlier career goals to become a professional athlete, pursuing instead a variety of professional endeavors that he hoped would be more meaningful and more valued use of his "miracle" survivorship. Almost 25 years after his original diagnosis, Jonathan was diagnosed with a second tumor, this time a primary colon cancer but late stage with liver metastasis. On his initial hospital admission, Jonathan confides in the social worker that he believes this second diagnosis is punishment from God since he never really "made anything of himself" after the miracle of his first cancer. He tells the social worker that he will decline any treatment for the new diagnosis, expressing that it is his destiny to die from cancer.

## *The Chronic, Seriously Ill Survivor*

Roberta is a 70-year-old woman diagnosed with stage IV ovarian cancer. Roberta is surrounded by a supportive family of children, grandchildren, and her husband, and she has far exceeded the original estimates for her survival. Over the years, Roberta has responded well to a number of chemotherapy regimens. Her disease has been kept under control and she has impressed the physicians by her response to a recent Phase I trial and intraperitoneal treatment.

Over the past few years Roberta has experienced numerous crises including a bowel obstruction, renal obstruction, pathological fracture, and numerous infections. The frequency of these crises has increased and on several occasions her condition has been quite serious. However, she has responded to treatment and has consistently expressed her desire for continued treatment, always supported in these decisions by her close supportive family.

During her current hospitalization, tests reveal that Roberta is now experiencing renal failure, likely related to toxicity from the latest trial. Her physician unfortunately recognizes that this will be very difficult to reverse and he has doubts about initiating dialysis given other emerging problems and her poor prognosis. An initial patient/family meeting is convened when it becomes evident that Roberta and her family are well prepared to face chronic and even serious health problems but are not at all prepared to address the possibility of death.

## Potential Solutions

In the IOM report, four essential components of patient-centered survivorship care and ten recommendations for improving the care provided to survivors were recognized [1]. The recommendations are broad and comprehensive and require the cooperation of health-care providers, researchers, government bodies, and policymakers if change is to be achieved. There are several potential solutions to correct the gaps in health-care delivery already identified. Early integration, psychological and spiritual care, and support for family caregivers are perhaps the areas where change would be most beneficial and needed for patients experiencing the final phase of cancer survivorship. Currently, much emphasis has been given to oncologists in taking responsibility for the continued care of the patient during survivorship. Oncologists are familiar with their patient's initial diagnosis and treatment, know the long-term effects of the treatments the patient received, and they have created a very important relationship of trust with their patient [7, 34].

Unfortunately, the field of oncology has not been able to sustain the numbers of professionals needed for the growing trend of cancer survivors. The IOM examined the oncology workforce issue in *Ensuring Quality Cancer Care through the Oncology Workforce: Sustaining Care in the 21st Century* based on a workshop on this subject [35]. It was noted that the current crisis in the workforce will continue to worsen as more oncologists are aging and retiring, and the number of cancer survivors will continue to grow. The report suggests that there will be a significant demand for oncologists to be available for those diagnosed or undergoing active treatment and that other models such as nurse practitioner-run survivorship clinics and involving primary care physician with survivorship care will be needed. While these solutions hold promise, primary care physicians often feel ill-equipped to continue the care the oncologist began [7]. Educating and increasing awareness of the oncology force on cancer survivorship particularly end-of-life care and involving an interdisciplinary team to address issues in palliative care in cancer survivors would address the problems seen with the current system.

Another major factor contributing to this problem has been the lack of communication between those involved in patient care. Jacobs [7], describing this gap in the continuum of care for cancer survivors, proposed development of treatment summaries and survivorship care plans that may serve as effective communication tools that will provide a focus for the evolving field of adult survivorship. As patient is being transitioned from their oncologist to their primary care physician, the patient's quality of care may become compromised due to the poor communication between oncologist and primary care physician and the primary care physician's limited ability to provide survivorship-specific care [7]. A survivorship care plan not only provides an effective communication tool and a clear roadmap for the patient leaving the protective environment in which they received initial care, but it must also address issues concerning palliative care and end of life. This will enable the early integration of palliative care into survivorship care as aspects of spiritual and palliative care will be offered to them as a protocol in their survivorship care plan. For the protocol to be successful in providing this well-rounded palliative and spiritual aspects of care, it is important to develop an interdisciplinary team that will address the biopsychosocial aspects of survivorship and in that model include end-of-life care education and support necessary to prepare patients and families for the possibility of recurrence and death.

Family caregivers, although profoundly impacted by a loved one's cancer diagnosis, have received only minimal attention by most health-care providers who are focused primarily upon the physical needs of the patient. Only recently, as attention has been expanded to the psycho-social-spiritual needs of the patient, has a body of literature been developed that begins to recognize the multidimensional needs of family caregivers throughout the continuum of the cancer experience [36–43]. The goals of support should be to enable family caregivers to maintain the patient's comfort, enhance the patient's quality of life, and to prevent or minimize unnecessary caregiver distress [36].

The oncology care team can play a significant role to reduce caregivers' anxiety, depression, and sense of frustration by identifying patients' home care needs, tailoring plans of care, and then instructing family members about how to implement them [36]. To be able to provide this support, it is important that a partnership be formed between the health-care professional and family caregivers around the patient's plan of care. To accomplish this, a patient family member-focused plan for care that recognizes the caregiver's capabilities should be developed [36]. Aside from establishing a focused partnership with the oncology health-care team, Given [36] also has identified three key interventions and strategies to support family caregivers (Table 12.3). The interventions address the caregivers' priority needs such as the need for information and education; the ability to mobilize formal and informal sources of assistance; and strategies for maintaining physical health, positive attitudes, and well-being. These areas must be tailored to the different levels of knowledge and skill, level of burden, level of care demand, and support received from other family members.

**Table 12.3** Intervention and strategies in support of family caregivers (Adapted from Given et al. [44] and Puchalski and Ferrell [45])

| | |
|---|---|
| *Information* | *Psychotherapeutic* |
| Family conferences | Support groups |
| Skills training | Psychologists/counselors |
| Problem-solving strategies | Psychiatric referral |
| Caregiver training | Counseling sessions |
| Books, videos, CD ROMs, Web pages | Telephone |
| Help sheets | In person |
| *Mobilizing resources* | *Spiritual* |
| Support groups | Spiritual counseling |
| Caregiver classes | Encourage utilization of established spiritual practices |
| Visiting nurses | |
| Chore services | Participation in spiritual or faith communities |

It is a common misconception of many individuals, including patients and medical personnel, that cancer patients with recurrent or progressive disease would be most concerned about pain, suffering, and dying. However, a few studies [46, 47] have illustrated that the patients' main concerns are centered around family and the prospect of becoming a burden. Therefore, addressing this issue benefits not only the caregiver but also the patient. The Clinical Practice Guidelines for Quality Palliative Care addresses this issue by emphasizing the need and involvement of an interdisciplinary team with patient-population-specific skills in the assessment and management of social and practical needs during the illness of the patient [5]. The team would be involved, for example, conducting routine patient and family meetings to assess understanding and address questions; provide information and help with decision making; discuss goals of care and advance care planning; determine wishes, preferences, hopes, and fears; provide emotional and social support; and enhance communication [5].

## Future Research to Test Proposed Approaches

To change systems and implement the potential solutions proposed, research is needed in end-of-life care for patients in their cancer trajectory. Much has yet to be learned and developed in transitional aspects in cancer care to prepare clinicians for the important issues related to helping patients and families face the end of life (Table 12.4). Both palliative care and end-of-life care are concepts that have expanded within the last decade to address the supportive care needs that accompany the occurrence of life-threatening disease. Each concept addresses different aspects in the trajectory of cancer. With the publication by the National Consensus Project (NCP) of Clinical Practice Guidelines for Quality Palliative Care, the view of palliative care within the trajectory of disease has changed [49].

**Table 12.4** Potential areas for research in end-of-life care (Adapted from Ferrell and Coyle [48])

| Critical areas of end-of-life (EOL) care | Example of area content | Example of potential areas of inquiry |
|---|---|---|
| 1. The concept of palliative care | A. Definition of palliative care<br>B. Important goals/characteristics of palliative care:<br>1. Dignity/respect<br>2. Relief of symptoms<br>3. Peaceful death<br>4. Ethical issues<br>5. Patient control/choices<br>C. Importance of interdisciplinary collaboration | • Refinement of definition/criteria for palliative care<br>• Descriptive studies of interdisciplinary involvement and related outcomes |
| 2. Quality of life (QOL) at the EOL | A. Recognition of multiple dimensions of QOL at the EOL<br>1. Physical well-being<br>2. Psychological well-being<br>3. Social well-being<br>4. Spiritual well-being | • Development/testing of QOL instruments for use in palliative care<br>• Refinement of research methods to decrease patient burden in QOL assessment<br>• Development/testing of QOL instruments for family caregivers |
| 3. Pain management at EOL | A. Definition of pain<br>B. Assessment of pain<br>C. Assessment of meaning of pain<br>D. Pharmacological management of pain at EOL<br>E. Physical pain vs. suffering<br>F. Principles of addiction, tolerance, and dependence | • Methods of assessing pain in the nonverbal or confused patient<br>• Refine methods for pain assessment to decrease patient burden<br>• Development of pain measurement that incorporate all dimensions of pain at EOL (e.g., spiritual pain)<br>• Development/evaluation of teaching programs for patient/families to decrease fears regarding pain management |
| 4. Other symptoms management at EOL | A. Assessment and management of common EOL symptoms<br>1. Dyspnea/cough<br>2. Nausea/vomiting<br>3. Dehydration/nutrition<br>4. Altered mental status/delirium/terminal restlessness<br>5. Anxiety/depression<br>6. Weakness/fatigue<br>7. Dysphagia<br>8. Incontinence<br>9. Skin Integrity<br>10. Constipation/bowel obstruction<br>11. Agitation/myoclonus | • Descriptive studies to better understand<br>• Symptom prevalence and patterns at EOL<br>• Development of patient/family caregiver education for symptom management, including pharmacological and non-pharmacological treatment<br>• Assessment and management |

(continued)

**Table 12.4** (continued)

| Critical areas of end-of-life (EOL) care | Example of area content | Example of potential areas of inquiry |
|---|---|---|
| 5. Communication with dying patients and families | A. Definition/goals of communication<br>B. Importance of listening<br>C. Barriers to communication<br>D. Delivering bad news/truth-telling<br>E. Recognizing family dynamics in communication<br>F. Sensitivity to culture, ethnicity, values, and religion<br>G. Discussion of option/decisions with patients/family<br>H. Communication among interdisciplinary team members/collaboration<br>I. Responding to request for assisted suicide | • Descriptive studies to better determine common areas of concern regarding communication at EOL<br>• Evaluation of protocols for delivering/reinforcing bad news<br>• Studies that explore cultural issues influencing communication<br>• Evaluation of methods that support communication (e.g., written materials, family conferences)<br>• Exploration of decision making my patients and family caregivers<br>• Exploration of causes for assisted suicide and preparation of nurses to respond to request |
| 6. Role/needs of family caregivers in EOL care | A. The importance of recognizing family and caregivers needs at EOL<br>B. Assessment of family needs<br>C. Family dynamics<br>D. Recognizing ethical/cultural influences<br>E. Coping strategies and support systems | • Descriptive studies to enhance understanding of the family caregiver perspective of terminal illness<br>• Studies that explore family dynamics and the family as a unit rather than focus only on single caregivers<br>• Exploratory studies to enhance understanding of cultural influences |
| 7. Care at the time of death | A. Death as a natural process<br>B. Recognizing signs/symptoms of impending death<br>C. Patient/family's fears associated with death<br>D. Preparing for death event<br>1. Health-care providers<br>2. Patient<br>3. Family caregivers<br>E. Physical care at the time of death<br>F. Spiritual care at the time of death | • Evaluation of educational/support approaches to enhance personal death awareness<br>• Evaluation of teaching approaches to prepare families for impending death<br>• Development and evaluation of protocols for care at the time of death, i.e., physical and spiritual care |

(continued)

**Table 12.4** (continued)

| Critical areas of end-of-life (EOL) care | Example of area content | Example of potential areas of inquiry |
|---|---|---|
| 8. Issues of policy, ethics, and law | A. Patient preferences/advance directives<br>B. Assisted suicide<br>C. Euthanasia<br>D. Withdrawing food/fluids<br>E. Discontinuing life support<br>F. Legal issues at the EOL<br>G. Need for changes in health policy<br>H. Confidentiality | • Evaluation of approaches to enhance use of advance directives<br>• Development and evaluation of protocols that promote patient comfort while discontinuing food/fluids and life support<br>• Identification of legal and regularly barriers to optimal EOL care |
| 9. Bereavement | A. Stages/process of grief<br>B. Assessment of grief<br>C. Interventions/resources | • Descriptive studies of grief by patients, families, and staff with attention to cultural considerations<br>• Refinement of efficient methods of grief assessment |

Palliative care is defined as "medical care provided by an interdisciplinary team, including the professions of medicine, nursing, social work, chaplaincy, counseling, nursing assistant, and other health care professions focused on the relief of suffering and support for the best possible quality of life for patients facing serious life-threatening illness and their families. It aims to identify and address the physical, psychological, spiritual, and practical burdens of illness [49]." As illustrated in Fig. 12.2, palliative care begins at the time of diagnosis of a serious disease, and continues throughout treatment, cure, or until death, and involves the family during the bereavement period. Many hospitals may currently have a palliative care program and a survivorship care program in place at their institution but they often exist as separate entities. Therefore, merging palliative care and survivorship care programs would be an area worth further research and investing to better understand and implement quality-of-life–specific care.

Due to the origins of the palliative care concept from the hospice movement in the 1960s [46], there is a strong association between palliative care hospice and end-of-life care. This common misconception has limited the ability of implementing palliative early care in the disease trajectory. Researchers at the City of Hope Medical Center are currently conducting a study, "Palliative Care for Quality of Life and Symptom Concerns in Lung cancer," that focuses on implementing palliative care at the time of initial diagnosis of lung cancer. The synergy of simultaneous research in Early Stage, Late Stage, and Family Caregiver perspectives and the interdisciplinary care plan developed to address holistically the patient's needs will advance the science of palliative care and add to the evidence base of quality of life in lung cancer [50].

Finally, there are barriers in the multiple transitions a patient is confronted with during their cancer trajectory that have not been addressed. As noted earlier, cancer

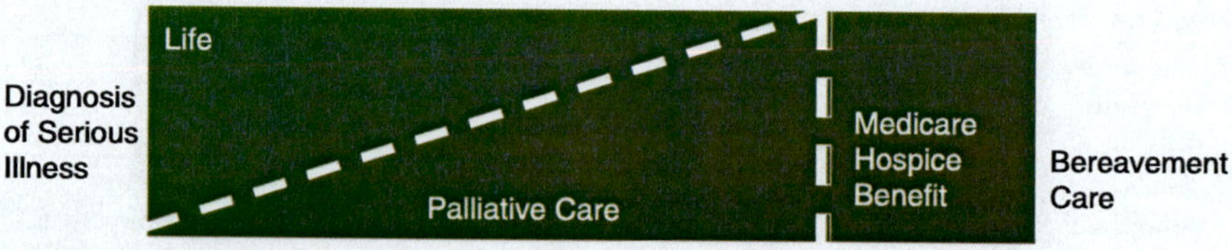


**Fig. 12.2** Palliative care

survivorship research is lacking greatly in the area of transitions. A limited amount of research has been done on the role of palliative care in patients transitioning from remission to recurrence and much less has been studied in the transition of recurrence to end of life. Barriers in transition can be appreciated now that the study of cancer survivorship is expanding. This is unfortunate as the population of cancer survivors grows and more is needed to explore the palliative needs through their trajectory. The multidimensional nature of care at the end of life and the vulnerability of the population are but two examples of factors that pose special challenges to this area of research. The challenge of nursing research in palliative care should be prefaced by a discussion of the benefits. Although even the mention of conducting research with dying patients and their burdened families immediately creates concerns, there are in fact many benefits to participants. Participating in research, even at this most vulnerable and sensitive time of life, provides the opportunity for research subjects to contribute to others. Research participation often provides an opportunity to derive meaning from illness and to feel that one's suffering will provide benefit to others [51–53].

## Implications for Policy, Practice, Reimbursement

End-of-life care is not just the concern of health-care professionals, patients, and families but it is also a concern for the public health and health policy [54]. There has been increasing interest and activity within the public policy arena at the state and federal levels of government that can create needed improvement in end-of-life care [55] (Table 12.5).

A major barrier to adequate palliative care has been the institutionalization of a system that focuses on either active therapy or palliative care and does not allow the appropriate integration between these two approaches [2]. This results in patients unfairly needing to choose between treatment and palliative care rather than integrating it with the treatment plan. This is unfortunate since patients with cancer, at all stages, identify substantial physical, psychological, functional, and spiritual needs [46]. The old paradigm of palliative care no longer fits [46]. The more recent view of palliative care suggests that both disease-oriented and palliative treatments should be available over the spectrum of disease stages, and that the availability of palliative care services should be based on need and not on life expectancy [46] (Fig. 12.2).

**Table 12.5** Policy recommendations for improving end-of-life care (Adapted from Field and Cassel [56], Jennings et al. [57], and America's Care of Serious Illness [58])

| Recommendations for: | | |
|---|---|---|
| Institute of Medicine | Approaching just access | Elected officials and policymakers |
| • Ask health-care professional to commit themselves to improving care for dying patients and to using existing knowledge effectively to prevent and relieve pain and other symptoms<br>• Address deficiencies in the health-care system through improved methods for measuring quality, tools for accountability by providers, revised financing systems to encourage better coordination of care, and reformed drug-prescribing laws<br>• Developing medical education to ensure that practitioners have the relevant attitudes, knowledge, and skills to provide excellent care for dying patients<br>• Make palliative care a defined are of expertise, education, and research | • Public policy should expand the scope of hospice services<br>• Policymakers should act immediately to bring about policy reform of the absolute application of an individual's prognosis as a primary criterion for reimbursement of services<br>• Access and delivery of hospice care should be expanded to dying persons residing in long-term care facilities<br>• Leaders in the hospice community and in mainstream medicine must promote hospice–hospital partnerships to meet current and projected needs of the rapidly expanding volume of chronically and terminally ill patients<br>• Educational programs should be developed to "reintroduce" hospice and palliative care to the public in light of their new capabilities, flexibility, and accessibility | • Fund palliative care team training and technical assistance for all hospitals in your state<br>• Include palliative care indicators in your state's quality programs for your state health plan and Medicaid programs<br>• Ensure the development of palliative care programs in public and sole community provider hospitals, as these hospitals provide care to the underserved and most vulnerable patient populations<br>• Promote and pass legislation requiring all hospitals to offer palliative care services as a condition of Medicare and Medicaid reimbursement<br>• Promote and pass legislation requiring all state-supported medical schools to have affiliations with hospital palliative care programs<br>• Create loan-forgiveness programs for nurses and physicians seeking postgraduate palliative care training<br>• Create a statewide resource center for promotion of access to quality palliative care services (see New York Palliative care Training Act-Public Health Law Article 28 at http://public.leginfo.state.ny.us/menuf.cgi)<br>• Support congressional initiatives that increase National Institutes of Health and Veteran's Health Administration funding for palliative care research<br>• For a state directory of hospital palliative care programs, visit http://www.getpalliativecare.org |

This change in thinking emerged from a new understanding that problems at the end of life have their origins at an earlier time in the trajectory of disease [59]. Symptoms not treated early at the onset become very difficult to manage in the last days of life [59]. Unfortunately that is not the current practice. The objective of palliative care is to provide the patient with comfort and enhance the quality of life rather than the quantity of life. By implementing at an early stage what is recommended by the Clinical Practice Guidelines for Quality Palliative Care, we may begin to address this problem. The guidelines cover a spectrum of areas in which the health-care professional, family, and patient can all benefit from and, more importantly, treat the patient's symptoms before it becomes difficult to manage (Table 12.6).

From its origins outside mainstream health care, palliative care is now emerging as an integrated part of mainstream health-care delivery. This process of integration is, however, not without difficulty. The traditional focus of medical care is in curing the disease and failure to do so may be perceived as failure. This inability to deal with death has often meant that dying patients and their families are marginalized, with their needs unrecognized and unmet [61]. This is very unfortunate, especially with guidelines available that would address and make this already very stressful and difficult situation a little bit easier to bear. Again the NCP Guidelines provide us with useful tools to offer optimal care. Palliative care is best achieved through close coordination and partnerships between palliative care and hospice programs and is operationalized through effective management of pain and other distressing symptoms

**Table 12.6** Physical aspects of care (Adapted from National Consensus Project Guidelines [60])

Guideline 2.1 Pain, other symptoms, and side effects are managed based upon the best available evidence, with attention to disease-specific pain and symptoms, which is skillfully and systematically applied

- Regular ongoing assessment of pain, nonpain symptoms (including but not limited to shortness of breath, nausea, fatigue and weakness, anorexia, insomnia, anxiety, depression, confusion, and constipation), treatment side effects, and functional capacities are documented through a systematic process. Validated instruments, where available, should be utilized. Symptom assessment in children and cognitively impaired patients should be performed by appropriately trained professionals with appropriate tools
- The outcomes of pain and symptom management is the safe and timely reduction of pain and symptom levels, for as long as the symptom persists, to a level that is acceptable to the patient or the family if the patient is unable to report distress
- Barriers to effective pain management should be recognized and addressed, including inappropriate fears of the risk of side effects, addiction, respiratory depression, and hasting of death in association with opioid analgesics
- Family understanding of the disease and its consequences, symptoms, side effects, functional impairment, and treatment is assessed. The capacity of the family to secure and provide needed care and to cope with the illness and its consequences is assessed with consideration of culture and development
- Treatment of distressing symptoms and side effects incorporates pharmacological, non-pharmacological, and complementary/supportive therapies. Approach to the relief of suffering is comprehensive, addressing physical, psychological, social, and spiritual aspects
- Family is educated and supported to provide safe and appropriate comfort measures to the patient. Family is provided with backup resources for response to urgent needs

while incorporating psychosocial and spiritual care with consideration of patient/family needs, preferences, values, beliefs, and culture [60]. Evaluation and treatment should be comprehensive and patient-centered with a focus on the central role of the family unit in decision making [60]. The NCP guidelines agreed on key elements in palliative care such as serving all patient population with a chronic or life-threatening disease, patient- and family-centered care, timing the start of palliative care at the time of diagnosis, comprehensive care, and the care consisting of an interdisciplinary team [60]. Implementing the NCP guidelines will help bridge the gap observed with health-care professionals and palliative care. Death and palliative care should not be seen as a failure if health-care providers change their definition of success and allow it to include the gratification that comes with providing these hurting families and patients with tools necessary to face this transition.

Understanding end-of-life concerns in what may seem a contradicting phase of the cancer survivorship trajectory is important as more patients, who initially responded to treatment, die from their disease. Moreover, research is needed to test the merging of survivorship and palliative care programs and early implementation of palliative care, to further explore barriers in transitions. Being able to offer patients the benefits of palliative care regardless of their stage of disease should be priority for quality oncology care.

## References

1. Hewitt M, Greenfield S, Ellen S. From cancer patient to cancer survivors: lost in transition. Washington, DC: The National Academies Press; 2006.
2. Foley K, Gelband H. Improving palliative care for cancer. Washington, DC: National Academy Press; 2001.
3. Petrelli NJ, Winer EP, Brahmer J, Dubey S, Smith S, Thomas C, et al. Clinical cancer advances 2009: major research advances in cancer treatment, prevention, and screening – A report from the American Society of Clinical Oncology. J Clin Oncol. 2009;27(35):6052–69.
4. Society AC. Cancer facts & figures 2009. Atlanta: American Cancer Society; 2009.
5. National Consensus Project for Quality Palliative Care. Clinical practice guidelines for quality palliative care. Second edition. 2009. http://www.nationalconsensusproject.org.117–128
6. Clark E, Stovall E, Leigh S, Siu A, Austin D, Rowland J. Imperatives for quality cancer care: access, advocacy, action, and accountability. Silver Springs: National Coalition for Cancer Survivorship (NCCS); 1996.
7. Jacobs LA, Palmer SC, Schwartz LA, DeMichele A, Mao JJ, Carver J, et al. Adult cancer survivorship: evolution, research, and planning care. CA Cancer J Clin. 2009;59(6):391–410.
8. LIVESTRONG™. Poll finds nearly half of people living with cancer feel their non-medical needs are unmet by the healthcare system. 2004. http://www.livestrong.org/site/apps/nlnet/content2.aspx?c=khLXK1PxHmF&b=2661081&ct=3756677. Accessed 17 Feb 2010.
9. Jemal A, Siegel R, Ward E, Murray T, Xu J, Thun MJ. Cancer statistics, 2007. CA Cancer J Clin. 2007;57(1):43–66.
10. Ng AK, Travis LB. Subsequent malignant neoplasms in cancer survivors. Cancer J. 2008;14(6):429–34.
11. Andersen BL, Shapiro CL, Farrar WB, Crespin T, Wells-DiGregorio S. Psychological responses to cancer recurrence. Cancer. 2005;104(7):1540–7.
12. Mahon S. Exploring the psychosocial meaning of recurrent cancer: a descriptive study. Cancer Nurs. 1997;20(3):178–86.

13. Lazarus RS, Folkman S. Stress, appraisal, and coping. New York: Springer; 1984.
14. Mahon S, Casperson D. Psychosocial concerns associated with recurrent cancer. Cancer Pract. 1995;3(6):372–80.
15. Kenne Sarenmalm E, Thoren-Jonsson A-L, Gaston-Johansson F, Ohlen J. Making sense of living under the shadow of death: adjusting to a recurrent breast cancer illness. Qual Health Res. 2009;19(8):1116–30.
16. Ferrell B. The quality of lives: 1, 525 voices of cancer. Oncol Nurs Forum. 1996;23(6):909–16.
17. Padilla G, Mishel M, Grant M. Uncertainty and quality of life. Qual Life Res. 1992;1(3):155–65.
18. Mishel M, Padilla G, Grant M, Sorenson D. Uncertainty in illness theory: a replication of the mediating effects of mastery and coping. Nurs Res. 1991;40(4):236–40.
19. Wenzel LB, Donnelly JP, Fowler JM, Habbal R, Taylor TH, Aziz N, et al. Resilience, reflection, and residual stress in ovarian cancer survivorship: a gynecologic oncology group study. Psycho Oncol. 2002;11(2):142–53.
20. Ekwall E, Ternestedt B, Sorbe B. Recurrence of ovarian cancer-living in limbo. Cancer Nurs. 2007;30(4):270–7.
21. Katie B, Beaver K, Kitchener H, O'Neill J, Farrell C. Women's experiences of information, psychological distress and worry after treatment for gynaecological cancer. Patient Educ Couns. 2005;56(2):225–32.
22. Mahon S, Cella D, Donovan M. Psychosocial adjustment to recurrent cancer. Oncol Nurs Forum. 1990;17(3):47–52.
23. Munkres A, Oberst M, Hughes S. Appraisal of illness, symptom distress, self-care burden, and mood states in patients receiving chemotherapy for initial and recurrent cancer. Oncol Nurs Forum. 1992;19(8):1201–9.
24. Weisman AD, Worden JW. The emotional impact of recurrent cancer. J Psychosoc Oncol. 1986;3(4):5–16.
25. Karen B, Lorraine R. Psychosocial impact of recurrent cancer. Eur J Oncol Nurs Off J Eur Oncol Nurs Soc. 2000;4(1):29–38.
26. Brennan J. Adjustment to cancer – coping or personal transition? Psychooncology. 2001;10(1):1–18.
27. Meleis A, Sawyer L, Im E, Messias DH, Schumacher K. Experiencing transitions: an emerging middle-range theory. Adv Nurs Sci. 2000;23(1):12–28.
28. Bridges W. Managing transitions: making the most of change. 2nd ed. London: Nicholas Brealy; 2006.
29. Schumacher K. Transitions: a central concept in nursing. Image J Nurs Scholarsh. 1994;26(2):119–27.
30. Goodman J, Schlossberg N, Anderson L. Counseling adults in transition: linking practice with theory. 3rd ed. New York: Springer; 2006.
31. Lunney JR, O'Mara A. The end of the survival journey. Semin Oncol Nurs. 2001;17(4):274–8.
32. Rowland JH. What are cancer survivors telling us? Cancer J. 2008;14(6):361–8.
33. Feuerstein M. Cancer survivorship: research, practice, and policy. In: Feuerstein M, editor. Handbook of cancer survivorship. New York: Springer; 2007. p. 483–94.
34. Building a bridge of continued care for cancer survivors. J Oncol Pract. 2006;2(2):77–82.
35. Patlak M, Levit L. Ensuring quality cancer care through the oncology workforce: sustaining care in the 21st century. Workshop summary. Washington, DC: National Academies Press; 2009.
36. Given BA, Given CW, Kozachik S. Family support in advanced cancer. Cancer J Clin. 2001;51(4):213–31.
37. Given B, Wyatt G, Given C, Sherwood P, Gift A, De Voss D, et al. Burden and depression among caregivers of patients with cancer at the end of life. Oncol Nurs Forum. 2004;31(6):1105–17.
38. Lewis F. The relational model of functioning with cancer: a family-focused framework for nursing practice. In: Miaskowski C, Buchesel P, editors. Cancer across health care sites. St Louis: Mosby; 1999. p. 319–31.
39. Marcus Lewis F. Family-focused oncology nursing research. Oncol Nurs Forum. 2004;31(2):288–92.

40. Northouse L, Kershaw T, Mood D, Schafenacker A. Effects of a family intervention on the quality of life of women with recurrent breast cancer and their family caregivers. Psychooncology. 2005;14:478–91.
41. Northouse LL, Walker J, Schafenacker A, Mood D, Mellon S, Galvin E, et al. A family-based program of care for women with recurrent breast cancer and their family members. Oncol Nurs Forum. 2002;29(10):1411–9.
42. Zhang AY, Siminoff LA. The role of the family in treatment decision making by patients with cancer. Oncol Nurs Forum. 2003;30(6):1022–8.
43. Eilers J. Family issues and perspectives. In: Whedon M, Wujik D, editors. Blood and marrow stem cell transplantation: principles, practice, and nursing insights. 2nd ed. Sudburg: Jones and Bartlett; 1997. p. 442–56.
44. Given BA, Given CW, Kozachik S. Family support in advanced cancer. CA Cancer J Clin. 2001;51(4):213–31.
45. Puchalski C, Ferrell B. Making health care whole: integrating spirituality into patient care. West Conshohocken: Templeton Press; 2010.
46. Dudgeon D. When does palliative care begin? A needs assessment of cancer patients with recurrent disease. J Palliat Care. 1995;11(1):5–9.
47. Silberfarb P. Psychosocial aspects of neoplastic disease: I. Functional status of breast cancer patients during different treatment regimens. Am J Psychiatry. 1980;137(4):450–5.
48. Ferrell B, Coyle N. Oxford textbook of palliative nursing. 3rd ed. New York: Oxford University Press; 2010.
49. NCP. Clinical practice guidelines for quality palliative care. 2004. http://www.nationalconsensusproject.org.
50. Ferrell B (Principle Investigator). Palliative care for quality of life and symptom concerns in lung cancer. P01 Funded by National Cancer Institute #P01 CA136396.
51. Kristjanson L, Coyle N. Qualitative research. In: Doyle D, Hanks G, Cherny NI, Calman K, editors. Oxford textbook of palliative medicine. 3rd ed. Oxford: Oxford University Press; 2004. p. 138–44.
52. Kuebler KK, Lynn J, Von Rohen J. Perspectives in palliative care. Semin Oncol Nurs. 2005;21(1):2–10.
53. David C, Betty F, Jane K, Levetown M, Merriman MP, Ramey M, et al. NHPCO Task Force Statement on the ethics of hospice participation in research. J Palliat Med. 2001;4(4):441–9.
54. Scanlon C. Public policy and end-of-life care: the nurse's role. In: Ferrell B, Coyle N, editors. Textbook of palliative nursing. 3rd ed. New York: Oxford University Press; 2010.
55. Schuster L, Kabcenell A. Improving care for the end of life: a source book for health care managers and clinicians. New York: Oxford University Press; 2000.
56. Field M, Casse C. Approaching death: improving care at the end of life. Washington, DC: National Academy Press; 1997.
57. Jennings B, Ryndes T, D'Onofrio C, Baily MA. Access to hospice care. Expanding boundaries, overcoming barriers. The Hastings Center report. 2003;Suppl:S3-7, S9-713, S715-71321 passim.
58. America's Care of Serious Illness: A State-by-State Report Card on Access to Palliative Care in our Nation's Hospital: Center to Advance Palliative Care and National Palliative Care Research Center; 2008.
59. Cecilia S, Amanda M, Tokuo Y, Andreas U. Palliative care: The World Health Organization's global perspective. J Pain Symptom Manage. 2002;24(2):91–6.
60. National Concensus Project. Clinical practice guidelines for quality palliative care. 2004. http://www.nationalconsensusproject.org.
61. Duncan W. Caring or curing: conflicts of choice. J R Soc Med. 1985;78(7):526–35.

# Chapter 13
# Building a Critical Mass of Health-Care Providers, Administrators, and Services for Cancer Survivors

**Marcia Grant and Denice Economou**

## Introduction

To build a critical mass of health-care providers, administrators, and services for cancer survivors, education about cancer survivorship and multidiscipline involvement in survivorship care activities is the initial and essential step. One cannot practice what one does not know. This education is most successful when developed by those with educational expertise. This chapter focuses on the initial definitions needed to begin an educational program in cancer survivorship care, approaches to define the content or curriculum needed, approaches to conducting educational needs assessments, how to formulate educational objectives, how to identify appropriate teaching methods, and will end with approaches to evaluations. Examples focused on cancer survivorship care are provided throughout.

Innovative educational efforts in survivorship care are beginning to emerge as a National Action Plan for Cancer Survivorship was identified along with the recommended content of a survivorship program (Table 13.1) [1]. Providing survivorship care in general requires an understanding of the overall picture of survivorship care and how this content applies to each discipline involved in this care. Curriculum has been developed to help medical schools and nursing schools improve the understanding of cancer survivorship for health-care professionals and anticipate their health needs for their future (Table 13.2). The Institute of Medicine (IOM) report on Cancer Survivorship (2006) defined the components of survivorship care. This report also included raising awareness of the needs of cancer survivors and recognizing that surviving cancer will change the patients' future health-care concerns and will affect their families and caregivers as well.

The definition of a cancer survivor varies across organizations, institutions, and settings. Survivorship according to the IOM report begins at the time of diagnosis and beyond and includes the family and caregivers. Other programs may refer to cancer survivors as patients who have completed cancer treatment, and still others

M. Grant (✉)
Nursing Research and Education, City of Hope National Medical Center, Duarte, CA, USA
e-mail: mgrant@coh.org

M. Feuerstein and P.A. Ganz (eds.), *Health Services for Cancer Survivors*,
DOI 10.1007/978-1-4419-1348-7_13, © Springer Science+Business Media, LLC 2011

**Table 13.1** A National Action Plan for Cancer Survivorship: Public health strategies (Adapted from IOM Box 4-7 Communication, education, and training, p. 246; [1])

| Administrators | Health professionals | Patients | Public | Components |
|---|---|---|---|---|
| Overview of survivorship care (SC)<br>Develop, test, maintain, and promote patient navigation systems for people living with cancer | Overview of SC. Educate HCP about issues from diagnosis through long-term treatment effects and end-of-life care | Empower with advocacy skills | Strategies to educate that cancer can be a chronic disease. People do survive | Physical |
| Educate policy and decision makers about the role and value of long-term follow-up care<br>Improved quality of life<br>Patient and staff satisfaction | Educate policy and decision makers about the role and value of long-term follow-up care<br>Quality-of-life issues<br>Legal needs<br>Access to clinical trials<br>Multidiscipline resources | Teach survivors how to access and evaluate available information<br>Multidiscipline management – referrals to psychosocial support programs, Occupational Rehabilitation/Physical therapy, Treatment Summary/ Survivorship Care Plan | Positive attitudes toward health maintenance and early diagnosis | Psychosocial |
| QoL | QoL | QoL, spiritual support | QoL | Spiritual |
| Legal needs | Legal needs | Legal needs | Accountability for health care | Coordination |
| Access to clinical trials, positive PR | Access to clinical trials. Positive PR Survival & pt. satisfaction | Positive outcomes – patient satisfaction and improved survival | Access to clinical trials. Positive outcomes – Health Promotion | Media/marketing |
| | | | | Public forums |

**Table 13.2** Professional education programs in cancer survivorship

| | | |
|---|---|---|
| American Society of Clinical Oncology (ASCO) | Education and training – survivorship focused programs | http://www.asco.org |
| Office of Cancer Survivorship | Educational tools and resources for patients and families | http://survivorship.cancer.gov |
| American Academy of Family Physicians | Educational programs related to adult survivors of childhood cancers and general education about cancer risk and improved outcomes | http://search.aafp.org |
| American Cancer Society | Educational resources for survivors after treatment | http://www.cancer.org |
| CancerCare | Resources to help health-care professionals stay informed of current cancer practice and issues in psychosocial oncology | http://www.cancercare.org/professionals/progressional_ed.php |
| Nurse Oncology Education Program (NOEP) | CNE programs for nurses in survivorship care | http://www.noeptexas.org/ |
| Oncology Nursing Society | Clinical practice resources and CNE offerings | http://www.ons.org/clinicalresources |

may define it related to the number of years posttreatment, that is, 5 years posttreatment. One of the first steps in developing a survivorship education program is to decide on a definition of survivorship and address professional and patients' needs related to that setting.

The deficits in education of survivors as well as health-care providers are related to a number of factors. Barriers to providing survivorship education include staffing and financial concerns effecting health-care systems in general today. Growing concerns about deficits in the future oncology workforce of physicians and nurses add to the challenge of providing patient and family education. Health-care providers must be aware of outside services and resources available for survivors and their families. A multidiscipline as well as multisystem approach will provide the most efficient methods for meeting the IOM recommendations for cancer survivorship care.

The IOM components of cancer survivorship care include the following parts: prevention/detection and surveillance, interventions, and coordination (Fig. 13.1). Defining educational activities within those components will be the focus of this chapter.

## *Prevention/Detection*

Prevention and detection are two very important areas for future education and research. This survivorship program component is defined as "prevention of recurrent and new cancers, and of other late effects." Promoting healthy lifestyles is

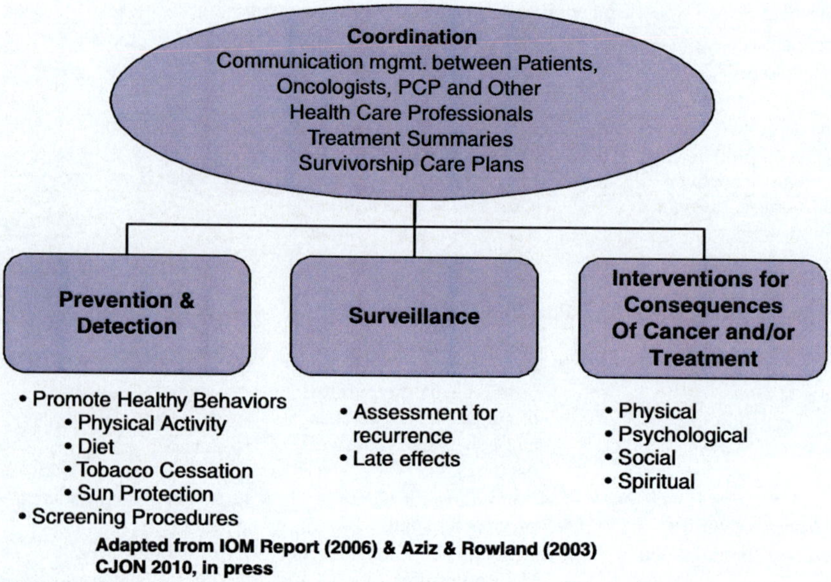


**Fig. 13.1** IOM components of survivorship care

important here and includes techniques that can prevent new cancers and reduce the risk of recurrence. Tobacco cessation is an excellent example of health promotion activities. Educating to provide this type of activity is most difficult because it involves changing behaviors. Changing behaviors involve changing an attitude toward these activities and even with education, improved knowledge does not always lead to behavior changes. In order to meet those challenges as health-care providers, the first step is to understand the attitudinal barriers to these activities and develop educational strategies toward changing those attitudes to promote changes in behavior [2].

Education about this component begins by understanding the population being served. Needs assessment can help gather facts regarding health promotion, smoking, and obesity attitudes. A questionnaire for patients, families, and caregivers can identify barriers to these activities and provide information needed to develop appropriate objectives for the instructional plan. Guidelines for prevention and detection strategies can be found through the American Cancer Society [3] and the National Comprehensive Cancer Network [4]. Once the objectives are identified then the lesson plan can be developed and the teaching methods to be used defined.

An example of a primary prevention program is an ongoing education program for adolescents and young adult cancer survivors on health, wellness, and cancer prevention. Within that program, attitudes toward health behaviors can be identified and promotional strategies incorporated into the education. Providing factual information along with motivational activities and modeling of these behaviors over the length of the course can lead to behavioral changes. Offering follow-up support and booster sessions through written references or electronic access to health professionals can improve outcomes. Behavioral change requires multiple methods to reinforce the desired outcomes. Combining the educational piece, with evidenced-based data on health promotion benefits, and providing guidelines for quality improvement activities to document changes in behavior round out a successful educational plan [5].

## Surveillance

Surveillance as a component of survivorship care involves observing for cancer spread, recurrence, or second cancers. It also includes assessment of medical and psychosocial late effects. Adult survivor guidelines for surveillance remain consensus focused using current evidenced-based studies as appropriate. Recommendations for surveillance postcancer treatment include American Society of Clinical Oncology (ASCO) and the National Coalition of Cancer Network (NCCN). The American Cancer Society (ACS) has been a keystone to teaching the general public on cancer risk and symptoms associated with cancer development. Examples of surveillance programs for cancer survivors may include implementing psychosocial screening for symptoms of distress and depression into follow-up practice; establishing adult surveillance and education programs for survivors of childhood leukemia; developing a resource program for patients and families recently completing treatment which includes information for surveillance follow-up care and testing, general treatment effects, and symptoms to be reported to the physician.

## Interventions

Interventions within survivorship care are focused on providing support for the consequences of cancer and its treatment related to patients and caregivers and supporting quality of life. Using the quality-of-life model related to cancer survivors [6], education can be organized around the four domains. Physical consequences of cancer and its treatment include programs developed around symptom management strategies. Programs related to lymphedema management, skin care, fatigue and pain management, as well as healthy lifestyle education and sexuality and fertility programs are examples of survivorship care needs that can be addressed in these programs. Psychological needs programs can be built around coping, stress management, and family and caregiver support programs. Social issues include issues related to employment, insurance, and disability. Spiritual support programs would include general spiritual guidance or ways to promote resilience, and restorative activities that provide an environment and guidance to deal with existential feelings or religious focused support. Interventions are developed around needs assessments to identify areas of concern within a specific population, late and long-term effects education, health promotion activities, and survivorship celebration days to provide educational events for patients and families.

## *Coordination*

Coordination of care among patients, specialists, and primary care providers to guarantee that survivors' needs are met is essential to the success of survivors' follow-up care. This requires multiple disciplines to work together from the health-care providers to the information technologists in a joint effort to retrieve necessary information, document it, and provide it to the patient and their health-care team. Treatment Summaries (TS) and Survivorship Care Plans (SCPs) fall into this category and have been recommended by the Joint Commission, IOM and the American Society of Clinical Oncology and European Society for Medical Oncology (ASCO-ESMO) for the promotion of quality cancer care [7]. These tools would serve to assess and support uncontrolled side effects, provide for early detection of recurrence or new cancers, and avert preventable consequences such as osteoporosis and heart failure. They provide the framework of communication for all educational activities.

Although this component of survivorship care has become a major challenge due to multiple medical records, multiple treatment sites, and the inability for electronic medical records to link with other electronic documentation programs, strides are being made. Online documentation programs available to everyone have allowed patients to access these tools and begin building their own personal TS and care planning tools. Providers who have limited staff to provide these tools within their practice can be most helpful by educating and supporting their survivors in accessing and completing these tools on their own. Examples of activities being done in this area include providing all newly diagnosed cancer patients with a treatment summary template to begin documenting their treatments starting at diagnosis. Educational classes or instruction sheets can be provided to new patients to assist them with gathering these data [8, 9].

## Assessing the Needs of Specific Education Audiences

Needs assessments are used to gather information about patients, providers, or settings. Assessments may include patients and caregivers but also administrators, health-care professionals, and public consumers. This information helps identify deficits or needs in care, education, or systems, and helps define how best to use resources. Needs assessments are used to plan education or interventions to meet the identified needs. They provide the what, how, and why of program planning. Multiple tools are available and electronic programs such as SURVEY MONKEY can be very helpful for developing a questionnaire that can be provided electronically and will coordinate the results to make using the information easy [10]. Assessment questions may be general to allow short answers and provide the educator with overall information on the population and the interests or concerns they have. Needs assessment tools can target specific areas such as healthy behavior education focused on lifestyles, diet, financial concerns, or health screenings and smoking cessation. Tools may be used as a learner self-assessment to rank the degree of competence staff may have for providing certain skills or interventions. Needs assessments are the first step in planning education that will be relevant to the population being served. Collecting needs assessments from a variety of survivorship populations can be done in different settings. Formal or informal meetings can be used to gather this information. Patients and caregivers can complete needs assessment tools during patient visits, be directed to hospital web sites, or during cancer patient events like a yearly survivorship celebrations. Satisfaction surveys can include open-ended questions regarding patients' wishes or requests that would provide assessment information as well. Examples of needs assessment tools can be found at the Pain & Palliative Care Resource Center, City of Hope (http://www.prc.coh.org). Needs assessments can be important tools for evaluating the knowledge level that administrators or health-care professionals have regarding survivorship care in an institution or setting. Without administrative support for survivorship care, efforts may be stunted or abandoned. Participating in committee meetings where administrators are attending is an important part of program building. Presenting the survivorship care–planned interventions is important, but must begin with the buy-in of the administrator.

Using survivorship care interventions including patient interviews or video programs, such as the IOM Cancer Survivorship video, helps non-health-care providers hear what patients are saying in their own voice. Recruiting support from administrators with experience in cancer either personally or from a family member or friend's knowledge can build understanding in the program's goals from a cognitive or emotional understanding. Assessing these populations is essential to build value for survivorship care and to bring them from casual acceptance to true commitment for the program. Defining the target audience for education is essential. Administrators, health-care professionals, patients, and public require different strategies. Administrators may be interested in physician satisfaction or systems satisfaction as in documentation systems or patient scheduling systems. They are generally interested in satisfaction results and cost-effectiveness of these programs. Health-care professionals need specific medically focused information to meet their needs. Using online educational programs or in-service type programs can provide detailed in-depth information for professionals. Patients need similar medical information that may be individualized but tempered with less detail. Public education is broader and provides more general information. Resources like the ACS, Cancer Care, and the Lance Armstrong Foundation have developed educational materials specifically for the public including caregivers and family focused information.

Additional information to consider when planning a program would include the information gained from the needs assessments as well as considering what the education program has to offer. Can you provide a new perspective for addressing the identified needs? Can you provide concrete answers to the problems or share information from a national perspective to help build new skills or assure the participants that they are providing the level of care needed?

## Developing Learning Objectives Related to Those Needs

Learning objectives define what the educator anticipates that the learner will gain from the activity. They communicate the educators' intent for the participants and provide details to help build the lesson plan. Based on Bloom's Taxonomy of Learning Domains, there are three types of learning: cognitive or knowledge building, affective or attitude growth, and psychomotor or skill building [2]. Learning objectives are developed to provide the specific actions necessary to promote learning in the subject [11].

Cognitive or knowledge-focused objectives provide facts about a specific subject. Objectives could include providing information to improve knowledge or providing new facts regarding a subject. An example of a knowledge objective would be to learn three disease-specific long-term or late effects related to breast cancer treatment. Teaching methods for this type of objective would not only include lecture or didactic format but also include web-based learning modules with posttest evaluations to verify the extent of knowledge improvement. Learning games and handouts to reinforce facts are very helpful.

Attitude objectives are meant to increase positive feelings or emotions around an area or to reinforce or provide new insights into the value placed on a concept by an organization or group. In survivorship, building the case for survivorship care and the phenomena of awareness of the needs associated with cancer survivorship and the long-term and late effects of treatment are essential to growing these programs. The IOM's 2006 report provided a video of patients discussing their needs, which elicits an emotional response in providers and patients who view this video [12]. The awareness of survivors' needs is made very visual. Objectives aimed at raising awareness and emphasizing values and behaviors that meet the organization's goals are attitudinal. An example of an attitude objective would be to assess personal feelings associated with providing survivorship information to your patients. Methods used to carry out this objective might include a general overview lecture, a Lunch & Learn, or a case study to help encourage a discussion about fears or knowledge deficits that may be hindering the action of providing survivorship information to patients. Opening up discussions and providing information regarding survivors' needs are essential and provide the basis for building a philosophy within an institution or setting.

Psychomotor objectives are aimed at improving specific skills. They are used to train staff in new techniques or procedures and are easily measured. An example of a psychomotor objective might be to demonstrate how to complete an SCP. Components of an SCP would be identified and a template might be provided or recommended. Small groups work well for achievement of these objectives. Posttesting, role play, or return demonstrations are important assessment features of psychomotor objectives. Examples of objectives are found in Table 13.3.

**Table 13.3** Objective examples in survivorship care

| Objective type | Sample objective |
|---|---|
| Attitude objectives – feelings, emotions, and values | Recognize the need for survivorship follow-up care for cancer patients |
| Knowledge objectives – facts, improved knowledge | Describe the survivorship programs available to patients and how to refer to those programs |
| Psychomotor objectives – improve skills | Conduct a survivorship follow-up visit and provide a treatment summary to the patient |

## Educational Methods

Many different and creative methods can be used to provide survivorship education to different populations. Based on the types of objectives set for a program, teaching methods can follow. For example, standard programs like lectures, live face-to-face, grand rounds, or Lunch & Learns are best when trying to convey general knowledge building principles or an overview of survivorship care. These provide factual information. Case study and self-study programs can also be effective. Providing these programs as web-based or online access may also improve participation. Health-care providers face many challenges for time; allowing access from home computers and flexibility of timing can help them access these educational programs. The amount of research data published today continues to be underused in practice. Connecting the information to the people who would benefit from it is difficult. For example, using electronic prompts can be useful in encouraging health promotion activities or prompting physicians on how often to order surveillance tests. One study found that using prompts called "provider reminders" to physicians increased preventive care activities by 13.1% [13]. Depending on your audience you would choose the appropriate providers or venue to convey the information. Using professional speakers is a recommended approach when attempting to deliver general information to physicians. Health-care professionals look for data associated with the information and are more likely to accept recommendations when they are presented from a scientific perspective. Administrators and patients benefit from that type of speaker as well but will also appreciate the personal perspective that a survivor or professional providing that care may share.

Attitude objectives require different approaches to reach successful results. Attitude objectives are focused on feelings or values and need time to be discussed, and reframed if necessary. Providing provocative questions to understand how someone may feel about the subject and sharing attitudes in small group discussions may be necessary. From an administrative or health-care provider standpoint, these changes in philosophy may have a significant impact in the daily provision of patient care. Modeling the benefit of survivorship care and the improvement in quality of life for these patients is important and is a crucial part of the process to allow for a transition in the type of care provided.

Psychomotor or skill-focused objectives require methods of instruction that require physical activity and written instructions. Methods include written guidelines, demonstration models, and return performance opportunities. Time must be provided to practice these new skills in a nonjudgmental environment. Examples in survivorship care activities might be teaching lymphedema massage or symptom assessment skills. This method requires an active learner and provides for learning new skills.

Survivorship days and large multiday education programs can be used to meet multiple needs for cancer survivors, health-care providers, and caregivers. In many settings, an annual recognition day for cancer survivors is provided. It allows for a positive celebration of survivorship for cancer survivors, families, and caregivers, and is an opportunity for community involvement and sharing resources with other cancer support services like the ACS, LIVESTRONG, and CancerCare to take place (http://www.cancercare.org). Institutions have partnered with community resources that provide psychosocial support, physical therapy, and nutritional services in their community to share the cost but also reach a greater number of participants. This is also a great venue for collecting needs assessments from the participants. These are usually programs that attract large numbers of cancer survivors, their families, and caregivers. They can be an excellent way to kick off a plan to provide survivorship care in a setting and gather the information needed to steer the educative components of a program in an appropriate way. Examples of programs to meet the essential content of survivorship training for health-care providers can be found in Table 13.4.

**Table 13.4** Survivorship training content and recommended programs (Adapted from IOM report Box 5-1 p. 327; [14])

| Essential content of survivorship training for health care providers | Recommended programs |
|---|---|
| Prevention of secondary cancers | Health promotion activities – smoking cessation, skin examinations, nutrition, and exercise recommendations |
| General discussion of survivorship | Survivorship day programs, support group formats, Lunch & Learn, grand rounds |
| Long-term/late effects of cancer and its treatment | Lymphedema, cardiac complications, psychosocial issues |
| Health-care systems/quality assurance/models of care | Patient and health-care professionals needs assessments. Overview of models of care, research, or clinical focused care |
| Rehabilitation services/ occupational therapy | Available programs and services offered within your setting or community |
| Quality-of-life issues in survivorship | Focus on improved quality of life within a setting or disease focus. Psychosocial support, occupational needs, and sexual issues |
| Detection of recurrent and secondary cancers | Surveillance programs – educate primary care physicians on detection and surveillance recommendations |
| Pain management | Educate health-care providers on managing pain. Provide access for patients to pain management programs |
| Palliative care/end-of-life care | Aggressive symptom management, access to palliative and hospice care as needed |
| Short-term complications | Acute symptom management clinics |
| Treatment of recurrent cancer | Easy referral back to oncologist and oncology program |

Multiday educational programs have been used to provide an educational curriculum to health-care providers or survivors. The curriculum is built to meet the needs of a particular population and may be related to general education for patients and families or to train health-care professionals in specifics of survivorship care. Survivorship Education for Quality Cancer Care was one of the first multidiscipline training programs funded by the NCI. The curriculum was developed with expert faculty input around the time the IOM report was published. Sessions defining the physical, psychological, social, and spiritual effects of cancer survivorship provided a guideline for program planning. Over the course of 5 years, four training programs were completed and 104 teams from cancer settings across the nation attended [15]. Goal analysis was used to evaluate the success of the training program. Data collected showed that participating institutions improved survivorship care in their settings. Evaluation of educational programs is necessary to justify the financial and time commitment of a program. Dissemination of information is essential but evaluating the extent that the training met its goal and provided the proposed information must come first.

## Evaluating Programs

Evaluation of training programs provides data that affirms the information taught was received as intended. Financial support of the program either from institutional support or NCI funding requires evaluation data. A formative evaluation focuses on the process of the educational program. It is an opportunity to evaluate the learning materials and teacher effectiveness as well as achievements throughout the development and application of the program. Summative evaluation evaluates a program at the end, so focuses on the outcome [16]. Evaluating training programs have been historically measured for effectiveness using the Kirkpatrick model [17]. It is useful because it uses four levels for evaluating effectiveness of the program based on different goals of the evaluation. The first level, reaction, is used most often. This is a basic evaluation of satisfaction with the program. Simple evaluation tools ask if the program met the program's objectives. The next level evaluates the extent to which the participants increased their knowledge or changed their attitudes. These would be measurable evaluations with scales rating the increase or change in attitude or knowledge. The next level, behavior evaluations, requires a more interactive evaluation. This level of evaluation measures the extent to which behavior has changed. These are usually done by supervisors or observers who either through interviews, chart audits, or direct observation can measure a change in behavior. For example, after providing an educational session, nurses are documenting patient education that includes survivorship care. Finally, the fourth level of evaluation is called results. Results evaluations determine the final results of training. They are similar to behavior evaluations by including a measurement of a changed behavior but go beyond that to include a philosophical change in attitude and practice. An example of results, evaluations in the Survivorship Education for Quality Cancer Care program described above involved a required Institutional Assessment that identified system areas that changed from baseline to 18 months post course. In this case, there were significant differences in the seven domains that included vision and management standards, practice standards, psychosocial and emotional standards, communication standards, quality improvement standards, patient and family education post cancer treatment, and community network and partnership standards [18]. Evaluations are necessary not only to help define the quality of a new program or the faculty providing it but also to justify the cost of the program either personally, administratively, or institutionally. The future of health care will be much more focused on outcomes data and tied to reimbursement. Changes in government monitoring and oversight are expected. Professional societies have been involved in evaluation of programs and patient care for quality. The Quality Oncology Practice Initiative (QOPI) is a project by the ASCO to collect data about the quality of care provided to patients in an effort to standardize care and establish indicators that compare performance [19]. Keeping track of the benefits of programs provided as they relate to the patient, the provider and the family will be essential for the future.

The recommendations for quality cancer care include survivorship care planning as part of the long-term follow-up plan for cancer patients [7]. Access to information as well as prevention services and pain and palliative care are included. How we provide this information is a challenge. Multidiscipline collaboration for providing education and resources to patients, health-care providers, families, and caregivers is essential. Multiple venues and methods of education require experts in additional areas beyond the physical components and development of survivorship education programs or materials. Information technologists, web masters, and template experts all contribute to the dissemination of survivorship knowledge. Creative methods reviewed have found that using venues appropriate to age-specific survivors can be effective. Participating programs have discussed using rooms associated with coffee houses, for instance, to meet young adults. They are off site and provide a low key area to meet and discuss issues affecting their lives. Another site that provides access to families and caregivers and provides an area to post general educational information or provide specific marketing information for a particular program is the local mall. Centers have been able to use empty storefront windows to post information and calendars of events for cancer survivors in their community. Hospitals have found those to be very cost effective and positive outcome expenditures for marketing dollars along with providing excellent public relations information. As people walk through the mall, they can read information on cancer prevention and detection, pick up information, or attend educational programs. Table 13.5 provides examples of additional education techniques.

## Future

An important part of survivorship education is helping patients build self-advocacy skills. Developing programs to help survivors learn skills to manage the many and ever-changing informational needs they experience is essential [20]. Innovative educational efforts for cancer survivorship care involve didactic and interactive

**Table 13.5** Educating objectives and related teaching methods

| Type of objectives | Teaching methods |
|---|---|
| Attitude – Feelings, attitudes, and values | Lectures |
| | Grand rounds |
| | Lunch & Learn |
| | Web-based learning modules |
| | Videos |
| | Discussions-small group |
| | Knowledge and attitude testing |
| | Role play modeling |
| | Case studies |
| | List values – prioritize/contrast different values, compare, and synthesize |
| | Listening exercises |
| Knowledge – providing facts and information | Handouts |
| | Posters |
| | Lectures |
| | Web-based learning modules |
| | Videos |
| | Games |
| | Pre- and posttesting |
| Psychomotor – techniques or procedures | Lecture – small groups with posttest or return method evaluation |
| | Modeling new procedure-role play |
| | Web-based learning modules with posttest or return evaluation |
| | Handouts describing technique or procedure |

programs along with media, online resources, and coordination of these efforts. Assessing the needs of the setting and developing appropriate activities aimed at motivating the participants, and providing the information needed is essential for providing successful educational programs. As survivorship care continues to be recognized as an essential part of quality cancer care, educating health-care professionals and support staff will be a necessary aspect of providing quality health care.

## References

1. Hewitt M, Greenfield S, Stovall E. From cancer patient to cancer survivor lost in transition. Washington, DC: Institute of Medicine; 2006.
2. Bloom BS. Taxonomy of educational objectives, handbook I; The cognitive domain. New York: David McKay; 1956.
3. American Cancer Society (ACS). http://www.cancer.org. Accessed 18 Mar 2010.
4. National Comprehensive Cancer Network (NCCN). http://www.nccn.org. Accessed 18 Mar 2010.
5. Smith AB, Bashore L. The effect of clinic-based health promotion education on perceived health status and health promotion behaviors of adolescent and young adult cancer survivors. J Pediatr Oncol Nurs. 2006;23(6):326–34.

6. Ferrell BR, Hassey DK, Grant M. Measurement of the quality of life in cancer survivors. Quality of Life Research, 1995;4:523–531
7. ASCO-ESMO. ASCO-ESMO consensus statement on quality cancer care. J Clin Oncol. 2006;24(21):2.
8. The Journey Forward Care Plan Builder. http://www.journeyforward.org. Accessed 17 Mar 2010.
9. LIVESTRONG Care Plan. http://www.livestrongcareplan.org. Accessed 17 Mar 2010.
10. Survey Monkey Web Site. http://www.surveymonkey.com/. Accessed 2 June 2010.
11. Pohl M. Learning to think, thinking to learn: models and strategies to develop a classroom culture of thinking. Cheltenham: Hawker Brownlow; 2000.
12. Institute of Medicine (IOM). Cancer Patient to Cancer Survivor-Lost in Transition. [Video]. 2005. http://www.youtube.com/watch?v=yhugWM3dNAw. Accessed 10 Feb 2010.
13. Balas EA, Weingarten S, Garb CT, Blumenthal D, Boren SA, Brown GD. Improving preventive care by prompting physicians. Arch Intern Med. 2000;160(3):301–8.
14. Ferrell BR, Virani R, Smith S, Juarez G. The role of oncology nursing to ensure quality care for cancer survivors: a report commissioned by the National Cancer Policy Board and Institute or Medicine. Oncol. Nurs. Forum 2003;30(1): E1–E11.
15. Grant M, Economou D, Ferrell B, Bhatia S. Preparing professional staff to care for cancer survivors. J Cancer Surviv. 2007;1(1):98–106.
16. Scriven M. The methodology of evaluation. In: Tyler RW, Gagne RM, Scriven M, editors. Perspectives of curriculum evaluation. Chicago: Rand McNally; 1967. p. 39–83.
17. Kirkpatrick DL. Evaluating training programs: the four levels. San Francisco: Berrett-Koehler; 1994.
18. Grant M, Economou D. An update on survivorship education for quality cancer care. Oncology. 2008;S11:1.
19. Neuss MN, Jacobson JO, McNiff KK, Kadlubek P, Eisenberg PD, Simone JV. Evolution and elements of the quality oncology practice initiative measure set. Cancer Control. 2009;16(4):312–7.
20. Stovall E. Cancer advocacy. In: Ganz PA, editor. Cancer survivorship today and tomorrow. New York: Springer; 2007. p. 283–5.

# Part IV
# Foundations for Improving Quality of Care

# Chapter 14
# Epidemiology of Cancer Recurrence, Second Primary Cancer, and Comorbidity Among Cancer Survivors

**Xinhua Yu**

## Introduction

Several definitions of cancer survivor have been proposed [1]. This chapter uses the modified National Cancer Institute (NCI) definition of cancer survivor as any one who has a history of cancer diagnosis and has completed the primary treatment. The long-term cancer survivors refer to those who have survived for 5 or more years.

According to 2003–2007 Surveillance, Epidemiology and End Results (SEER) data, the 5-year relative survival rate is about 66% for all cancers [2]. The rates are 89%, 65%, and 99% for female breast cancer, colorectal cancer, and male prostate cancer, respectively. Early stage cancers usually have 95% or higher 5-year relative survival rates. Survivors of these three cancers account for 64% of the over 11 million people who have a history of cancer diagnosis.

The increasing number of cancer survivors and longer survival of common cancers testify to the effectiveness of cancer prevention, cancer screening, and medical treatment. Meanwhile, they impose an increasing pressure on the US health-care system. At issue is how to optimally care for the cancer survivors to facilitate and maximize changes in health, function, and well-being consistently over time.

One key component in assessing the quality of care is to understand the disease burden among cancer survivors. Health-related burdens specifically relevant to cancer survivors are the risk of recurrence of the original cancer and the development of a second primary cancer. Even among patients with an early stage cancer, so-called "curative treatments" do not completely eliminate the possibility of recurrence. The life expectancy of many cancer survivors, especially those with an early stage cancer, is similar to those without a history of cancer diagnosis [2]. However, the risk of a second primary cancer among cancer survivors is similar to, and, in some cases, higher than among individuals without a cancer diagnosis [3].

X. Yu (✉)
Division of Epidemiology and Biostatistics, School of Public Health,
University of Memphis, Memphis, TN 38152, USA
e-mail: xyu2@memphis.edu

M. Feuerstein and P.A. Ganz (eds.), *Health Services for Cancer Survivors*,
DOI 10.1007/978-1-4419-1348-7_14, 

Cancer treatments such as radiation and alkylating agents, as well as inherent genetic predispositions often increase the risk of second primary cancers.

Another key issue that influences the quality of care among cancer survivors is comorbidity. Cancer survivors have more comorbidities than those without cancer [4–6]. Some comorbidities may be due to the long-term side effects and complications of cancer treatments, some may be due to the overall decrease of health status with age [5, 7].

The risk of cancer recurrence and a second primary cancer, together with the impact of comorbidity, have complicated the disease management among cancer survivors. As depicted in the framework in Fig. 14.1, which is derived from the shared care model [8], primary care physicians and specialists such as medical oncologists should coordinate the follow-up cancer care and the management of comorbidities. The overall health care of cancer survivors are also affected by health-care system factors. Note that the framework only addresses the factors that are related to quality of care, in particular regarding the cancer recurrence, second primary cancer, and comorbidity. The goal is to minimize the risk of cancer recurrence and a second primary cancer and to improve quality of care among cancer survivors.

In this chapter, the epidemiology of cancer recurrence and a second primary cancer will be reviewed first. Common cancers such as female breast cancer, colorectal cancer, and male prostate cancer will be used as examples to illustrate the complexity of assessing cancer recurrence and the relevance to the quality of care among cancer survivors. The discussion on the second primary cancer will

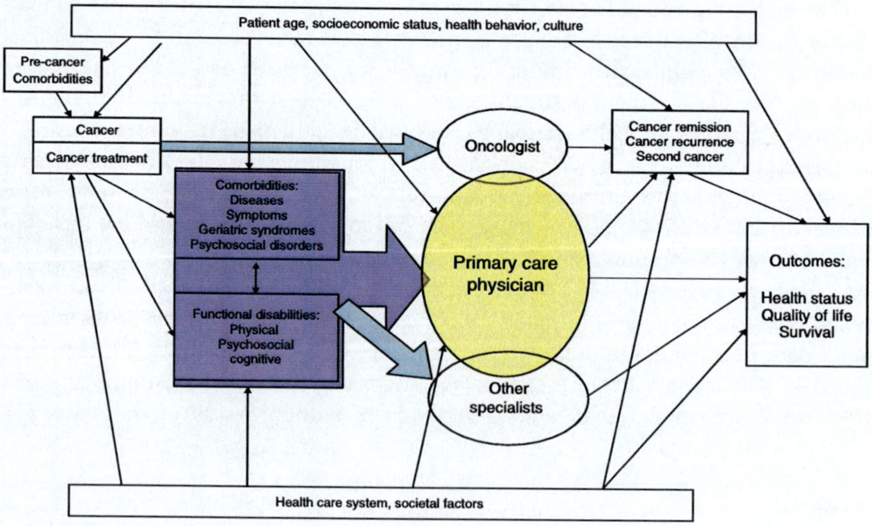


**Fig. 14.1** Relationship among cancer, cancer treatment, cancer recurrence, second primary cancer, comorbidity, and functional disabilities

also be limited to these cancer types. Studies on the cancer recurrence, second primary cancer, and chronic conditions among childhood cancer survivors have shed many new lights on cancer survivorship research. However, because childhood cancer survivors consist of many heterogeneous groups and account for a relatively small percent of total cancer survivors in the USA, this chapter will be limited to adult cancer survivors. Information on childhood cancer survivors can be found in other reports [9, 10] and the special issue of *Journal of Clinical Oncology* [11]. In addition, for an overview of cancer survivorship and follow-up issues for specific cancer type, readers are referred to Feuerstein [12] and Ganz [13].

## Cancer Recurrence

### *Definition*

Recurrence is defined as the return of any sign or symptom of cancer after remission, which is actual evidence that the cancer has physically returned and can be palpated, imaged, or biochemically detected. There are two types of recurrence: local or regional recurrence refers to the recurrence at the same site or nearby regions, and distant or systemic recurrence refers to the recurrence in other locations. The recurrence could occur in the same organ or different organs. Recurrences in different organs or at different locations are examples of cancer metastasis. With intensive cancer follow-up, usually managed by medical oncologists or other specialists, cancer recurrence can be detected earlier. With effective treatment, patients with local recurrence may have similar overall survival to those without recurrence. However, distant recurrence is more ominous, especially for solid tumors. Prognosis of distant recurrence is often poor.

### *Detecting Cancer Recurrence*

Methods to detect cancer recurrence are evolving rapidly. The common practice is to use cancer screening tests regularly for an extended period. For example, regular mammography has been used to detect local recurrence of breast cancer and second primary cancer in the ipsilateral and/or contralateral breast. One issue of using repeated screening tests such as repeated mammography is the high–false-positive rate. Modern mammography usually has about 75–90% sensitivity and 90–95% specificity [14]. However, repeated annual mammography may lead to a false-positive rate of more than 40% over 10 years. For female breast cancer survivors who will have more intensive cancer screening than non-cancer women, more than 40% of them will have to go through additional diagnostic tests to rule out the cancer recurrence within the first 10 years.

Biochemical tests have been used in detecting cancer recurrence as well. For example, in addition to regular colonoscopy, serial carcinoembryonic antigen (CEA) testing has been used to detect the recurrence of colorectal cancer. The sensitivity and specificity of CEA test depend on the cutoff criteria but generally lower (about 36% for sensitivity and 85% for specificity for a single test) [15]. Similarly, serial prostate-specific antigen (PSA) testing, in which a single PSA test has sensitivity of 35% and specificity of 63% in the general population [16], is also used to detect the recurrence of prostate cancer. One particular issue of the PSA test is that the criteria of positive serial PSA testing depend on the initial cancer treatment. After radical prostatectomy, there is no prostate tissue left and a detectable serum PSA level indicates a possible recurrence, either local or systemic. After radiation therapy in which some prostate tissue remains, a continuous increase of PSA level and/or a shorter PSA doubling time indicate the recurrence of prostate cancer. This also suggests the need for additional research on how to best use the serial biochemical tests to detect cancer recurrence.

## *Epidemiology of Cancer Recurrence*

Since a long follow-up is required to obtain a cancer recurrence rate, the recurrence rate from the published literature reflects the effectiveness of treatments that occurred 5–10 years ago. The recurrence rates under the current treatment regimens may be lower than the published results but they are unlikely to be zero. In addition, patterns of recurrence differ among different cancers. The following discussions only use common cancers as examples to illustrate the key issues in monitoring cancer recurrence. As also illustrated in the examples, different cancer treatments will lead to different recurrence rates.

For female breast cancer, within 10 years after the cancer diagnosis, as high as 20% of patients had local, regional, or distant recurrence [17]. More importantly, recurrence can occur much later. More than half of cancer recurrence and cancer-related death occur after 5 years from diagnosis among women with estrogen receptor (ER)–positive breast cancer [18]. As shown in Fig. 14.2 [19], for women with early stage breast cancer who had survived into the second decade after the initial treatment, the risk of recurrence was still high. It is of note that, as shown in Fig. 14.2, despite that women who received no radiation therapy had a significantly higher recurrence rate than those who did receive radiation therapy, the overall survival rate difference was smaller than that of recurrence difference [19].

For colon cancer, 12% of stage I colon cancer patients may have a recurrence within 5 years [20], and 40% of patients with stage II or III colon cancer may eventually have a recurrence [21]. For prostate cancer, on average 15% of patients may have a recurrence within 5 years after a radical prostatectomy, with a lower recurrence rate for early stage cancer [22].

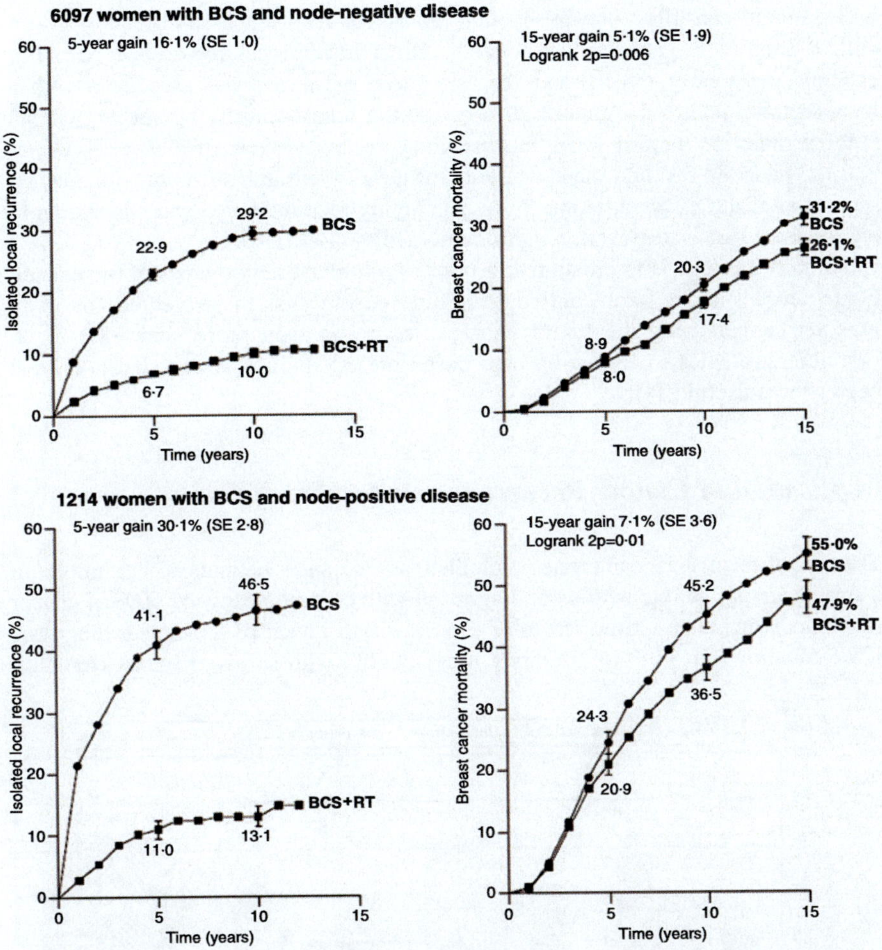


**Fig. 14.2** Effect of radiotherapy (RT) after Breast Conserving Surgery (BCS) on local recurrence and on breast cancer mortality – 15-year probabilities (data from ten trials). *Vertical lines* indicate 1 SE above or below the 5-, 10-, and 15-year percentages (Adapted from Clarke, M et al. for Early Breast Cancer Trialists' Collaborative Group (EBCGCG). In Effects of radiotherapy and of differences in the extent of surgery for early breast cancer on local recurrence and 15-year survival: an overview of the randomised trials. The Lancet; 2005;366:2087–2106. With permission from Elsevier) [19]

## *Determinants of Cancer Recurrence*

Factors such as tumor characteristics, clinical presentation, treatment modality, and quality of treatment may affect the recurrence rate [23]. The most important factor is tumor characteristics. Early stage cancer has a much lower recurrence rate than late stage cancer, as demonstrated in the recurrence patterns in breast cancer [17, 18].

Treatment can affect the probability of cancer recurrence significantly. More radical surgery is generally associated with a lower local recurrence rate. For example, with early stage female breast cancer, mastectomy is associated with a local/regional recurrence rate of 14%, while the breast-conserving surgery (BCS) without radiation therapy has a local/regional recurrence rate of 39% [17]. Given that the possible residual cancer (either invasive or intraductal, micro- or macroscopic) after the BCS, radiation therapy is highly recommended and has shown to reduce local cancer recurrence significantly (Fig. 14.2) [19].

Another strategy is to create risk groups to estimate the prognosis of the cancer. For example, a risk score called Vul/Hun scoring system is created for male prostate cancer using the tumor characteristics, Gleason score, and PSA level. Different strategies to follow-up care based on risk groups are needed and have been shown useful [24].

## *Implication of Cancer Recurrence on Quality of Care*

The fear of recurrence can cause much distress for cancer patients. For example, in a survey among people who were diagnosed with common cancers, 60% of cancer survivors worried about the return of cancer within 1 year of the cancer diagnosis [25]. As shown in Fig. 14.3, among older people who survived breast (female),

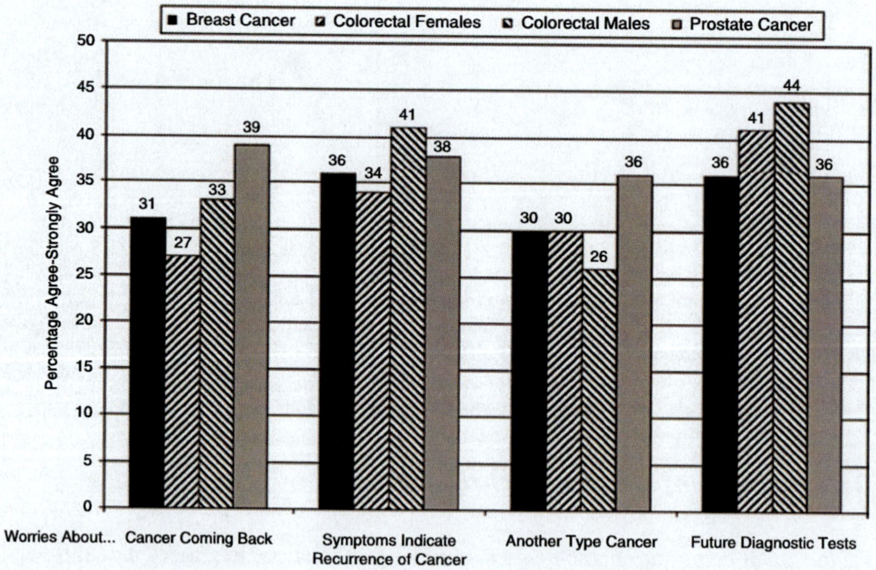


**Fig. 14.3** Cancer-related worries by cancer type and gender. *Note*: Sample size for female breast cancer, 133; colorectal cancer, 96; and male prostate cancer, 92 (Adapted from Deimling et al. (2006). "Cancer-related health worries and psychological distress among older adult, long-term cancer survivors." Psychooncology 15(4): 306–320. With permission from Wiley) [26]

colorectal (both genders), and prostate (male) cancers for more than 5 years, about one third of them still worried about the return of cancer [26].

Even among patients with early stage cancer who received extensive treatment, the possibility of cancer recurrence is not zero. The overall survival rate may be excellent, but the recurrence of cancer can change the prognosis significantly. For instance, breast cancer survivors who developed regional recurrence had much worse survival than those who had ipsilateral recurrence [27]. Nevertheless, it is possible to effectively treat local recurrence and still retain the overall survival benefits. Even for distant recurrence, it is still possible to treat effectively by chemotherapy. However, for some cancers such as prostate cancer, early detection of distant recurrence (metastatic cancer) may have no discernible benefit in overall survival, partly due to poor prognosis of late stage of cancer and metastatic cancer [28].

The nontrivial risk of recurrence even among long-term cancer survivors suggests that cancer follow-up care should be maintained until very late in life. Although more intensive surveillance may provide moderate or no survival or quality of life benefit among colorectal cancer survivors compared to regular physical exam [29], early detection of local or regional recurrence may still provide an opportunity for a more effective treatment, in particular for breast cancer. Thus, intensive cancer follow-up is highly recommended for cancer survivors during the first 5 years after the initial cancer treatment, and regular cancer follow-up care is also recommended [30]. As recommended by Institute of Medicine cancer survivorship report [8, 31], coordinating patient care between primary care physicians and medical oncologists is essential to ensure higher quality of care among cancer survivors.

## Second Primary Cancer

### *Definition*

A second primary cancer refers to the occurrence of a new cancer after a patient has survived the original cancer. The new cancer is not an extension, recurrence, or metastasis of the original cancer. The second primary cancer can be the same type, for example, a new breast cancer in the contralateral breast, or a different type, for example, breast cancer among colorectal cancer survivors. The occurrence of the second primary cancer can be within a short time period of the original cancer (e.g., within 6 months), that is, synchronous multiple primary cancer. More often, the second primary cancer occurs after a long period of surviving the first primary cancer.

### *Epidemiology of Second Primary Cancer*

A comprehensive report on the incidence of new malignancies following the original cancer has been published by NCI based on 1973–2000 SEER data [3].

Several recent reviews also addressed this issue [32–34]. This section discusses the key issues that are relevant to the quality of care among cancer survivors.

Currently, about 16% of newly diagnosed cancer cases have a second or higher order (third, fourth, etc.) cancer [3, 35]. Of the total 11 million cancer survivors, about 8% of them have a diagnosis of two or more cancer types. Of these second or higher order cancers, over 80% of new malignancies occur at different organs or sites, except for breast cancer in which local or contralateral cancer sites are the most common second malignancy sites.

The risk of having another cancer is 14% higher among cancer survivors than the general population [3]. The most common second primary cancers are breast cancer among female cancer survivors, prostate cancer among male cancer survivors, and lung cancer and colorectal cancer among both genders. Gynecological cancer and leukemia are also common second primary cancers. Younger age at the time of first primary cancer diagnosis is related to a greater risk of developing a second primary cancer, partly due to longer survival among younger cancer survivors and competing causes of death among older survivors. For example, after taking account of the incidence of the original cancer at different ages, the greatest burden of having a second primary cancer is among age group 30–59, a period when most cancer types start to appear. Compared with the general population, the excess absolute risk is 32–39 per 10,000 person years for this age group [3].

The risk of new malignancies is highest in the first 5 years after the diagnosis of original cancer [3]. This may be due to the intensive surveillance during the follow-up care. The cancer treatment and shared etiology are also the reasons for the close occurrence between the first and second primary cancers. In addition, long-term cancer survivors, for example, testicular cancer survivors, may still have 1.9 (95% CI: 1.8–2.1) times higher risk of a second primary cancer 10 years after the original cancer [36].

## *Etiology of Second Primary Cancer*

From the etiological perspective, the second primary cancers can be classified into three groups: treatment related, syndromic and genetic predisposition, and shared environmental factors [32].

### Treatment-Related Cancers

Radiation therapy and chemotherapy are known risk factors that may cause new cancers. The patient's age at cancer diagnosis and treatment, the duration of treatment, the dose of radiation and chemotherapy, and the types of chemotherapy agents are all related to the risk of new cancers. For example, leukemia following chemotherapy for Hodgkin lymphoma is well documented [34, 37]. Of note is the platinum-based chemotherapy that can increase the risk of leukemia significantly among other cancers. Radiation therapy may induce solid tumors such as cancer of breast and thyroid. A high radiation dose at >40 Gy may be related to eightfolds higher risk of breast cancer among women with Hodgkin lymphoma [32]. Radiation of cervical cancer may lead to a 30% increased risk to develop cancers at nearby tissue sites such as colon, rectum, and bladder [38]. In a recent systemic review on the risk of breast cancer among women who had chest radiation for pediatric or young adult cancer, there is a linear association between radiation doses and the risk of breast cancer [39]. In addition, chest radiation at younger age itself can increase the risk of breast cancer.

#### Cancer Syndromes and Genetic Susceptibility

Certain patients are at an increased risk of multiple related cancers because of the genetic mutations. For example, *BRCA-1* and/or *BRCA-2* are known genetic mutations that are related to an increased risk of breast cancer and ovarian cancer. Some breast cancer patients have elected to remove their ovaries to eliminate the risk of the ovarian cancer. The risk of uterine cancer among breast cancer survivors is also elevated partly due to shared etiological factors, and partly due to treatment such as Tamoxifen [40], despite that Tamoxifen can prevent the recurrence or second primary of breast cancer [18].

#### Shared Environmental Factors

The shared environmental factors include not only lifestyles but also the social and physical environment. The environmental factors are particularly important in preventing both second primary cancer and cancer recurrence among cancer survivors. For example, tobacco use is a common risk factor for lung cancer and cancers of upper aerodigestive tract. Endocrine imbalance has been well documented, linking breast cancer and ovarian cancer. In addition, obesity, unhealthy diet, and physical inactivity are also related to a number of cancers such as colon, renal cell, and prostate. Weight gain among adult women may be related to the increased risk of breast cancer [41], and obesity (Body Mass Index ≥ 30 kg/m [2]) is related to twofolds increased risk of colon and endometrial cancer [42].

### *Implication of Second Primary Cancer for Quality of Care*

Given the elevated risk of second primary cancer among cancer survivors, prevention and early detection of a second primary cancer are of high priority. Lifestyle changes and intensive cancer screening should be emphasized for both patients and physicians.

Lifestyle changes such as smoking cessation, weight loss, dietary change, and increasing physical activity have been shown to reduce the risk of cancer recurrence and second primary cancer [43]. Particularly, tobacco smoking is an established risk factor for lung cancer, oral cancer, and gastrointestinal cancer. Smoking cessation may have greater benefits in cancer survivors than general population.

For some cancers such as breast and ovarian cancer that share the same biological etiology, chemoprevention can be used to reduce the risk of a second primary cancer, for example, using selective estrogen receptor modulators (SERMs) or oral contraceptive therapy [40]. In addition, the most common second primary cancers such as female breast, colorectal, and male prostate cancer all have effective screening tools. The relative survival rates of these cancers are excellent, particularly if detected at an early stage with effective treatment.

Including these prevention measures and intensive cancer screening increases the demands on both physicians and cancer survivors. Evidence-based clinical guidelines should be developed regarding the preventing and screening for a second primary cancer among cancer survivors, particularly among elderly cancer survivors for whom the cost-benefit of cancer screening is debatable [44, 45]. Finally, because most prevention and cancer screenings are likely recommended by primary care physicians, how to coordinate patient care between primary care physicians and medical oncologists should be studied.

## Comorbidity

### *Definition*

The concept of comorbidity, introduced by Dr. Alvan Feinstein in 1970, refers to any coexisting diseases among patients with a particular index disease such as cancer [46]. However, it was not until the 1990s that the importance of comorbidity has become fully recognized in clinical research. No consensus exists about the practical definition of comorbidity that can be used in epidemiologic and health services research. The original definition limits itself to clinical diseases. To accommodate specific research purposes, researchers have begun to use coexisting health conditions in the comorbidity definition to encompass the functional disabilities and clinical symptoms that may also significantly affect the health outcomes [47, 48]. Therefore, in the context of cancer survivorship research, this chapter adopts a broad definition of comorbidity, namely, any existing health condition other than the original cancer diagnosis.

A related concept, multiple chronic conditions, or multimorbidities, is often used in health services research [49]. This is slightly different from the concept of comorbidity in that there is no index disease in the multiple chronic conditions framework. Clearly, comorbidity among cancer survivors already fits into the definition of multiple chronic conditions, that is, two or more chronic conditions.

In practice, comorbidity and multiple chronic conditions are often used interchangeably among cancer survivorship research. Both concepts are useful to describe overall disease burden among cancer survivors.

Our comorbidity definition includes functional disabilities and clinical symptoms in accordance with the framework of multiple chronic conditions. Specifically, disability refers to difficulty or dependency in carrying out activities essential for independent living. The dimensions of functional disabilities include physical, psychological, and social difficulties. Another related concept is "frail elderly," which is often used to describe elderly people who are weak in general. The concept of frailty refers to people's overall vulnerability of health status due to physiological change and debilitative consequence of chronic diseases [49]. Our definition of comorbidity, when used in elderly people, captures parts of the frailty construct as well.

## *Comorbidity Measure*

Comorbidity can be assessed in many ways. The most common measure is a composite score of weighted sum of disease counts such as Charlson Index [50]. This index is a weighted summary score of 19 disease status in which weights are based on the ability of predicting 1 year mortality after the hospital discharge. The main advantage of Charlson Index is its simplicity and high validity and reliability in predicting mortality [51]. The disadvantage is that the weights are not based on disease severity but on the impact of the diseases on total mortality. For research whose outcomes are not mortality, a comorbidity measure incorporating disease severity would be preferable. A few other composite scoring methods have been developed. For example, the National Institute on Aging (NIA)/NCI comorbidity measure includes disease severity, time of diagnosis, and state of medical management into the weights [5]. However, this method requires medical chart review, thus limiting its usefulness in large population-based research.

In small-scale studies, accurate comorbidity measures may be constructed using medical chart review or personal interview during the clinical encounters. However, cancer survivorship research is often focused on large population-based studies. Detailed clinical information may not be available or infeasible to obtain. The assessment of comorbidity is particularly problematic when using SEER-Medicare linked data to study the effectiveness of treatment, health-care utilization, and patterns of cancer care among elderly cancer survivors. Modified Charlson Index based on ICD-9 diagnosis is often used [51]. However, administrative data is considered as the weakest data source for constructing comorbidity measures because disease severity is not available on the claims. In addition, regardless of disease severity, because health-care providers may over-record coexisting disease diagnosis or under-record some disease diagnoses, to justify or increase the payment rate, such comorbidity measures will be inaccurate.

Furthermore, the existing comorbidity composite measures are not comprehensive and do not consider the interactions among comorbidities [52, 53]. In the area of risk adjustment for predicting health-care costs, several comprehensive systems have been developed. For example, the CMS Hierarchical Condition Categories (HCC) risk adjustment system classifies over 15,000 diseases into 804 clinically relevant groups and hierarchically summed up into 189 or fewer condition categories [54]. Coefficients (weights) for disease by race/ethnicity and age groups are updated regularly based on national Medicare claim datasets. These coefficients can be used to adjust disease severity when comparing health-care costs among health-care providers. Similarly, Agency for Healthcare Research and Quality (AHRQ) has developed the Clinical Classifications Software (CCS) based on over 14,000 ICD-9 disease diagnoses and 3,900 procedure codes [55]. These diagnosis codes are grouped into 285 clinically relevant and mutually exclusive categories, and procedure codes are grouped into 231 categories. In addition, a four-level hierarchical system is also constructed to further group the disease diagnoses according to the clinical relevance. There is no predefined weight for these groups. Rather, when comparing health-care costs or quality of care, these groups enter the analytic models as covariables. Quality of care research in cancer survivorship could adopt similar comprehensive strategies to capture the large spectrum of comorbidity [47].

## *Causes of Comorbidity Among Cancer Survivors*

The etiology of comorbidity among cancer survivors is less well understood. Some issues among cancer survivors warrant specific considerations. For instance, some comorbidities may exist before the cancer diagnosis. They will affect the choice of cancer treatment and patient's prognosis. Patients with heart disease or kidney disease may not be appropriate for chemotherapy. Furthermore, comorbidities can be due to the cancer itself and/or the cancer treatment. Radiation to the left chest wall may increase the risk of heart disease. Some chemotherapy agents may also increase the risk of heart disease and/or cognitive impairment. Female breast cancer survivors may have conditions such as lymphedema, sexual dysfunction, and cognitive impairment because of cancer treatment. A summary of late effects of cancer treatments are presented in Table 14.1. For a detailed discussion on the treatment-related morbidities, readers are referred to Earle [12] and Ganz [31].

In addition, cancer and cancer treatment can cause the decrease of overall health status and induce clinical symptoms such as anemia, fatigue, pain, and weight loss. Chronic pain can not only be caused by cancer and/or its treatment but also influence the treatment. Furthermore, being diagnosed with cancer is also a significant life change which can cause depression and anxiety. The increased risk of depression may last well into the later follow-up period because of the fear for recurrence, a second primary cancer, and death.

**Table 14.1** Common long-term and late effects of cancer treatment (Adapted from Earle CG. Quality of care. In: Handbook of Cancer Survivorship, edited by Feuerstein M. Springer Science+Business Media, LLC, New York; 2007; 25; with permission) [12]

| Surgery | Radiation | Systemic therapy |
|---|---|---|
| Cosmetic effects | Second malignancies | Second malignancies (myelodysplasia and leukemia) |
| Functional disability from removal of a limb or organ | Neurocognitive deficits | "Chemo brain" |
| Damage to an organ (bowel, bladder, sexual organs) | Xerophthalmia, cataracts | Cardiomyopathy |
| Pain | Xerostomia, dental caries | Renal toxicity |
| Scarring/adhesions | Hypothyroidism | Premature menopause |
| Incisional hernia | Pneumonitis, pulmonary fibrosis | Infertility |
| Lymphedema | Coronary artery, valvular, conduction, cardiomyopathic, and pericardial disease | Osteoporosis |
| Systemic effects (removal of endocrine organs, infection risk postsplenectomy) | Bowel stricture | Neuropathy |
| | Radiation proctitis | |
| | Bladder scarring | |
| | Infertility, impotence, premature menopause | |
| | Lymphedema | |
| | Bone fractures | |

Finally, comorbidity can occur independently of cancer. Many such comorbidities may be caused by common genetic predisposition, biological risk factors, health behaviors and lifestyle, social environment, physical environment, and demography [56]. Given that over 60% of cancer survivors were age 65 or older at diagnosis, aging is one key factor that causes many age-related comorbid conditions. For example, hypertension, dyslipidemia, and diabetes are three common chronic conditions among people aged 65 or older [57]. They are also among the most common chronic conditions in elderly cancer survivors.

## *Epidemiology of Comorbidity Among Cancer Survivors*

Cancer survivors have a higher prevalence of many chronic conditions than people without cancer [4, 6, 7]. For example, using National Health Interview Survey (NHIS), Yabroff et al. found that 58% of cancer survivors, defined as anybody who had a history of cancer diagnosis, had one or more comorbidities while only 45% of non-cancer controls did [4]. Cancer survivors had significantly higher prevalence of arthritis/rheumatism, back/neck problem, hypertension, and lung/breath problems. Using other years of NHIS data, Hewitt et al. and Mao et al. examined the impact of age on the prevalence of comorbidity among cancer survivors and also found similar differences [7, 58]. Hewitt et al. found that among cancer survivors, 52% of those aged 65 or older had reported one or more comorbidities as listed in the survey questionnaires, compared with 44% of the non-cancer participants [7]. Cancer survivors were also more likely to report psychological problems than non-cancer people, and the difference was higher among the younger age group than the older group (6.1% vs. 3.1% for cancer survivors vs. non-cancer people among age group 45–64, and 3.6% vs. 2.5% among age group 65 or older). Furthermore, Mao et al. found that the rates of ongoing pain, psychological distress, and insomnia in the NHIS survey were 34%, 26%, and 30%, respectively, among cancer survivors compared with 18%, 26%, and 30% among people without a history of cancer diagnosis [58]. Similar to other studies [59], Yu et al. found that among elderly cancer survivors who survived for more than 5 years, the most common comorbidities are cardiovascular diseases, chronic obstruct pulmonary disease, diabetes, hypertension, dyslipidemia, and cognitive impairment [6].

Functional disabilities such as emotional and physical disabilities among cancer survivors were less studied. Studies from childhood cancer survivors suggest that cancer survivors generally had more chronic conditions [9], more physical limitations [60], and were less likely to be married [61] than non-cancer siblings. Studies from elderly cancer survivors show that functional limitations depend on comorbidities [62]. For example, in the Duke Established Populations for Epidemiologic Studies of the Elderly study [62], cancer survivors who self-reported having one or more comorditities (stroke, diabetes, hypertension, and myocardial infarction) were more likely to have functional disabilities. Recent reports from Iowa Women's Health Study found that elderly women with cancer were more likely to have comorbidities such as diabetes, rheumatoid arthritis, and hypertension than women without cancer [63]. Cancer survivors were also more likely to report increased bodily pain and decreased general health, physical functioning, vitality, and emotional and social functioning compared with women with no cancer. Furthermore, among women who had survived cancer for 5 or more years, 42% reported they were unable to perform heavy household work, while 31% of non-cancer elderly women had such complains [64]. Long-term female cancer survivors were also more likely to be unable to walk long distance, or go up- or downstairs compared with non-cancer controls. Breast cancer survivors reported the largest increased rates of functional limitations.

The burden of comorbidity differs among socioeconomic and racial/ethnical groups. For example, using SEER-Medicare data, of 77 adverse comorbidities defined using disease diagnoses that had significantly increased the risk of death (hazard ratio $\geq 1.2$ in the Cox regression for total mortality) or clinically important diseases [65], 61% of black female breast cancer survivors had two or more adverse comorbidities while only 57% white cancer survivors did; 26% of black cancer survivors had diabetes with or without complications, while only 9.5% of white cancer survivors did. Similarly, 63% of black cancer survivors had hypertension compared with only 36% of white cancer survivors. Although no difference was found in breast cancer–specific deaths between blacks and whites, black breast cancer survivors were more likely to die of competing causes than white cancer survivors.

It should be noted that cancer survivors may have higher use of health services than non-cancer controls [6]. For example, female colorectal cancer survivors had a slightly higher rate of mammography use than non-cancer controls. In addition, when comorbidity is assessed based on disease diagnosis using administrative data, detection bias may also exist. Cancer survivors are more likely to have more disease diagnoses because of more frequent visits to physicians [6] and more willingness to seek care for minor disorders such as heart burn.

## *Implication of Comorbidity in Quality of Care Among Cancer Survivors*

In clinical research, the purpose of measuring comorbidity is to profile the patient's overall health status, although the comorbidity measured can be the exposure, confounder, effect modifier, and outcome [66]. In quality of care research among cancer survivors, comorbidity introduces the complexity in patient care that needs to be addressed.

Better comorbidity measures for quality of care research in cancer survivorship are needed. The comorbidity measure should go beyond the composite measure for the traditional purpose in clinical research and encompass clinical symptoms and functional disabilities that are relevant to cancer survivors. Disease severity should also be considered in the comorbidity measure [47]. In addition, given that population-based studies often utilize existing data such as SEER-Medicare data and insurance claims, research is needed to develop methods similar to the NIA/NCI comorbidity measure [5] using administrative data.

Comorbidity may have different effects during the cancer care trajectory. Interactions among comorbidities and between comorbidities and cancer also exist. Specific cancer sites may require researching on specific comorbidities due to the anatomic location of cancer, biological behavior, and cancer treatment. For example, people who had chest radiation may need more intensive follow-up regarding heart health, while people who had abdominal radiation may need more attention to gastrointestinal illness. In addition, young cancer survivors may have issues regarding reproductive health and sexual functions [61].

On the other hand, certain comorbidities such as psychosocial disorders may affect cancer care in unique ways. Cancer survivors have been shown to have higher prevalence of mental disorders and psychological problems such as distress and insomnia compared with non-cancer controls [58]. People with rheumatoid arthritis had increased use of cancer screening while people with dementia had decreased use of cancer screening [45]. Cancer patients with depression had worse prognoses of cancer and decreased use of many other health services during the follow-up as well [67]. In addition, cancer survivors who fear the recurrence of cancer may avoid cancer follow-up care, thus missing the opportunity of detecting the local recurrence early.

The concordance between comorbidity and cancer care is also important. For example, common comorbidities such as hypertension, dyslipidemia, and diabetes are often managed together by primary care physicians [68]. Clinical symptoms such as fatigue, chronic pain, and sleep problems are also managed by primary care physicians although they may be related to cancer and cancer treatment among cancer survivors. Therefore, it is important to examine the pattern of comorbidities and how the different patterns affect cancer care and overall health care. Furthermore, the higher prevalence of comorbidity in cancer survivors causes competing priorities in the disease management [69]. During the limited time of an office visit, both patient and physician have to prioritize the treatments of different diseases [6]. In addition, specialists such as medical oncologists may ignore the non-cancer care, while the primary care physicians may defer the cancer care to medical oncologists. This fragmented health-care model leaves patients disorganized and sometimes confused, particularly among elderly cancer survivors who may have limited ability and resources to move around.

The patient-centered medical home model has been revived recently [70]. In this model, primary care physicians will be the main coordinator of the care regarding the disease management, while specialties can serve as the neighbors of the medical home. For example, medical oncologists may send a summary of cancer treatment and recommendations for follow-up cancer care to primary care physicians. The primary care physicians will incorporate the cancer care into the overall disease management plan for the patients. This model is similar to the shared care model recommended by Institute of Medicine cancer survivorship report [8]. This process will be greatly facilitated with the implementation of electronic health records to communicate effectively among different health-care providers.

## Future Research

The increasing overall cancer survival rates result in more than 11 millions of cancer survivors today [2]. Due to nontrivial probability of recurrence and increased risk of second primary cancer, regularly visiting an oncologist is recommended. The goal of follow-up care with an oncologist is to detect recurrence (some of which are potentially curable) and second primary cancer early, and screen and monitor cancer treatment–related complications.

In addition, comorbidity not only affects the cancer survivors' abilities to remain highly functional in work and families, but also imposes challenges for health care among both patients and physicians [8]. Comorbidity complicates the disease management and demands more time and efforts from both physicians and patients. But the time of an office visit is always limited and competing priorities exist. In addition, providing efficient care for cancer survivors and coordinating care between primary care physicians and specialists requires the advancement in both technology and disease management strategy.

From the epidemiological perspective on the risk of cancer recurrence and second primary cancer, and the complex care for comorbidity, more research is needed in the following areas to improve the quality of care among cancer survivors:

1. Developing a theoretical framework that includes cancer care, pathophysiological and psychosocial causes of comorbidities and functional disabilities, and health-care system and organizational factors. The framework should explain how specific elements impact the quality of care among cancer survivors. In particular, this framework should reflect the dynamics and multilevels of patient care. How do the changes of comorbidities affect functional status? How do these changes affect the patient's outcomes? How do patients' socioeconomic status, race/ethnicity, health behavior, and culture impact on care for comorbidity and cancer? Multilevel and longitudinal research is needed to incorporate characteristics of patients and physicians, factors of health-care system and society, and dynamic changes of disease process and management.
2. Updating clinical guidelines to include recommendations for comorbidity care among cancer survivors. Current guidelines are mostly disease specific. Few of them provide recommendations on how to manage comorbidity. For example, an empirical evaluation of current guidelines on a typical patient with diabetes, osteoporosis, and heart disease revealed that physicians were not able to meet the guideline recommendations [71]. Because of the cancer and cancer treatment, cancer survivors may experience both medical and often symptom comorbidities such as fatigue, pain, and functional changes over a long period. These will make disease management even more complex. Clinical guidelines that target these comorbidities should be created and tested among both young and old cancer survivors. In addition, given that many cancer survivors can survive for many years, clinical guidelines should also consider the long-term follow-up of the cancer survivors and the efficiency of providing care for them.
3. Finally, coordinating cancer care between primary care physicians and specialists for caring cancer survivors, as suggested in the shared care model or patient-centered medical home model [8]. For cancer survivors, particularly for long-term cancer survivors, medical oncologists will not play a central role in overall patient care. Rather, primary care physicians should be responsible for coordinating the overall health care, while cancer-related care such as monitoring recurrence and second primary cancer is managed by oncologists. Therefore, to develop a better care plan for cancer survivors, both primary care physicians and medical oncologists should not only update their knowledge on follow-up cancer care and primary care but also communicate more efficiently.

## References


1. Feuerstein M. Defining cancer survivorship. J Cancer Surviv. 2007;1(1):5–7.
2. Altekruse S, Kosary C, Krapcho M, Neyman N, Aminou R, Waldron W, Ruhl J, Howlader N, Tatalovich Z, Cho H, Mariotto A, Eisner M, Lewis D, Cronin K, Chen H, Feuer E, Stinchcomb

D, Edwards Be. SEER Cancer Statistics Review, 1975–2007, National Cancer Institute, Bethesda, MD. http://seer.cancer.gov/csr/1975_2007/, based on November 2009 SEER data submission, posted to the SEER web site, 2010.
3. Curtis R, Freedman D, Ron E, Ries L, Hacker D, Edwards B, Tucker M, and Fraumeni JJe. New malignancies among cancer survivors: SEER Cancer Registries, 1973–2000. Bethesda, MD: National Cancer Institute. NIH Publ. No. 05-5302; 2006.
4. Yabroff KR, Lawrence WF, Clauser S, Davis WW, Brown ML. Burden of illness in cancer survivors: findings from a population-based national sample. J Natl Cancer Inst. 2004;96(17):1322–30.
5. Yancik R, Wesley MN, Ries LA, Havlik RJ, Edwards BK, Yates JW. Effect of age and comorbidity in postmenopausal breast cancer patients aged 55 years and older. JAMA. 2001;285(7):885–92.
6. Yu X, McBean AM, Virnig BA. Physician visits, patient comorbidities, and mammography use among elderly colorectal cancer survivors. J Cancer Surviv. 2007;1(4):275–82.
7. Hewitt M, Rowland JH, Yancik R. Cancer survivors in the United States: age, health, and disability. J Gerontol A Biol Sci Med Sci. 2003;58(1):82–91.
8. Hewitt M, Greenfield S, Stovall E, editors. From cancer patient to cancer suvivor: lost in transition. Washington, DC: The National Academies Press; 2006.
9. Oeffinger KC, Mertens AC, Sklar CA, Kawashima T, Hudson MM, Meadows AT, et al. Chronic health conditions in adult survivors of childhood cancer. N Engl J Med. 2006;355(15):1572–82.
10. Landier W, Bhatia S. Cancer survivorship: a pediatric perspective. Oncologist. 2008; 13(11):1181–92.
11. Robison LL, Armstrong GT, Boice JD, Chow EJ, Davies SM, Donaldson SS, et al. The Childhood Cancer Survivor Study: a National Cancer Institute-supported resource for outcome and intervention research. J Clin Oncol. 2009;27(14):2308–18.
12. Feuerstein M, editor. Handbook of cancer survivorship. New York: Springer; 2007, xix, 504 p.
13. Ganz PA, editor. Cancer survivorship, today and tomorrow. 1st ed. New York: Springer; 2007.
14. Mandelblatt JS, Cronin KA, Bailey S, Berry DA, de Koning HJ, Draisma G, et al. Effects of mammography screening under different screening schedules: model estimates of potential benefits and harms. Ann Intern Med. 2009;151(10):738–47.
15. Fakih MG, Padmanabhan A. CEA monitoring in colorectal cancer. What you should know. Oncol Williston Park. 2006;20(6):579–87. discussion 588, 594, 596 passim.
16. Crawford E, Leewansangtong S, Goktas S, Holthaus K, Baier M. Efficiency of prostate-specific antigen and digital rectal examination in screening, using 4.0 ng/ml and age-specific reference range as a cutoff for abnormal values. Prostate J. 1999;38(4):296–302.
17. Fisher B, Anderson S, Bryant J, Margolese RG, Deutsch M, Fisher ER, et al. Twenty-year follow-up of a randomized trial comparing total mastectomy, lumpectomy, and lumpectomy plus irradiation for the treatment of invasive breast cancer. N Engl J Med. 2002;347(16):1233–41.
18. Early Breast Cancer Trialists' Collaborative Group (EBCTCG). Effects of chemotherapy and hormonal therapy for early breast cancer on recurrence and 15-year survival: an overview of the randomised trials. Lancet. 2005;365(9472):1687–717.
19. Clarke M, Collins R, Darby S, Davies C, Elphinstone P, Evans E, et al. Effects of radiotherapy and of differences in the extent of surgery for early breast cancer on local recurrence and 15-year survival: an overview of the randomised trials. Lancet. 2005;366(9503):2087–106.
20. Manfredi S, Bouvier AM, Lepage C, Hatem C, Dancourt V, Faivre J. Incidence and patterns of recurrence after resection for cure of colonic cancer in a well defined population. Br J Surg. 2006;93(9):1115–22.
21. Figueredo A, Rumble RB, Maroun J, Earle CC, Cummings B, McLeod R, et al. Follow-up of patients with curatively resected colorectal cancer: a practice guideline. BMC Cancer. 2003;3:26.
22. Han M, Partin AW, Piantadosi S, Epstein JI, Walsh PC. Era specific biochemical recurrence-free survival following radical prostatectomy for clinically localized prostate cancer. J Urol. 2001;166(2):416–9.
23. Kerlikowske K, Molinaro A, Cha I, Ljung BM, Ernster VL, Stewart K, et al. Characteristics associated with recurrence among women with ductal carcinoma in situ treated by lumpectomy. J Natl Cancer Inst. 2003;95(22):1692–702.

24. Evans CP. Follow-up surveillance strategies for genitourinary malignancies. Cancer. 2002;94(11):2892–905.
25. Baker F, Denniston M, Smith T, West MM. Adult cancer survivors: how are they faring? Cancer. 2005;104(11 Suppl):2565–76.
26. Deimling GT, Bowman KF, Sterns S, Wagner LJ, Kahana B. Cancer-related health worries and psychological distress among older adult, long-term cancer survivors. Psychooncology. 2006;15(4):306–20.
27. Anderson SJ, Wapnir I, Dignam JJ, Fisher B, Mamounas EP, Jeong JH, et al. Prognosis after ipsilateral breast tumor recurrence and locoregional recurrences in patients treated by breast-conserving therapy in five National Surgical Adjuvant Breast and Bowel Project protocols of node-negative breast cancer. J Clin Oncol. 2009;27(15):2466–73.
28. Nielsen HM, Overgaard M, Grau C, Jensen AR, Overgaard J. Study of failure pattern among high-risk breast cancer patients with or without postmastectomy radiotherapy in addition to adjuvant systemic therapy: long-term results from the Danish Breast Cancer Cooperative Group DBCG 82 b and c randomized studies. J Clin Oncol. 2006;24(15):2268–75.
29. Renehan AG, Egger M, Saunders MP, O'Dwyer ST. Impact on survival of intensive follow up after curative resection for colorectal cancer: systematic review and meta-analysis of randomised trials. BMJ. 2002;324(7341):813.
30. Snyder CF, Earle CC, Herbert RJ, Neville BA, Blackford AL, Frick KD. Trends in follow-up and preventive care for colorectal cancer survivors. J Gen Intern Med. 2008;23(3):254–9.
31. Ganz PA. Survivorship: adult cancer survivors. Prim Care. 2009;36(4):721–41.
32. Travis LB. The epidemiology of second primary cancers. Cancer Epidemiol Biomark Prev. 2006;15(11):2020–6.
33. Travis LB, Rabkin CS, Brown LM, Allan JM, Alter BP, Ambrosone CB, et al. Cancer survivorship–genetic susceptibility and second primary cancers: research strategies and recommendations. J Natl Cancer Inst. 2006;98(1):15–25.
34. Ng AK, Travis LB. Second primary cancers: an overview. Hematol Oncol Clin North Am. 2008;22(2):271–89. vii.
35. Mariotto AB, Rowland JH, Ries LA, Scoppa S, Feuer EJ. Multiple cancer prevalence: a growing challenge in long-term survivorship. Cancer Epidemiol Biomark Prev. 2007;16(3):566–71.
36. Travis LB, Fossa SD, Schonfeld SJ, McMaster ML, Lynch CF, Storm H, et al. Second cancers among 40, 576 testicular cancer patients: focus on long-term survivors. J Natl Cancer Inst. 2005;97(18):1354–65.
37. Tward J, Glenn M, Pulsipher M, Barnette P, Gaffney D. Incidence, risk factors, and pathogenesis of second malignancies in patients with non-Hodgkin lymphoma. Leuk Lymphoma. 2007;48(8):1482–95.
38. Chaturvedi AK, Engels EA, Gilbert ES, Chen BE, Storm H, Lynch CF, et al. Second cancers among 104, 760 survivors of cervical cancer: evaluation of long-term risk. J Natl Cancer Inst. 2007;99(21):1634–43.
39. Henderson TO, Amsterdam A, Bhatia S, Hudson MM, Meadows AT, Neglia JP, et al. Systematic review: surveillance for breast cancer in women treated with chest radiation for childhood, adolescent, or young adult cancer. Ann Intern Med. 2010;152(7):444–55. W144-54.
40. Fisher B, Costantino JP, Redmond CK, Fisher ER, Wickerham DL, Cronin WM. Endometrial cancer in tamoxifen-treated breast cancer patients: findings from the National Surgical Adjuvant Breast and Bowel Project (NSABP) B-14. J Natl Cancer Inst. 1994;86(7):527–37.
41. Huang Z, Hankinson SE, Colditz GA, Stampfer MJ, Hunter DJ, Manson JE, et al. Dual effects of weight and weight gain on breast cancer risk. JAMA. 1997;278(17):1407–11.
42. Bergstrom A, Pisani P, Tenet V, Wolk A, Adami HO. Overweight as an avoidable cause of cancer in Europe. Int J Cancer. 2001;91(3):421–30.
43. Kushi LH, Kwan ML, Lee MM, Ambrosone CB. Lifestyle factors and survival in women with breast cancer. J Nutr. 2007;137(1 Suppl):236S–42.
44. Walter LC, Covinsky KE. Cancer screening in elderly patients: a framework for individualized decision making. JAMA. 2001;285(21):2750–6.
45. Walter LC, Lewis CL, Barton MB. Screening for colorectal, breast, and cervical cancer in the elderly: a review of the evidence. Am J Med. 2005;118(10):1078–86.

46. Feinstein AR. The pre-therapeutic classification of co-morbidity in chronic disease. J Chron Dis. 1970;23(7):455–68.
47. Boyd CM, Weiss CO, Halter J, Han KC, Ershler WB, Fried LP. Framework for evaluating disease severity measures in older adults with comorbidity. J Gerontol A Biol Sci Med Sci. 2007;62(3):286–95.
48. Valderas JM, Starfield B, Sibbald B, Salisbury C, Roland M. Defining comorbidity: implications for understanding health and health services. Ann Fam Med. 2009;7(4):357–63.
49. Fried LP, Ferrucci L, Darer J, Williamson JD, Anderson G. Untangling the concepts of disability, frailty, and comorbidity: implications for improved targeting and care. J Gerontol A Biol Sci Med Sci. 2004;59(3):255–63.
50. Charlson ME, Pompei P, Ales KL, MacKenzie CR. A new method of classifying prognostic comorbidity in longitudinal studies: development and validation. J Chron Dis. 1987;40(5):373–83.
51. Deyo RA, Cherkin DC, Ciol MA. Adapting a clinical comorbidity index for use with ICD-9-CM administrative databases. J Clin Epidemiol. 1992;45(6):613–9.
52. Satariano WA, Silliman RA. Comorbidity: implications for research and practice in geriatric oncology. Crit Rev Oncol Hematol. 2003;48(2):239–48.
53. Karlamangla A, Tinetti M, Guralnik J, Studenski S, Wetle T, Reuben D. Comorbidity in older adults: nosology of impairment, diseases, and conditions. J Gerontol A Biol Sci Med Sci. 2007;62(3):296–300.
54. Pope GC, Kautter J, Ellis RP, Ash AS, Ayanian JZ, Lezzoni LI, et al. Risk adjustment of Medicare capitation payments using the CMS-HCC model. Health Care Financ Rev. 2004;25(4):119–41.
55. Elixhauser A, Steiner C, Palmer L, Clinical classifications software (CCS), 2010. U.S. Agency for Healthcare Research and Quality. Available: http://www.hcup-us.ahrq.gov/toolssoftware/ccs/ccs.jsp.
56. Gijsen R, Hoeymans N, Schellevis FG, Ruwaard D, Satariano WA, van den Bos GA. Causes and consequences of comorbidity: a review. J Clin Epidemiol. 2001;54(7):661–74.
57. Wolff JL, Starfield B, Anderson G. Prevalence, expenditures, and complications of multiple chronic conditions in the elderly. Arch Intern Med. 2002;162(20):2269–76.
58. Mao JJ, Armstrong K, Bowman MA, Xie SX, Kadakia R, Farrar JT. Symptom burden among cancer survivors: impact of age and comorbidity. J Am Board Fam Med. 2007;20(5):434–43.
59. Keating NL, Norredam M, Landrum MB, Huskamp HA, Meara E. Physical and mental health status of older long-term cancer survivors. J Am Geriatr Soc. 2005;53(12):2145–52.
60. Ness KK, Hudson MM, Ginsberg JP, Nagarajan R, Kaste SC, Marina N, et al. Physical performance limitations in the Childhood Cancer Survivor Study cohort. J Clin Oncol. 2009;27(14):2382–9.
61. Janson C, Leisenring W, Cox C, Termuhlen AM, Mertens AC, Whitton JA, et al. Predictors of marriage and divorce in adult survivors of childhood cancers: a report from the Childhood Cancer Survivor Study. Cancer Epidemiol Biomark Prev. 2009;18(10):2626–35.
62. Garman KS, Pieper CF, Seo P, Cohen HJ. Function in elderly cancer survivors depends on comorbidities. J Gerontol A Biol Sci Med Sci. 2003;58(12):M1119–24.
63. Lazovich D, Robien K, Cutler G, Virnig B, Sweeney C. Quality of life in a prospective cohort of elderly women with and without cancer. Cancer. 2009;115(18 Suppl):4283–97.
64. Sweeney C, Schmitz KH, Lazovich D, Virnig BA, Wallace RB, Folsom AR. Functional limitations in elderly female cancer survivors. J Natl Cancer Inst. 2006;98(8):521–9.
65. Tammemagi CM, Nerenz D, Neslund-Dudas C, Feldkamp C, Nathanson D. Comorbidity and survival disparities among black and white patients with breast cancer. JAMA. 2005;294(14):1765–72.
66. Lash TL, Mor V, Wieland D, Ferrucci L, Satariano W, Silliman RA. Methodology, design, and analytic techniques to address measurement of comorbid disease. J Gerontol A Biol Sci Med Sci. 2007;62(3):281–5.
67. Earle CC, Neville BA, Fletcher R. Mental health service utilization among long-term cancer survivors. J Cancer Surviv. 2007;1(2):156–60.

68. Kerr EA, Heisler M, Krein SL, Kabeto M, Langa KM, Weir D, et al. Beyond comorbidity counts: how do comorbidity type and severity influence diabetes patients' treatment priorities and self-management? J Gen Intern Med. 2007;22(12):1635–40.
69. Jaen CR, Stange KC, Nutting PA. Competing demands of primary care: a model for the delivery of clinical preventive services. J Fam Pract. 1994;38(2):166–71.
70. National Committee for Quality Assurance (NCQA). Patient-Centered Medical Home. [cited 2010 05/07]; Available from: http://www.ncqa.org/tabid/631/Default.aspx.
71. Boyd CM, Darer J, Boult C, Fried LP, Boult L, Wu AW. Clinical practice guidelines and quality of care for older patients with multiple comorbid diseases: implications for pay for performance. JAMA. 2005;294(6):716–24.

# Chapter 15
# Health Economics and Cancer Survivorship

**Emile Tompa, Jennifer Lund, and Robin Yabroff**

## Introduction

In this chapter, we review both the methodology of economic evaluation and evidence from the literature to advance the understanding of the role of economic considerations in evaluating health care in general and program options to improve the quality of cancer survivorship. Some might say that it is imperative to consider the economics because the scarcity of resources obliges individuals, organizations, and societies to select only a small subset of all health-care intervention and program possibilities. Essentially, economic analysis provides invaluable information for short- and long-run policy decision making at the national and local levels, for cancer survivors and their families, for insurers and health-care providers, for employers, and for society as a whole.

In the next section, we review the roots of economic evaluation and the measures that have been developed to value health. This is followed by a background on burden studies in cancer. The third section provides an overview of economic evaluation methods followed by a review of the literature on the economic evaluation of cancer treatment options, with colorectal cancer as the exemplar. The next section covers special topics in the economic evaluation of cancer survivorship, specifically socioeconomic status, health insurance, bankruptcy, and the high costs of new biologic therapies. The final section reviews the gaps in burden and economic evaluation studies with a focus on future directions for research.

E. Tompa (✉)
Institute for Work & Health, Toronto, ON, Canada
e-mail: etompa@iwh.on.ca

M. Feuerstein and P.A. Ganz (eds.), *Health Services for Cancer Survivors*,
DOI 10.1007/978-1-4419-1348-7_15, © Springer Science+Business Media, LLC 2011

## Valuing Health in Economics

### Roots of Economic Evaluation

The valuation of health outcomes for use in economic evaluation has its roots in a subdisciplinary area known as welfare economics. Welfare economics is focused on an abstract concept known as utility to measure values placed on alternatives by individuals. The utility construct is translated into measures of the value of health in different ways.

### Measures Used to Value Health

#### Willingness-to-Pay

One utility-based measure of health is known as willingness to pay (WTP). This method is also termed contingent/stated valuation because individuals are asked directly about the values they ascribe to alternatives. WTP identifies the maximum amount an individual would pay to acquire a benefit such as a health improvement. If the sum of WTP of all affected individuals exceeds the costs of implementing an alternative, then the program is worth undertaking based on its resource implications.

The key shortcoming of WTP measure is that it is sensitive to the ability to pay. Thus, programs benefiting those with more disposable income may be given priority over programs benefiting those of more modest means. Other concerns include whose preferences to elicit, and how broadly or narrowly to cast the questions about valuation. A narrow WTP question that inquires only on health outcomes would require capturing non-health outcomes such as earnings and productivity implications of an intervention in monetary terms through other means in order to be comprehensive.

#### Human Capital

Another monetary method used to value health is known as the human capital approach [1]. This approach assumes that the only value flowing from good health is productive time. Health gains/losses are translated into a money metric using the wage rate and work hours gained/lost due to health changes. For lifetime health gains or losses, the wage rate can be assumed fixed or adjusted for lifetime earnings growth. For nonwage work, the opportunity cost of time or replacement cost approach might be used to estimate potential productivity losses in nonwork roles. Because the human capital approach takes a very narrow view of the value of health, it is not commonly used as the sole outcome measure in program evaluation.

There are four key concerns regarding the human capital approach. First, wage rates may not accurately reflect the value of output of a worker due to market imperfections. Second, its focus on labor-market output as the only source of health-related utility is too narrow by many accounts. Third, the approach explicitly places greater value on the time of individuals with greater earnings, and lesser value on the time of individuals with lesser earnings. Fourth, a strong assumption commonly made when using this metric is that societal productivity losses due to an individual's long-term health condition are enduring.

## Health-Related Units and Quality-of-Life Measures

Because welfare economics is limited to measures of utility, economists have developed an alternative approach often labeled extra-welfarist that entails the inclusion of a broader set of considerations in the measurement process [2]. Rather than maximizing utility as measured in monetary terms, health becomes the maximand in the extra-welfarist paradigm.

Economic evaluations of health-care programs that fall under the rubric of extra-welfarist use a range of intermediate and final outcome measures, which we term "health-related units," to value health changes associated with programs [1]. These include pain, discomfort, symptoms, general health status, cases of particular health conditions, disability days, life expectancy, and survival rates. The measures found in such studies can be classified as specific to a particular disease or a measure of general health. They may also be categorized as intermediate or final, that is, intermediate proxies for downstream health outcomes or direct measures of end-state and ultimate outcomes. The choice of measure to use depends on the outcome of most relevance to the intervention options being evaluated.

One of the key concerns with intermediate and final health measures is the limitations on comparability. Even when studies use apparently similar outcomes, they may not be fully comparable due to the use of different measurement protocols, for example, fatigue being measured using different questionnaires with different scales. General health measures such as the SF-36 are more broadly applicable and comparable and have been tested for construct validity and reliability. However, such general health measures may be less responsive to the interventions than purpose-specific measures, particularly in the short run. Furthermore, non-health outcomes need to be captured through other, preferably monetary measures, if they are to be included in an analysis. Another issue is the need for an external yardstick to assess the monetary value of a unit of health outcome.

An alternative to measuring health outcomes with program-specific health-related units is to use health-related quality-of-life measures that combine quality (i.e., level of morbidity) and quantity (i.e., length of time in a health state) of health [1, 3]. These include Quality-Adjusted Life-Years (QALYs) and variants such as Healthy Year Equivalents (HYEs), and Disability-Adjusted Life-Years (DALYs). Preference-based multi-attribute health status classifications systems, such as Quality of Well-Being, and Health Utility Index (HUI) can be used as weights in conjunction with data on the length of time in health state to estimate QALYs.

Also overlooked in most health maximization approaches is a consideration of the value of health outcomes for individuals other than the recipient. In economics, these are termed health externalities. They are associated with contagious diseases and sentiments, such as altruism and parentalism (e.g., the value one places on good health for others). In most studies, values associated with externalities are not captured in analyses. Furthermore, as a society we may place different values on good health for other individuals, depending on their demographic characteristics and contextual factors (e.g., a year in good health for a child may be of greater value than for an adult because the child has not yet experienced many years of life), but this is not considered in the standard approach to measuring the value of good health. This issue is related to distributional equity, which we discuss later in this chapter.

Table 15.1 provides a summary of measures used to value health and some implications of their use for studies of cancer survivorship.

## Measuring Cost and Consequences in Economics

### *Categories of Costs and Consequences*

The costs of alternatives considered in an economic evaluation of health care or program options can be subdivided into several categories, including overhead costs for clinical/office space, capital expenditure/equipment purchase or upgrade costs; clinician time for providing services; patient time for received services, and the time of other individuals who assist with patient care in the community.

Health changes and associated productivity implications are best conceptualized as consequences. Good health has intrinsic value to individuals, but good health also makes it possible for individuals to fulfill various social roles. In its abstract form, productivity might be thought of as social role functioning. A key social role is engagement in the labor market (i.e., work), which individuals undertake to earn a livelihood. Other important social roles include domestic responsibilities, parenting, community participation, involvement in religious activities, and leisure. To ensure the various health and productivity consequences are captured requires explicitly considering how best to measure them. As noted above, the convention is to measure work-related productivity consequences separately from health. The health measure would then capture the intrinsic value of health as well as its value for the fulfillment of all social roles other than work. Labor-market productivity implications can then be captured separately in monetary terms.

There may be other consequences not captured by the health and work-productivity measures described above. These may include changes in family time use and future health-care costs. Such consequences are best captured separately, if possible, and preferably in monetary terms. If these consequences are known to be significant in magnitude but difficult to quantify, it is good practice to, at a minimum, report them in an analysis.

**Table 15.1** Summary of measures used to value health

| Paradigm | Measure | Details | Issues | Implications for cancer survivorship program evaluation |
|---|---|---|---|---|
| Welfarist | Willingness to pay/receive | Monetary value of health states ascribed to alternatives by directly asking individuals about their willingness to pay/receive | – Sensitive to ability to pay/receive<br>– Clarity needed on what to consider in the valuation | – Programs for higher income earners and individuals with more wealth may be given greater value than that for lower income earners and poorer individuals.<br>– The quality of an evaluation will depend on how well the alternatives are described to respondents of the contingent. |
| | Human capital approach | Monetary value of health states determined by multiplying the wage rate by work hours associated with alternatives | – Narrow view of the value of health<br>– Wage rates may not accurately reflect the marginal product of a worker<br>– Strong assumption regarding long-term societal productivity losses | – Programs that improve health for individuals in the labor force may be given greater value than those for individuals out of the labor force.<br>– Programs for higher income earners may be given greater value than that for lower income earners<br>– Programs for younger individuals may be given higher value than for older individuals.<br>– Outcome other than earnings would not be captured. |

(continued)

**Table 15.1** (continued)

| Paradigm | Measure | Details | Issues | Implications for cancer survivorship program evaluation |
|---|---|---|---|---|
| Extra-welfist | Natural units | Value of health states measured in natural units that reflect intermediate and final health outcomes | – Only studies using similar measures can be compared<br>– Generic measures may be less responsive to the interventions than purpose-specific measures<br>– Non-health outcomes (e.g., worker time costs, productivity) need to be captured through other measures<br>– Health externalities not considered<br>– Need monetary value of a unit of health outcome to make decisions | – Many aspects of health improvements and their variation across options may not get captured in the evaluation.<br>– Program-specific measures may make it impossible to compare interventions for different kinds of cancers or programs for different stages of recovery.<br>– Earnings, productivity, and other non-health outcomes may not be considered in the analysis unless efforts explicit made to measure them.<br>– Value of an individual's good health to family and community will not be captured. |
| | Quality-adjusted life-years | Value of health states measure in health quality–adjusted time units | – Quality and quantity assumed separable and divisible<br>– Underlying axioms violated in practice<br>– Non-health outcomes (e.g., worker time costs, productivity) need to be captured through other measures<br>– Health externalities not considered<br>– Need monetary value of a unit of health outcome to make decisions | – Good health treated would have the same value regardless of the recipients and the distribution of gains.<br>– Earnings, productivity, and other non-health outcomes may not be considered in the analysis unless efforts explicitly made to measure them.<br>– Value of an individual's good health to family and community will not be captured. |

### *Adjustments for Time Preference and Uncertainty*

Over time, nominal monetary values are typically affected by inflation. Values drawn from different years are therefore generally not directly comparable. It is standard practice in economics to remove the inflationary component by adjusting prices from different years to a base year using price indices. These are available from national statistical agencies. There are often separate indices for different categories of goods and services because they can have different rates of inflation. Hence, it is important to use indices appropriate for the goods and services under consideration.

In general, money and resources (including good health) in the future are worth less than the same quantity today. The phenomenon of preference for the timing of cost and benefits is known as "time preference." Adjusting resource flows for time preference is particularly relevant if the trajectory of costs and consequences over the assessment period differs substantially between the alternatives, but even if they do not it is standard practice to discount all flow (for details see [1, 3]). For example, though cancer survivorship and good health are important across the life span, years of good health in the near future are of greater value than similar years of good health many years into the future.

## Background on Burden of Disease Studies and Examples from the Cancer Literature

### *Burden Studies and Their Role*

Burden of disease studies measure the total loss of healthy time (i.e., morbidity and mortality) from a particular disease, the costs of treating individuals with the disease, and the impact of the disease in terms of undesirable consequences such as lost productivity to society. They are often cited in news articles to emphasize the magnitude of a particular disease burden, as the following quote exemplifies: "The global burden of cancer is increasing, hitting hardest the developing countries .... By 2010, cancer will become the leading cause of death worldwide – replacing AIDS, tuberculosis, and malaria combined as the main health challenge in low-resource countries ..." [4]. Though burden of disease studies do not measure the probability of success of treatment options or the opportunity costs of interventions that might be undertaken to reduce the burden, these types of studies serve an important information role. They provide insights into the magnitudes of the health loss and the cost of a disease to society. This information can be used to assess how the burden may have changed over time or how it compares to the burden of other diseases. It can also help health authorities with priority setting. Burdens that appear particularly onerous may bring attention to the need to (1) increase funding for intervention options known to reduce the burden; (2) evaluate the merits (both in terms of health and resource implications) of burden reduction resulting from known treatment options that have not yet been evaluated; and (3) invest in research to discover treatment options to reduce the burden in cases where no new alternatives currently exist.

Burden of disease estimates are typically reported for a specific calendar year, and are based on costs in that year for all individuals diagnosed with or living with that disease. These aggregate costs are also referred to as prevalence costs, because they encompass costs for individuals across the disease trajectory, including the newly diagnosed, long-term survivors, as well as those at the end of life. Burden studies can also report health-care costs longitudinally, starting from diagnosis, and only include newly diagnosed patients. The time period for these longitudinal or incidence cost studies ranges from several months to the patient lifetime following diagnosis. These two general types of burden studies are not directly comparable, because of differences in the time periods measured and patient inclusion.

One method of modeling health-care costs for a particular health condition is the phase-of-care approach. This approach divides services and costs following diagnosis into distinct periods or phases (e.g., initial, continuing, last year of life) and can be used to estimate either incidence or prevalence costs. When phase-of-care–specific cost estimates are applied to survival probabilities from an incident cohort, the result is analogous to an incidence cost estimate. When phase-of-care–specific cost estimates are applied to phase-specific person-years of survival within a specific year, the result is a prevalence cost estimate.

## *Burden of Cancer Studies*

The burden of cancer is expected to increase in the future for a number of reasons. Cancer prevalence is increasing due to population changes in the USA [5] and most developed countries [6]. Further, survival following diagnosis and treatment for many cancers has also improved. As a result of these trends, a larger prevalence of cancer survivorship is expected in the future [7, 8]. Based on increased prevalence alone, the economic burden of cancer is expected to increase [9]. Other trends, including increasing costs and, in particular, expensive new chemotherapy drugs for treatment, make measuring and projecting the burden of cancer an important issue for policy makers as well as for cancer survivors and their families.

Most studies of the burden of cancer focus on a single component of cost (i.e., health care, productivity loss, and patient and caregiver time) in their analyses, so we review these dimensions separately. We focus on colorectal cancer because it is a common cancer that affects both men and women, and effective cancer control interventions for prevention, screening, and treatment are available.

Health care costs of cancer post-diagnosis are based on services that patients receive, such as hospitalizations, surgery, physician visits, chemotherapy, radiation therapy, home health care, and hospice care. Some cancer-related health-care costs can be outside of the formal health care system, such as gym and yoga membership.

Historically, economic evaluations have focused on health-care treatment options, so costs have focused on specific service categories, such as hospitalizations or chemotherapy. In 2006, the health-care costs of cancer care for all cancer survivors were estimated to be approximately $US 104.1 billion in the USA alone (in 2006 dollars) [10]. Similar estimates from other countries by Koopmanschap et al. [11] also suggest that the health-care cost burden of cancer is substantial.

When measured longitudinally, the costs of cancer care vary across the trajectory of care, and are highest in the initial period following diagnosis, and among those that die from their disease, at the end of life [12–15]. Costs are lowest in the period between the initial and end-of-life periods, following a "u-shaped" curve. Figure 15.1 illustrates the distribution of expenditures for cancer care in prevalent cancer survivors by cancer site and phase of care in 2006.

Other costs of cancer include time spent seeking health care for patients and caregivers, time lost from work or other usual activities, and lost productivity due to premature death (productivity losses). In the few studies that measure both productivity losses and health-care costs, productivity loss estimates are generally at least the equivalent of the health-care costs [16–19]. Because these lost opportunities are not typically reflected in monetary transactions, a critical component of these studies is the method for valuing lost time. As described previously, the two main approaches for valuing time are the human capital approach and the WTP approach. Because cancer incidence and mortality rates are highest in the elderly, a population less likely to be in the workforce than their younger counterparts, comparison of

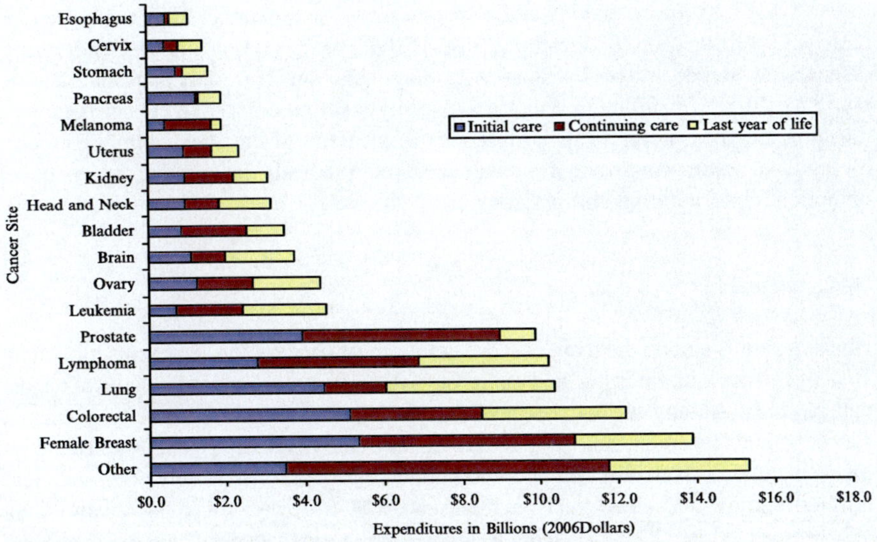


**Fig. 15.1** Estimates of US national expenditures for cancer care in 2006 by cancer site and phase of care

these two approaches is particularly relevant for evaluating the burden of cancer. For example, cancer productivity losses in the USA in 2000 have been reported to range from $US 115.8 billion based on the human capital approach (in 2006 dollars) [20] to $US 960.6 billion based on the WTP approach using a constant value for a year of life (i.e., $US 150,000) [21]. Differences in these estimates are based only on the methods used for valuing the opportunity cost associated with premature mortality.

Patient and caregiver time data are not routinely collected, and as a result, few studies have estimated time costs [22]. Time spent traveling to and from care, waiting for appointments, in consultation with providers, and receiving services or procedures represents time not spent pursuing usual activities, including work and leisure. These time costs can be substantial. Recently, patient time costs during the first year following diagnosis (incidence cost) in the elderly with the eleven most common cancers were estimated to be approximately $US 2.3 billion in the USA (in 2002 dollars) [23]. Other studies suggest that caregiver time costs may be of a similar magnitude [24, 25]. These studies use patient or caregiver surveys or modeled approaches for patient time that combine health-care service (e.g., hospitalizations, physician visits, chemotherapy administration) frequencies with estimates of time for specific services [26].

## *Burden of Cancer: Focus on Colorectal Cancer*

### Overall Costs

In 2006, the colorectal cancer–related health-care costs in the USA were estimated to be $US 12.1 billion, making it the second most costly cancer after breast cancer ($US 13.9 billion) (in 2006 dollars) (Fig. 15.1). These estimates reflect underlying disease prevalence, stage distribution at diagnosis, survival, and patterns of care. Burden estimates from other countries also suggest that colorectal cancer is among the most costly cancers [27]. Differences in systems of care and reimbursement, methods of estimating cancer prevalence, and methods for estimating costs do complicate international comparisons.

### Hospitalizations

Hospital care is among the main cost drivers for most cancers and represents more than 70% of net costs in the initial and last-year-of-life phases of care for colorectal cancer patients [15]. Among the approximately 80% of newly diagnosed elderly colorectal cancer patients receiving cancer-directed surgery in the USA, mean total Medicare payments were $US 24,910 in 2002 (in 2004 dollars) [28]. Approximately 40% had other hospitalizations, and mean total payments were $US 18,455 (in 2004 dollars) [28]. When projected to 11 and 25 years following diagnosis, cancer-related hospital costs are highest for patients with early-stage cancers and lowest for patients with later-stage cancers, reflecting shorter survival among patients with more advanced disease [29].

### Chemotherapy

In the USA, the mean Medicare payment for chemotherapy-related care in newly diagnosed elderly cancer patients was $US 12,972 in 2002, and the total Medicare payment was $US 331 million (in 2004 dollars) [28]. These estimates include all care related to an episode of chemotherapy. When restricted to the costs of specific chemotherapy agents in common regimens, there are multiple methods for estimating costs and each may lead to a wide range of estimates. Estimates also vary by country, reflecting different systems of care, structure of care delivery, methods of price setting, and other factors related to patterns of care. Despite these differences, the longtime standard of care for patients with metastatic disease, 5-FU/folinic acid, is dramatically less expensive than newer regimens which include irinotecan, oxaliplatin, bevacizumab, and cetuximab [30]. For example in 2004, per-patient drug costs for 8 weeks of treatment with 5-FU/folinic acid were estimated to be $US 63 compared to $US 9,381 for 5-FU/folinic acid/irinotecan (FOLFIRI), $US 21,399 for FOLFIRI/bevacizumab, and $US 30,675 for FOLFIRI/cetuximab (in 2004 dollars) [31]. Notably, these newer agents are used with existing therapies, and are likely to add to existing costs rather than serve as a substitute. Further, with increased chemotherapy toxicity, the use of additional supportive agents, such as erythropoiesis stimulating agents and G-CSF has increased, also leading to increased chemotherapy-related costs. Thus, measuring the cost (and cost-effectiveness) of these novel chemotherapeutic agents is an important area for additional research.

### Productivity Losses

Colorectal cancer productivity losses are among the highest of all cancers, regardless of the methods used to measure the value of lost output from years of life lost. Using the human capital approach, colorectal cancer is second only to lung cancer, with an estimated $US 12.8 billion in 2010 (in 2006 dollars) [20]. Although there are fewer colorectal cancer deaths than breast cancer deaths each year, colorectal cancer affects both women and men, and more of these deaths occur in those under the age of 65 [8], reflecting a population with higher labor-market earnings. The value of life lost to premature death from colorectal cancer was much higher ($US 112.0 billion) using a constant value for a year of life (i.e., $US 150,000) than the human capital approach [21], but because this method values all life years equally, colorectal cancer was the third most costly following lung and breast cancers.

### Colorectal Patient and Caregiver Time Costs

Mean patient time costs associated with colorectal cancer care have been reported to be approximately $US 309 per month in the initial phase of care and $US 359 per month in the last-year-of-life phase of care (in 2002 dollars) [23]. Mean monthly time costs are approximately 19% and 37% of health-care costs in the initial and last-year-of-life phases of care, respectively [26]. In the 2 years following patient diagnosis with colorectal cancer, informal care giving time cost estimates have been reported to range from $US 27,235 to $US 48,498 depending on the method used for valuing time (in 2002 dollars) [25].

## Overview of Economic Evaluations and Review of Methodological Components

### *Economic Information in Health Care and Program Evaluation*

Various intervention options to treat cancer and its impact on health and function may come into play at different points in time over the course of treatment, recovery, and return to role functioning. Shortly after the identification of an illness, the focus is on interventions to eliminate the disease or arrest its advancement and minimize its impact on health. Intervention options at this stage are generally cancer type specific. There are large literatures that report on evaluation studies of the effectiveness and cost-effectiveness of health-care treatment options for specific types of cancers.

Further down the road, the focus may turn to minimizing the impact of a health condition on role functioning through rehabilitation and other forms of disability management and prevention. Also in the long run, cancer survivors have special health-care needs including screening for recurrence. Intervention options for disability management and prevention are generally not disease-specific, because many individuals with chronic conditions have common needs, regardless of the underlying health condition. Disability management and prevention, particularly in the area of work, are multidisciplinary fields in which much research has been done to identify the most effective approaches. In general, the application of economic evaluation methods is less developed in these areas compared to the health-care treatment area.

Below we review the key methodological components of economic evaluations. To assist with the quality assessment of evaluations, several authors have developed checklists, and others guidelines for good practice. Checklists for health-care evaluations have been developed by Drummond et al. [1] and Evers et al. [32], and for the health and safety literature by Culyer and Sculpher [33].

### *Study Design Issues*

Conceptually, economic evaluation follows an effectiveness evaluation and the information it provides on resource implications is relevant only if the intervention is found to be effective. Dependence on the effectiveness evaluation is not only conceptual; data on the magnitude of health and other consequences are generally taken from the effectiveness evaluation. Naturally, the quality of evidence on health and other consequences is very much dependent on the appropriateness of the study design used to evaluate an intervention. The merits of different epidemiological designs are well documented (see [34–36]). Most researchers would argue that randomized controlled trials are the design of choice, but nonrandomized controlled studies, interrupted time series, and simple before–after studies can also provide valuable information if well executed.

## *Types of Economic Evaluations and Decision Rules*

The underlying purpose of economic evaluation is to identify efficiency-enhancing reallocations of resources to ensure that individuals, organizations, and society get the greatest amount of valued output from the use of scarce resources. Information from an economic evaluation can assist decision makers with reallocation decisions where a choice is to be made between a known set of alternatives. In economic evaluations, inputs/costs and output/consequences are generally measured in monetary terms. The money metric is a widely used and familiar measure of value. But for some consequences, such as health, it is not seen as a good measure. As a result, economists have developed and rely on other measures, which we described earlier in this chapter.

There are four broad categories or types of economic evaluations that can be used to evaluate health interventions (see [1, 37] for details). The difference between the four is primarily the metric used to measure health consequences. The first, cost–benefit analysis (CBA), is an economic analysis in which health consequences are measured in monetary units. The second, cost-effectiveness analysis (CEA) is a form of economic evaluation in which health consequences are measured in health-related units. For example, a treatment program for a particular type of cancer might focus on increasing life expectancy. A CEA using this metric would then compare alternative treatment options in terms of the cost per life year gained (LYG). The third type of analysis is called cost-utility analysis (CUA). With this approach, health is valued in QALYs. In health-care technology assessments, CUA is the most commonly used economic evaluation method. The final type of economic evaluation is known as cost-minimizing analysis (CMA). In CMA, the only measure of interest is the difference in cost between alternatives. Health and possibly other key consequences such as productivity gains are assumed to be the same across alternatives being considered, so they are not explicitly measured or considered in the analysis.

Each of the four types of economic evaluation requires a decision rule by which to choose between alternatives. For CBA, several options exist. The most commonly prescribed approach is to maximize monetary returns by choosing the alternative with the highest net present value (the sum of discounted costs and consequences), on the condition that the value is positive. Since alternatives are being compared, it is customary to consider the incremental net present value of each new alternative relative to the standard treatment alternative. For CEA and CUA, the decision rule is more complex because one needs to consider incremental costs and incremental consequences that are measured in different units. For details on the decision rule for CUA see [1] or [37]. For CMA, the decision rule is to select the alternative with the lowest cost. Table 15.2 provides a summary of the four types of evaluations and their characteristics.

## *Perspective of an Economic Evaluation*

The perspective of an economic evaluation refers to the decision viewpoint adopted by the analyst. For example, the perspective of an analysis can be the patient, hospital, system, insurer, employer, or society. The perspective defines the scope and character of the costs and consequences considered, as well as other critical features such as the discount rate used. With interventions that are focused on the health of individuals and populations, there is a strong argument for considering a broad, societal perspective since good health is seen as an outcome with special status, different from consumer goods and services. But more than one perspective can be presented in a study. As well, presentation of the disaggregated costs and consequences can provide valuable information on the distribution of burdens and benefits. In fact, one of the shortcomings of many economic evaluations in the health-care area is the failure to explicitly consider distributional issues/equity and procedural issues/equity. The National Institute for Health and Clinical Excellence (NICE), an independent UK organization that makes public health-care coverage recommendations to the UK National Health Service (NHS), considers social values (including impact on equity) when making coverage decisions. Culyer and Tompa [38] provide a review of several well-known equity constructs found in the literature. Some have been considered in the economics literature, and specifically in health economics, whereas others come from other disciplines. Some approaches provide guidance on how to embody equity in a decision-making algorithm, as through the use of weights to adjust health or utility values based on the characteristics of recipients. Others provide guidance on how equity concerns can be incorporated alongside evidence into the decision-making process itself in order to afford an opportunity for decision makers to delve more deeply by considering the individuals that are likely to gain or lose from an intervention and the nature of their gains or losses. However, additional methods for incorporating equity perspectives into cost-effectiveness analysis are needed [39].

**Table 15.2** Summary of types of economic evaluation

| Type of evaluation | Health valuation | Details | Issues |
|---|---|---|---|
| Cost-benefit analysis (CBA) | Monetary terms | Health is valued in monetary terms through human capital, willingness to pay, or contingent valuation. | – Comparability within and across sectors is facilitated since monetary metric is widely used<br>– Value of health may not be adequately captured in monetary terms<br>– May be difficult to explicitly identifying what is captured in the health measure |
| Cost-effectiveness analysis (CEA) | Natural units | Health is measured in natural units relevant to the specific health condition. | – Not possible to directly compare studies unless they use the same natural units<br>– Not all units of the same type are of the same quality<br>– Need an external marker of the monetary value of the unit of health<br>– Need to capture productivity and other consequences in monetary terms and include them with costs |
| Cost-utility analysis (CUA) | Quality-adjusted life-years | Morbidity level and time in a health state are valued in terms of equivalent time in perfect health. | – Can only directly compare studies that measure health in terms of QALYs<br>– Need an external marker of the monetary value of QALY<br>– Need to capture productivity and other consequences in monetary terms and include them with costs |
| Cost-minimizing analysis (CMA) | Health not measured | Consequences are assumed to be the same across alternatives, so only the costs of alternatives are measured and compared. | – Can only compare alternatives that have the same consequences<br>– Consequences may not be the same across alternatives<br>– Distributional issues are difficult to expressly consider since only data on costs are collected |

## Application of Economic Analyses for the Evaluation of Cancer Care

### *Economic Evaluations of Cancer Care*

In a recent review of published studies included in the Tufts Medical Center Cost-Effectiveness Analysis Registry (http://www.cearegistry.org) from 1976 to 2007, Greenberg et al. identified 242 cancer-related CUAs. Figure 15.2 illustrates the steady increase in the number of cancer CUAs over time. The number of cancer-related CUAs published in the health economic literature has increased from 1976 to 2007, although the proportion of cancer CUAs relative to CUAs focused on other diseases has remained fairly constant. Overall, cancer CUAs have focused primarily on breast (36%), colorectal (12%), and hematological cancers [40]. The vast majority of CUAs (72%) were conducted for treatment compared to only 19% for screening and 8% for prevention (e.g., vaccination). Studies examining pharmaceutical interventions were most common (53%), while health-care procedures (18%) and screening programs (16%) contributed fewer studies. There was substantial variation in the methods used for the analyses with only 13% utilizing information captured alongside clinical trials and 23% focusing on a societal perspective. Notably, there were no studies evaluating survivorship management or end-of-life programs, which highlight a major gap in the current evaluation literature.

Economic evaluation studies of interventions for improving cancer outcomes can be used to examine trade-offs in resource allocations across the trajectory of care for a specific cancer, including surgery, chemo- and radiation therapy, follow-up care, palliative treatment, and end-of-life care. A review conducted by Tappenden et al. examined the economic evidence for the detection, diagnosis, treatment, and follow-up of colorectal cancer in the UK [41]. Of the 47 studies identified, 55% utilized a modeling framework such as Markov models or decision trees (based on extrapolated data from trials or the literature), with the

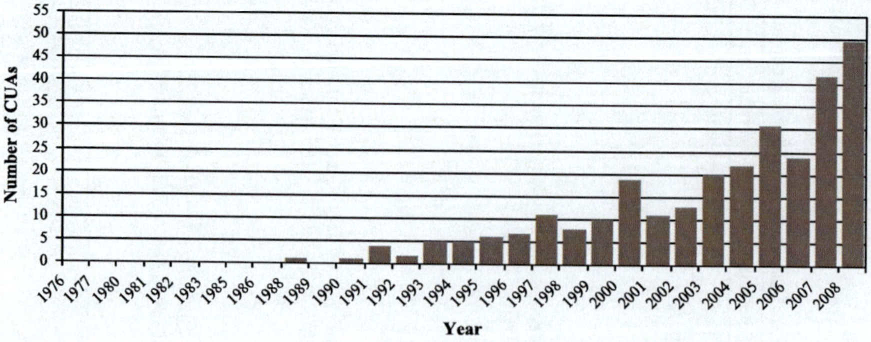


**Fig. 15.2** Growth of the cost-utility analysis (CUA) literature pertaining to cancer over time (Based on Greenberg et al. [40])

remainder relying on prospectively collected data from clinical trials. Over 40% of all studies were CEA or CUA, reporting cost per LYG or QALYs. The number of studies varied by phase of diagnosis or treatment as follows: screening [42], diagnostic technology [40], surgery [43], adjuvant chemotherapy [40], non-metastatic follow-up [41], curative treatment for metastatic disease [41], and palliative treatments (including chemotherapeutic treatment studies of metastatic disease) [44]. The review cited a number of between-study differences both in methodology (e.g., analytic tools, measure of effectiveness) and scope (e.g., population of interest, stage of disease). Further, a number of gaps were identified by the review such as management of patients with hereditary colorectal cancer. Two studies examined follow-up care for patients after curative treatment. However, no studies examined end-of-life interventions.

## *Economic Evaluations of Cancer Survivorship*

The period of transition from active cancer care to survivorship care has been identified as a critical but understudied area for improving the quality of cancer care [45]. Rehabilitation in cancer survivors emphasizes return to maximal functioning, including disability prevention and health promotion, performance improvement, and palliation [46]. Increasingly counseling [47], diet, and physical activity interventions [48] are conducted in randomized controlled trials of cancer survivors, but the cost and cost-effectiveness of these interventions are rarely evaluated. Examples of economic evaluation studies from the cardiac rehabilitation literature may have implications for evaluating long-term interventions in cancer survivorship [49, 50]. In one of the few economic evaluations of interventions to improve adjustment to cancer survivorship, Mandelblatt and colleagues assessed the costs associated with psychoeducational interventions conducted in breast cancer survivors [51].

More work has been conducted in palliation. For example, a cost-effectiveness study conducted by a UK group compared the use of cetuximab/irinotecan versus active/best supportive care (ASC/BSC) for the treatment of patients diagnosed with metastatic colorectal cancer, after having failed prior chemotherapeutic regimens [52]. The investigators included active chemotherapeutic treatment in ASC as part of the comparator arm. However, best supportive care (BSC) only included the use of analgesics, transfusions, antibiotics, corticosteroids, low-dose radiation (at palliative levels), and any other symptomatic therapy. Head-to-head trial information for this comparison did not exist, so modeling using indirect clinical trial data was necessary. Costs included in the analysis related to the study of drug and administration, palliative chemotherapy and administration, and non-chemotherapy resource use. The incremental cost per LYG for cetuximab/irinotecan compared to ASC/BSC was £42,975 and the incremental cost per QALY was £57,608 (in 2004 pounds). To account for uncertainty in the costs and outcomes utilized in the models, sensitivity analyses were conducted. Results of this analysis concluded that, if £50,000 (in 2004 pounds) was accepted as a reasonable value for an additional life-year, the likelihood of cetuximab/irinotecan being a cost-effective intervention is greater than 90%. However, after examining all available evidence, NICE concluded that cetuximab, either as a second-line or a subsequent-line treatment for metastatic colorectal cancer, would not be a cost-effective use of the UK NHS resources.

**Challenges to Economic Evaluation of Long-Term Survivorship Interventions**

Few economic evaluations of survivorship programs have been conducted, particularly for long-term interventions. Primary challenges to these analyses are related to acceptability and meaningfulness of the intermediate outcomes and the lack of standardized collection of long-term follow-up data among cancer survivors. Unlike treatment-related costs, which are often captured longitudinally through health-care utilization, clinical trials, and claims data over a finite period of time, long-term costs tend to occur across a broad spectrum of domains (i.e., health care, household, workplace, etc.) and periods of time. As such, the quantification of these costs is complex but feasible. Further discussion of this issue is noted in the section entitled, "Gaps in Cancer Burden Studies and Economic Analysis and Future Directions."

## Special Economic Issues in Cancer Survivorship

### *Impact of Population Trends on Burden of Cancer*

Recent technological developments have increased life expectancies for individuals diagnosed with cancer. Yet, the cost of these technologies coupled with a demographic shift in the overall age distribution has placed a substantial burden upon health-care systems worldwide. Populations in most industrialized countries, including the USA, are aging [53]. In many countries, the size of the population is growing as well. Because cancer incidence increases with age [8], these population trends will ultimately result in a larger population of newly diagnosed cancer patients. Additionally, improvements in cancer treatment are associated with an observed survival improvement following diagnosis. Thus, the number of cancer survivors will increase as a result of improvements in cancer treatment as well. These increases in cancer prevalence will also impact the economic burden of cancer. For example, projections of the cost of colorectal cancer care in the elderly in the USA between 2000 and 2020 are expected to increase by 53% from $US 7.49 billion to $US 11.43 billion based on population trends alone (in 2002 dollars) [54]. When current trends of decreasing colorectal cancer incidence, improving survival, and increasing costs of care are considered, projected costs are estimated to increase by 89% to $US 14.02 billion in 2020 (in 2002 dollars). Similarly, projections of the productivity losses associated with premature deaths due to cancer in the USA are also strongly associated with aging and growth of the population [20, 21]. Similar evaluations in other countries will be an important area for comparative research.

## *Socioeconomic Status, Health Insurance and Bankruptcy*

### Socioeconomic Status, Cancer Screening, and Outcomes

Lower socioeconomic status is associated with lower levels of cancer screening in the general population [55]. Among cancer patients, lower socioeconomic status is associated with later stage of disease at diagnosis, poorer survival following diagnosis, and higher cancer mortality [56, 57]. These socioeconomic relationships with cancer outcomes have been reported in countries with single-payer systems as well as in the USA, which has employment-based health insurance for most individuals of working age, the Medicare program for the elderly, and Medicaid for low-income women, children, and the disabled [56, 57]. In 2008, approximately 15.4% of the US population was uninsured, equivalent to 46.3 million people [58]. The greatest prevalence of uninsured was in the lowest income groups. Many others are "underinsured" and spend a large portion of their family income on health care [59]. Independent of socioeconomic status, health insurance coverage is associated with cancer stage at diagnosis [60]. Individuals without health insurance or with Medicaid coverage are more likely to be diagnosed with late-stage disease than individuals with private health insurance [60]. Additionally, because health insurance is predominantly employment-based in the USA, its relationship with cancer outcomes is complex. Cancer survivors who are unable to work may risk losing insurance coverage for themselves and their families. If they do not qualify for Medicaid, cancer survivors may not be able to purchase insurance independently, since it can be prohibitively expensive. In some cases their policy may have a preexisting condition exclusion for cancer care (this should change in the US under the new health care laws).

### Cost of Cancer Care by Socioeconomic Status

Few studies have examined the cost of cancer care by socioeconomic status or, in the USA, included details about health insurance status. Among elderly beneficiaries in the Medicare program, costs associated with cancer care are generally higher for patients diagnosed with advanced compared to localized disease within phase of care [15]. Because individuals of lower socioeconomic status are more likely to be diagnosed with advanced rather than localized disease, it is likely that the costs of cancer care are greater for this group as well. The majority of longitudinal data sources in the USA with information about the cost of care are from insurance claims [61] and, as a result, little is known about the trajectory of cancer-related costs by type of health-care insurance.

### Costs of Cancer Care and Bankruptcy

Cancer is one of the most costly health-care conditions in many industrialized countries [11, 19, 62–64]. Among patients in the USA, having a cancer history or being actively treated for cancer is associated with higher out-of-pocket costs compared to similar individuals without cancer [65], and the uninsured have more out-of-pocket expenditures than the insured despite less health care use [66]. In the past decade, health-care costs and insurance premiums have increased and a substantial proportion of families have health-care debt [67, 68]. Further, health-care expenses are reported to be the underlying reason for many bankruptcies, with cancer as a leading cause [69, 70]. Many of those filing for bankruptcy had health insurance. High patient cost-sharing (i.e., deductibles, co-payments, and coinsurance), limits on annual and lifetime benefits, and waiting periods for public programs contribute to the financial burden for cancer patients [71, 72]. Even with health insurance, some cancer patients may delay treatment or not seek care because of cost and concerns about health-care debt. Cancer survivors of lower socioeconomic status, or who are uninsured or underinsured are particularly vulnerable to the financial impact of cancer care, particularly in light of increasingly expensive cancer therapies. Regardless of insurance or socioeconomic status, cancer survivors may incur substantial out-of-pocket costs, and as a result, can experience financial difficulties.

## *High Costs of Cancer Therapies*

The price of newly developed cancer treatments has increased dramatically in the past decade [31, 73]. Adoption of these therapies, primarily biologics, has begun to impose a significant burden on both health-care payers and patients. Currently, ten monoclonal antibodies are approved by the US Food and Drug Administration (FDA) for the treatment of cancer [74]. To illustrate the magnitude of cost for treatment with these therapies, a 1-month treatment of bevacizumab for the treatment of metastatic colorectal cancer may cost more than $US 9,000 (in 2009 dollars), of which 20% is likely to be covered through patient out-of-pocket expenditures and not health insurance [75]. The average duration for a completed course of treatment in clinical trials was about 9 months, leading to a total cost in excess of $US 75,000 (in 2009 dollars) [76]. Many new biologic drugs are used to treat patients with advanced stage disease who are unresponsive to other available and less costly therapies. Because life expectancy for these patients is short and other treatment options have been exhausted, patients and their families may be desperate and willing to try high-cost and potentially high-risk treatments [77].

In order to understand whether the costs of these new biologic treatments are "worth" it, the therapeutic benefit of treatment must be evaluated. Results from recent clinical trials have reported relatively small benefits (e.g., only a few months of life) associated with the use of a number of newer chemotherapies [78]. Further, many biologics are effective only in specific subsets of patients, such as cetuximab for colorectal cancer patients with wild-type KRAS tumors [79].

Given such marginal benefits shown in clinical trials, how should payers decide whether or not to provide coverage for high-priced cancer drugs? In countries with single-payer systems such as the UK, Australia, and Canada, coverage decisions take into account the costs of treatment often by conducting cost-effectiveness analyses and calculating incremental cost-effectiveness ratios (ICER), a measure assessing the increased cost required by an intervention to obtain one additional year of life. Based on data from a clinical trial, the ICER associated with cetuximab treatment for advanced colorectal cancer is in excess of $CAD 150,000 (in 2007 dollars) per life year saved [80]. In contrast, the ICER estimates associated with colorectal cancer screening range from about $US 10,000 to $US 25,000 per life-year saved (in 2000 dollars) [81]. NICE often cites a range of £20,000–£30,000 (or $US 33,000–$US 49,000) as a threshold to inform coverage decisions which represents "good value." Currently, cetuximab is not covered by the NHS in the UK. In the USA, cost is not explicitly considered by the FDA or the Centers for Medicare and Medicaid Services for drug approval or coverage decisions, although the American Society of Clinical Oncology has recently endorsed a "critical role" for oncologists in addressing the cost of care with their patients [82].

## Impact of Personalized Medicine

Recent scientific advances have identified genetic mutations that identify individuals who are unlikely to respond to treatment. For example, researchers have found that individuals diagnosed with metastatic colorectal cancer carrying KRAS mutations do not respond to treatment with cetuximab [83] or panitumumab [84]. Limiting the use of these expensive drugs to patients without KRAS mutations will increase the likelihood of response to therapy and save health-care payers' and patients' money. A study by Mittmann et al. examined the impact of restricting cetuximab treatment to advanced colorectal cancer patients with KRAS wild-types and estimated an ICER of approximately $CAD 80,000 (in 2007 dollars) per life year less than when the entire population is treated [80].

Policy makers are now faced with identifying ways to control the costs of drugs and long-term care for cancer survivors. The methods commonly used by single-payer systems to evaluate treatment coverage decisions should be applied to long-term survivorship programs in order to identify interventions that represent an efficient use of resources.

## Cancer Burden Studies and Economic Analysis

### *Development of Data Resources*

Many estimates of the costs of cancer care in the USA are based on specific insured populations, such as elderly Medicare beneficiaries, or from cross-sectional surveys. Estimates based on insured populations do not include costs from other payers and exclude cancer patients without health insurance, who may have very different care and cost experiences. In the case of studies using data from Medicare, private payer (i.e., supplemental insurance), Medicaid, Veterans Health and Administration (VA), patient out-of-pocket payments are not included and must be estimated separately if they are to be included. Efforts are underway to improve data sources for producing nationally representative estimates for cancer survivors of all ages using the Medical Expenditure Panel Survey (MEPS). Data linkage efforts, such as those combining state- or province-level cancer registries with hospital discharge data, Medicare, and Medicaid as well as employer-based data are ongoing [85, 86]. Resulting estimates can be used in burden studies and in economic evaluations of specific treatment options.

### *Standardization of Measures*

Statistical methods for estimating cancer prevalence by phase of care for use in aggregate cost estimates require registry data and active follow-up of survival [9]. The availability and quality of these data vary considerably by country. Further, differences in burden estimates across countries reflect differences of health-care systems, distribution of cancer stage at diagnosis, survival, and patterns of care. A recent review found considerable heterogeneity across studies of the burden of cancer, with regard to study settings, populations studied, types of services included, measurement of costs, and study methods [87]. Greater documentation and reporting of patient characteristics that influence outcomes and costs (e.g., stage at diagnosis) and methods used to identify the sample of cancer survivors and treatment classification, address censored or missing data, and skewed distribution of cost data will be important for future efforts. Although standards for conducting cost-effectiveness analyses have been published [3], we were not able to identify any published standards for conducting and reporting burden of disease studies. Such standardization will improve the quality of burden studies as well as international comparisons of burden.

Even with guidelines for standardized reporting of economic evaluations, recommendations are often not implemented because of lack of consensus on standards and lack of appreciation on the value of standardized reporting. Other factors affecting comparability include the underlying health risks of different populations, differences in reimbursement schemes, and differences in health-care delivery systems also impact economic evaluations. These variations also complicate international comparisons. Improved standardization and future international research collaborations may provide harmonization of methods and new approaches for comparing studies across countries.

## *Comprehensive Measures of Cost*

Another limitation in burden and economic evaluation studies is the lack of comprehensive measures of cost. Although important in burden studies and routinely recommended for inclusion in economic evaluations, measures are generally limited to health-care costs, frequently excluding productivity costs and patient and community caregiver time costs [3, 25, 88]. Ignoring these important costs underestimates the burden of cancer and favors the adoption of interventions that use more patient and community time [88]. For example, the cost per QALY associated with a screening colonoscopy ignoring patient time costs is only $US 13,100 compared to $US 42,600 when time costs are considered (2006 dollars) [89]. A focus on the collection of patient and caregiver time costs alongside clinical trials and other long-term costs would greatly enhance the precision of future economic evaluations. As described previously, use of service frequencies, combined with estimates of service time and value of time, can also be used to estimate time costs. Although there is no consensus about the single best method for valuing patient and caregiver time, use of multiple methods can be assessed with sensitivity analysis.

## *Improving Methods*

Many of the evaluations of cancer treatment options utilize decision analytic or simulation modeling software packages such as TreeAge® to conduct their analyses. Many researchers rely upon this software because it is easy to use, but it may simplify important inputs and ignore contextual characteristics, resulting in biased results. Greenberg et al. reported that less than 30% of all cancer CUAs included in their review included a probabilistic sensitivity analysis which, given the inevitable uncertainty in many models, is an area in need of attention [40]. Further, sensitivity analysis is typically performed only for model inputs, not assumptions about natural history of disease or model structure. Consortiums of modelers, such as the National Cancer Institute supported Cancer Intervention and Surveillance Modeling Network (CISNET) [44], can use similar model inputs with different models to gain better understanding about the impact of model structure. Currently, CISNET groups are evaluating cancer control interventions for breast, colorectal, prostate, and lung cancers. Ongoing efforts in these cancer sites as well as newer efforts for other cancers will be important. Details of model structure, parameters, and results are available for researchers in a standardized format referred to as a model profile (http://cisnet.cancer.gov/profiles/). Modeling efforts can also be used for projections to help policy makers understand the potential impact of cancer control interventions, particularly in settings with constrained resources.

### *Long-Term Survivorship*

Several studies have reported that cancer survivors have poorer health outcomes than similar individuals without cancer, even many years after cancer diagnosis [93, 94]. However, a recent review of the cost of cancer care studies conducted in the USA found that many studies focused on the first year following diagnosis or in the initial phase of care and in the last year of life, but fewer studies have addressed the costs associated with long-term survivorship [87]. The few studies that have been conducted suggest that long-term survivorship is an important component of cancer burden. Also it is this long-term survivorship that will become increasingly important to optimize the use of a range of economically sensitive approaches. We need to better align our economic efforts with the bulk of people surviving as they go through life.

Compared to similar individuals without cancer, cancer survivors are more likely to report not being able to work or having limitations in their work because of health, and experience more work days lost [90, 91]. Cancer survivors are also more likely to report fair or poor health compared to similar individuals without cancer [90, 91]. Thus, preventing disability and improving quality of life are important goals for cancer survivors. Disability prevention studies focus on minimizing the impact of health conditions on labor-force participation. Unfortunately, disability prevention studies are lacking in the cancer literature and should be a priority area for future research. A key focus of these studies is the productivity consequences of alternatives, both in the form of work absences and lower levels of engagement while at work (known as presenteeism).

## Summary and Conclusions

Economic analyses are likely to provide an important source of data related to resource allocation. This may be even more the case in the future as populations in many countries continue to age, changes in health patterns continue to unfold, and the cost of new therapies continue to increase. Information on the burdens and resource implications of alternatives are invaluable for policy decision making at the local and national levels. By necessity, we must choose amongst more alternatives than are possible to support. Because choices must be made, decision makers have a moral imperative to ensure they are made in a way that brings the greatest good to the greatest number. But economic information is useful only if one can discern the nature and quality of the evidence and the transferability/generalizability of the findings reported in studies. This chapter emphasizes the importance of economic evaluation in decision making when considering health care and program options to improve the quality of cancer survivorship. In our review of the measures and methods of economic evaluation, we have sought to provide the needed foundations useful in understanding and interpreting economic evaluation studies in this area.

## References

1. Drummond M, Sculpher M, Torrance GW, O'Brien BJ, Stoddart GL. Methods for the economic evaluation of health care programmes. Oxford: Oxford University Press; 2005.
2. Culyer AJ. The normative economics of health care finance and provision. In: McGuire A, Fenn P, Mayhew K, editors. Providing health care: the economics of alternative systems of finance and delivery. Oxford: Oxford University Press; 1991. p. 65–98.
3. Gold MR, Siegel JE, Russell LB, Weinstein MC. Cost-effectiveness in health and medicine. New York: Oxford University Press; 1996.
4. Fiore K. Global burden of cancer is increasing [document on the Internet]. Medpage Today. December 10, 2008 [cited 2010 Mar 3]. Available from: http://www.medpagetoday.com/HematologyOncology/OtherCancers/12094.
5. Mariotto AB, Yabroff KR, Shao Y, Feuer EJ, Brown ML. Projections of the cost of cancer care in the U.S.: 2010–2020. 2011; JNCI 103(2):117–128.
6. Kamangar F, Dores GM, Anderson WF. Patterns of cancer incidence, mortality, and prevalence across five continents: defining priorities to reduce cancer disparities in different geographic regions of the world. J Clin Oncol. 2006;24(14):2137–50.
7. Edwards BK, Howe HL, Ries LA, Thun MJ, Rosenberg HM, Yancik R, et al. Annual report to the nation on the status of cancer, 1973-1999, featuring implications of age and aging on U.S. cancer burden. Cancer. 2002;94:2766–92.
8. Ries LAG, Melbert D, Krapcho M, Stinchcomb DG, Howlader N, Horner MJ, et al., editors. SEER cancer statistic review, 1975–2005. Bethesda, MD: National Cancer Institute; 2008.
9. Mariotto AB, Yabroff KR, Feuer EJ, De Angelis R, Brown M. Projecting the number of patients with colorectal carcinoma by phases of care in the US: 2000–2020. Cancer Causes Control. 2006;17:1215–26.
10. National Cancer Institute. Cancer trends progress report. [document on the Internet]. 2007 [cited 2010 Jul 19]. Available from: http://progressreport.cancer.gov/2007/.
11. Koopmanschap MA, van Roijen L, Bonneux L, Barendregt JJ. Current and future costs of cancer. Eur J Cancer. 1994;30A:60–5.
12. Riley GF, Potosky AL, Lubitz JD, Kessler LG. Medicare payments from diagnosis to death for elderly cancer patients by stage and diagnosis. Med Care. 1995;33:828–41.
13. Taplin SH, Barlow W, Urban N, Mandelson MT, Timlin DJ, Ichikawa L, et al. Stage, age, comorbidity, and direct costs of colon, prostate, and breast cancer care. J Natl Cancer Inst. 1995;87:417–26.
14. Fireman BH, Quesenberry CP, Somkin CP, Jacobson AS, Baer D, West D, et al. Cost of care for cancer in a health maintenance organization. Health Care Financ Rev. 1997;18:51–76.
15. Yabroff KR, Lamont EB, Mariotto A, Warren JL, Topor M, Meekins A, et al. Cost of care for elderly cancer patients in the United States. J Natl Cancer Inst. 2008;100:630–41.
16. Rice DP, Hodgson TA. Social and economic implications of cancer in the United States: vital and health statistics. DHHS publication no. PHS81-1404. Washington, DC: US Government Printing Office; 1981. Vol. 3, No. 20.

17. Max W, Rice DP, Sung H-Y, Michel M, Breuer W, Zhang X. The economic burden of prostate cancer, California, 1998. Cancer. 2002;94:2906–13.
18. Max W, Rice DP, Sung H-Y, Michel M, Breuer W, Zhang X. The economic burden of gynecologic cancers in California, 1998. Gynecol Oncol. 2003;88:96–103.
19. Lidgren M, Wilking N, Jonnson B. Cost of breast cancer in Sweden in 2002. Eur J Health Econ. 2007;8:5–15.
20. Bradley CJ, Yabroff KR, Dahman B, Feuer EJ, Mariotto A, Brown ML. Productivity costs of cancer mortality in the United States: 2000-2020. J Natl Cancer Inst. 2008;100(24):1763–70.
21. Yabroff KR, Bradley CJ, Mariotto AB, Brown ML, Feuer EJ. Estimates and projections of value of life lost from cancer deaths in the United States. J Natl Cancer Inst. 2008;100(24):1755–62.
22. Brown ML, Yabroff KR. Economic impact of cancer in the United States. In: Schottenfeld D, Fraumeni JF, editors. Cancer epidemiology and prevention. 3rd ed. New York, NY: Oxford University Press; 2004. p. 202–16.
23. Yabroff KR, Davis WW, Lamont EB, Fahey A, Topor M, Brown ML, et al. Patient time costs associated with cancer care. J Natl Cancer Inst. 2007;99:14–23.
24. Hayman JA, Langa KM, Kabeto MU, Katz SH, DeMonner SM, Chernew ME, et al. Estimating the cost of informal caregiving for elderly patients with cancer. J Clin Oncol. 2001;19:3219–25.
25. Yabroff KR, Kim Y. Time costs associated with informal caregiving for cancer survivors. Cancer. 2009;115(18 Suppl):4362–73.
26. Yabroff KR, Warren JL, Knopf K, Davis WW, Brown ML. Estimating patient time costs associated with colorectal cancer care. Med Care. 2005;43:640–8.
27. Economist Intelligence Unit. Breakaway: the global burden of cancer-challenges and opportunities [document on the Internet]. 2009 [cited 2010 Apr 1]. Available from: http://graphics.eiu.com/marketing/pdf/EIU_LIVESTRONG_Global_Cancer_Burden.pdf.
28. Warren JL, Yabroff KR, Meekins A, Topor M, Lamont EB, Brown ML. Evaluation of trends in the cost of initial cancer treatment. J Natl Cancer Inst. 2008;100:888–97.
29. Etzioni R, Ramsey SD, Berry K, Brown M. The impact of including future medical care costs when estimating the costs attributable to disease: a colorectal cancer case study. Health Econ. 2001;10:245–56.
30. Jansman FG, Postma MJ, Brouwers JR. Cost considerations in the treatment of colorectal cancer. Pharmacoeconomics. 2007;25(7):537–62.
31. Schrag D. The price tag on progress–chemotherapy for colorectal cancer. N Engl J Med. 2004;351(4):317–9.
32. Evers S, Goossens M, de Vet HC, van Tulder M, Ament A. Criteria list for assessment of methodological quality of economic evaluations: consensus on health economic criteria. Int J Technol Assess Health Care. 2005;21(2):240–5.
33. Culyer AJ, Sculpher M. Chapter 4: Lessons from health technology assessment. In: Tompa E, Culyer AJ, Dolinschi R, editors. Economic evaluation of interventions for occupational health and safety: developing good practice. Oxford: Oxford University Press; 2008. p. 51–70.
34. Lilienfeld DE, Stolley PD. Foundations of epidemiology. New York: Oxford University Press; 1994.
35. Rothman KJ, Greenland S. Modern epidemiology. Philadelphia: Lippincott-Raven; 1998.
36. Shadish WR, Cook TD, Campbell DT. Experimental and quasi-experimental designs for generalized causal inference. Boston: Houghton Mifflin; 2002.
37. Hoch J, Dewa C. Chapter 9: Kind of analysis and decision rule. In: Tompa E, Culyer AJ, Dolinschi R, editors. Economic evaluation of interventions for occupational health and safety: developing good practice. Oxford: Oxford University Press; 2008. p. 147–64.
38. Culyer AJ, Tompa E. Chapter 13: Equity. In: Tompa E, Culyer AJ, Dolinschi R, editors. Economic evaluation of interventions for occupational health and safety: developing good practice. Oxford: Oxford University Press; 2008.
39. Wailoo A, Tsuchiya A, McCabe C. Weighting must weight: Incorporating equity concerns into cost-effectiveness analysis may take longer than expected. Pharmacoeconomics. 2009;27(12):983–9.

40. Greenberg D, Earle C, Fang CH, Eldar-Lissai A, Neumann PJ. When is cancer care cost-effective? A systematic overview of cost-utility analyses in oncology. J Natl Cancer Inst. 2010;102(2):82–8.
41. Tappenden P, Chilcott J, Brennan A, Pilgrim H. Systematic review of economic evidence for the detection, diagnosis, treatment, and follow-up of colorectal cancer in the United Kingdom. Int J Technol Assess Health Care. 2009;25(4):470–8.
42. Koperna T, Semmler D. Innovative chemotherapies for stage III colon cancer: a cost-effectiveness study. Hepatogastroenterology. 2003;50(54):1903–9.
43. Dahlberg M, Stenborg A, Pahlman L, Glimelius B. Cost-effectiveness of preoperative radiotherapy in rectal cancer: results from the Swedish Rectal Cancer Trial. Int J Radiat Oncol Biol Phys. 2002;54(3):654–60.
44. National Cancer Institute. Cancer intervention and surveillance modeling network [homepage on the Internet]. [cited 2010 Feb 8]. Available from: http://cisnet.cancer.gov/.
45. Hewitt M, Greenfield S, Stovall E, editors. From cancer patient to cancer survivor, Lost in transition. Washington, DC: The National Academies Press; 2006.
46. DeLisa JA. A history of cancer rehabilitation. Cancer. 2001;92(4 Suppl):970–4.
47. Stanton AL, Ganz PA, Kwan L, Meyerowitz BE, Bower JE, Krupnick JL, et al. Outcomes from the Moving Beyond Cancer psychoeducational, randomized, controlled trial with breast cancer patients. J Clin Oncol. 2005;23(25):6009–18.
48. Morey MC, Snyder DC, Sloane R, Cohen HJ, Peterson B, Hartman TJ, et al. Effects of home-based diet and exercise on functional outcomes among older, overweight long-term cancer survivors: RENEW. JAMA. 2009;301:1883–91.
49. Inglis SC, Pearson S, Treen S, Gallasch T, Horowitz JD, Stewart S. Extending the horizon in heart failure: effects of multi-disciplinary, home-based intervention relative to usual care. Circulation. 2006;114:2466–73.
50. Dennis D, Houston-Miller N, Schwartz RG, Ahn DK, Kraemer HC, Gossard D, et al. Early return to work after uncomplicated myocardial infarction. Results of a randomized trial. JAMA. 1998;260(2):214–20.
51. Mandelblatt JS, Cullen J, Lawrence WF, Stanton AL, Yi B, Kwan L, et al. Economic evaluation alongside a clinical trial of psycho-educational interventions to improve adjustment to survivorship among patients with breast cancer. J Clin Oncol. 2008;26(10):1684–90.
52. Starling N, Tilden D, White J, Cunningham D. Cost-effectiveness analysis of cetuximab/irinotecan vs active/best supportive care for the treatment of metastatic colorectal cancer patients who have failed previous chemotherapy treatment. Br J Cancer. 2007;96(2):206–12.
53. World population ageing: 1950-2050 [document on the Internet]. The Population Division of the Department of Economic and Social Affairs of the United Nations. 2009 [cited 2010 Mar 3]. Available at: http://www.un.org/esa/population/publications/worldageing19502050/.
54. Yabroff KR, Mariotto AB, Feuer E, Brown ML. Projections of the costs associated with colorectal cancer care in the United States, 2000-2020. Health Econ. 2008;17(8):947–59.
55. Breen N, Wagener DK, Brown ML, Davis WW, Ballard-Barbash R. Progress in cancer screening over a decade: results of cancer screening from the 1987, 1992, and 1998 national health interview surveys. J Natl Cancer Inst. 2001;93:1704–13.
56. Kogevinas M, Porta M. Socioeconomic differences in cancer survival: a review of the evidence. IARC Sci Publ. 1997;138:177–206.
57. Faggiano F, Partanen T, Kogevinas M, Boffetta P. Socioeconomic differences in cancer incidence and mortality. In: Kogevinas M, Pearce N, Susser M, Boffetta P, editors. Social inequalities and cancer. IARC Sci Publ. 1997;138:65–176.
58. DeNavas-Walt C, Proctor BD, Smith JC. Income, poverty, and health insurance coverage in the United States: 2008 [document on the Internet]. US Census Bureau: Current Population Reports. 2009 [cited 2010 Mar 3]. Available from: https://www.census.gov/prod/2009pubs/p60-236.pdf.
59. Banthin JS, Bernard DM. Changes in financial burdens for health care: national estimates for the population younger than 65 years, 1996 to 2003. JAMA. 2006;296:2712–9.

60. Halpern MT, Ward EM, Pavluck AL, Schrag NM, Bian J, Chen AY. Association of insurance status and ethnicity with cancer stage at diagnosis for 12 cancer sites: a retrospective analysis. Lancet Oncol. 2008;9:222–31.
61. Lund JL, Yabroff KR, Ibuka Y, Russell LB, Barnett PG, Lipscomb J, et al. Inventory of data sources for estimating health care costs in the United States. Med Care. 2009;47:S127–42.
62. Meerding WJ, Bonneux L, Polder JJ, Koopmanschap MA, van der Maas PJ. Demographic and epidemiological determinants of healthcare costs in Netherlands: cost of illness study. BMJ. 1988;317:111–5.
63. Howard DH, Molinari N-A, Thorpe KE. National estimates of medical costs incurred by nonelderly cancer patients. Cancer. 2004;100:883–91.
64. Kim SG, Hahm MI, Choi KS, Seung NY, Shin HR, Park EC. The economic burden of cancer in Korea in 2002. Eur J Cancer Care. 2008;17:136–44.
65. Langa KM, Fendrick AM, Chernew ME, Kabeto MU, Paisley KL, Hayman JA. Out-of-pocket health care expenditures among older Americans with cancer. Value Health. 2004;7:186–94.
66. Thorpe KE, Howard D. Health insurance and spending among cancer patients. Health Aff (Web exclusive). 2003;W3:189–98.
67. Seifert RW, Rukavina M. Bankruptcy is the tip of a medical-debt iceberg. Health Affairs. 2006;25:w89–92.
68. Cunningham PJ. Trade-offs getting tougher: problems paying medical bills increase for U.S. families, 2003–2007. Track Report. 2008;21:1–5.
69. Himmelstein DU, Thorne D, Warren E, Woolhandler S. Medical bankruptcy in the United States, 2007: results of a national study. Am J Med. 2009;122:741–6.
70. Himmelstein DU, Warren E, Thorne D, Woolhandler S. Illness and injury as contributors to bankruptcy. Health Affairs. 2005;24:w63–73.
71. Schwartz K, Claxton G, Martin K, Schmidt C. Spending to survive: cancer patients confront holes in the health insurance system [document on the Internet]. Kaiser Family Foundation and American Cancer Society (#7934). 2009 [cited 2010 Mar 3]. Available from: http://www.kff.org/insurance/7851.cfm.
72. Schwartz K, Martin K, Finan S. Patients under pressure: profiles of how families affected by cancer are faring in the recession [document on the Internet]. Kaiser Family Foundation and American Cancer Society (#7934). 2009 [cited 2010 Mar 3]. Available from: http://www.kff.org/insurance/7934.cfm.
73. Bach PB. Limits on Medicare's ability to control rising spending on cancer drugs. N Engl J Med. 2009;360(6):626–33.
74. American Cancer Society. Monoclonal antibodies [document on the Internet]. 2009 [cited 2009 Dec 02]. Available from: http://www.cancer.org/docroot/ETO/content/ETO_1_4X_Monoclonal_Antibody_Therapy_Passive_Immunotherapy.asp?sitearea=ETO.
75. Kolata G. Costly cancer drug offers hope, but also a dilemma. The New York Times. 2008 July 6.
76. National Institute for Health and Clinical Excellence. NICE guidance on bortezomib (velcade) is a win-win solution for multiple myeloma patients and the NHs. Press release [document on the Internet]. 2007 [cited 2010 Mar 3]. Available from: http://www.nice.org.uk/media/eB7/14/2007056BortezomibformultiplemyelomaAppv2.pdf.
77. Gaskin DJ, Kong J, Meropol NJ, Yabroff KR, Weaver C, Schulman KA. Treatment choices by seriously ill patients: the Health Stock Risk Adjustment model. Med Decis Making. 1998;18(1):84–94.
78. Pirker R, Pereira JR, Szczesna A, von Pawel J, Krzakowski M, Ramlau R, et al. Cetuximab plus chemotherapy in patients with advanced non-small-cell lung cancer (FLEX): an open-label randomised phase III trial. Lancet. 2009;373(9674):1525–31.
79. Karapetis CS, Khambata-Ford S, Jonker DJ, O'Callaghan CJ, Tu D, Tebbutt NC, et al. K-ras mutations and benefit from cetuximab in advanced colorectal cancer. N Engl J Med. 2008;359(17):1757–65.
80. Mittmann N, Au HJ, Tu D, O'Callaghan CJ, Isogai PK, Karapetis CS, et al. Prospective cost-effectiveness analysis of cetuximab in metastatic colorectal cancer: evaluation of National

Cancer Institute of Canada Clinical Trials Group CO.17 trial. J Natl Cancer Inst. 2009;101(17):1182–92.
81. Pignone M, Saha S, Hoerger T, Mandelblatt J. Cost-effectiveness analyses of colorectal cancer screening: a systematic review for the U.S. Preventive Services Task Force. Ann Intern Med. 2002;137(2):96–104.
82. Meropol NJ, Schrag D, Smith TJ, Mulvey TM, Langdon RM, Blum D, et al. American Society of Clinical Oncology guidance statement: the cost of cancer care. J Clin Oncol. 2009;27(23):3868–74.
83. Khambata-Ford S, Garrett CR, Meropol NJ, Basik M, Harbison CT, Wu S, et al. Expression of epiregulin and amphiregulin and K-ras mutation status predict disease control in metastatic colorectal cancer patients treated with cetuximab. J Clin Oncol. 2007;25(22):3230–7.
84. Amado RG, Wolf M, Peeters M, Van Cutsem E, Slena S, Freeman DJ, et al. Wild-type KRAS is required for panitumumab efficacy in patients with metastatic colorectal cancer. J Clin Oncol. 2008;26(10):1626–34.
85. Bradley CJ, Given CW, Luo Z, Roberts C, Copeland G, Virnig BA. Medicaid, Medicare, and the Michigan Tumor Registry: a linkage strategy. Med Decis Making. 2007;27:352–63.
86. Schrag D, Virnig BA, Warren JL. Linking tumor registry and Medicaid claims to evaluate cancer care delivery. Health Care Financ Rev. 2009;30:61–73.
87. Yabroff KR, Warren JL, Brown ML. Costs of cancer care in the USA: a descriptive review. Nat Clin Pract Oncol. 2007;4:643–56.
88. Russell LB. Completing costs: patients' time. Med Care. 2009;47(7 Suppl 1):S89–93.
89. Jonas DE, Russell LB, Sandler RS. Value of patient time invested in the colonoscopy screening process: time requirements for Colonoscopy Study. Med Decis Making. 2008;28:56–65.
90. Yabroff KR, Lawrence WF, Clauser S, Davis WW, Brown ML. Burden of illness in cancer survivors: findings from a population-based national sample. J Natl Cancer Inst. 2004;96:1322–30.
91. Dowling E, Yabroff KR, Mariotto AB, McNeel T, Zeruto C, Buckman D. Burden of illness in adult survivors of childhood cancers: findings from a population-based national sample. Cancer. 2010;116:3712–21.

# Chapter 16
# Human Factors Engineering: Targeting Systems for Change

**Mary E. Sesto, Amye J. Tevaarwerk, and Douglas A. Wiegmann**

## Introduction

In 2003, the National Cancer Institute (NCI) Office of Cancer Survivorship estimated that cancer survivors represented nearly 4% of the US population. This number is expected to grow dramatically over time [1, 2]. As a group, cancer survivors represent a disparate population. Survivors include a broad range of ages (infants to octogenarians), disease types (acute leukemias to neuroendocrine tumors), disease severity (localized versus metastatic), and treatments received (observation, surgery, chemotherapy, radiotherapy, immunotherapy, stem cell transplant, etc.). However, certain challenges are universal: cancer treatment is generally complex, extends over long periods of time, may have persistent long-term and late effects, and often requires follow-up surveillance. These characteristics necessitate close attention to coordination and transfers of care.

The 2006 IOM report [3] recognized that many survivors did not receive routine or necessary primary care following active treatment. This may stem from inadequate provider-to-provider and provider-to-patient communication, but little literature exists to support or refute this claim. However, the extant literature does support the claim that the coordination of care for cancer survivors remains suboptimal. Nearly one-third of survivors are unsure which physician will direct follow-up care [4], and primary care providers (PCPs) generally rate the transition from oncologic to primary care as fair or poor [5].

Nationally, efforts are ongoing to improve systems of care for cancer survivors. However, evidence-based models and methods are needed for delivery of coordinated, interdisciplinary survivorship care in diverse communities and across different systems of care. The models and methods from Human Factors Engineering (HFE), a field focused on optimizing the performance of systems that involve interaction with people, may offer valuable lessons that can be applied to improve systems of

M.E. Sesto (✉)
Division of Physical Therapy, Department of Orthopedics,
Department of Industrial and Systems Engineering,
University of Wisconsin, Madison, WI, USA
e-mail: msesto@wisc.edu

M. Feuerstein and P.A. Ganz (eds.), *Health Services for Cancer Survivors*,
DOI 10.1007/978-1-4419-1348-7_16, © Springer Science+Business Media, LLC 2011

care for cancer survivors. By applying lessons learned from other complex systems, including aviation, nuclear power, and health care safety, we hope to illustrate how the cancer survivorship system may benefit from HFE models and methods.

First, readers will be introduced to HFE, and how HFE has already been applied to improve certain areas of health care. Second, we will make a case for why cancer survivorship fits into the care models for which HFE has already been successfully implemented. Third and lastly, we will provide a framework for how HFE could be applied to improve care for cancer survivors. Throughout the chapter, we will focus on breast cancer as a disease example. However, this process could be readily applied to other cancer types.

## Human Factors Engineering

### *What Is Human Factors Engineering?*

Human Factors Engineering (HFE) (also referred to as ergonomics or human factors) is a science and practice discipline that seeks to enhance human performance [6]. The role of human factors grew substantially in the US during World War II when it was realized that the design of equipment, such as airplane cockpits, had to account for human limitations while capitalizing on human capabilities. Until this point, attention was focused on personnel selection and training. However, despite selection and extensive training, even the best and most highly trained individuals were making critical errors that jeopardized safety and performance: even the best pilots were still crashing airplanes. As the limits of human capacity were reached, the focus shifted to improving the design of controls, displays, equipment, and teams to improve performance.

As a science, HFE investigates human capabilities, limitations, behaviors, and other characteristics. In practice, this information is used to design tools, technology, tasks, equipment, organizations, procedures, and environments to achieve productive, safe, and effective human use. Above all, HFE focuses on effectively integrating the human element into system design. Human factors engineers design system components to fit the people who live, work, and use these systems. A goal of HFE system design is to fit the needs, abilities, and limitations of people who interact with the system [6–8]. Consequently, use of HFE system design is prominent in many safety critical systems, especially in regulated industries such as aviation and nuclear energy production [9–18].

Six features [19] that characterize HFE and distinguish it from other applied fields are listed in Table 16.1. Notably, these characteristics are generally in direct contrast to traditional thinking which often expects the individual to fit the system rather than designing the system to fit the individual.

Recently, the tools, techniques, and principles of HFE have been applied to health care. HFE has been closely involved in the development of medical devices,

**Table 16.1** Characteristics of Human Factors Engineering and Design

| | |
|---|---|
| 1. | Devices, machines, and technologies are built to serve people and must be designed with the end user(s) in mind. |
| 2. | Recognition that individual variability in physical and cognitive capabilities and limitations exists and affects design. |
| 3. | Knowledge that the design of all things (e.g., tools, technologies, and organizations) influences human behavior, performance, and well-being. |
| 4. | Emphasis on evaluation and empirical data throughout the design process. |
| 5. | Use of evaluation, empirical data, and the scientific method to test hypotheses and evaluate results about human behavior and performance. |
| 6. | Reliance on a system-oriented approach and recognizing that people do not exist in isolation and that effective design must take into account technologies, tools, equipment, procedures, processes, environments, and organizations, and the interactions across these elements. |

[20–24] enhancing effectiveness and usability of health information technology [25–29] and aiding improvements in patient safety [27, 28, 30–37]. Application of HFE can improve the design and control of complex health care systems and technology resulting in improved quality of care, clinical process efficiency, and effectiveness of decision support systems [38, 39] ultimately enhancing the quality of care and satisfaction of patients and clinicians.

Systems of care for cancer survivors may derive similar benefits. For instance, a common frustration in clinical practice is the volume of records generated by any patient encounter, as well as the variability of records accompanying any transfer of care. A medical record often regurgitates data in an unorganized fashion. Generally, records consist of pages of potentially unhelpful and unnecessary labs and medications, interspersed with a few valuable bits of information such as surgery reports, pathology reports, and radiology reports. This unorganized avalanche of data is generated without any standardization or clear method for transfer. An HFE approach to this problem could be used to identify methods that effectively present, organize, and transfer information to optimize the usability of medical records and improve patient care.

The IOM [40] has emphasized the need for collaboration between health care and engineering: "… it is time to … establish a vigorous new partnership between engineering and health care and hasten a transition to a patient-centered 21st century health care system" [40]. The committee recognized that engineering tools and methods have transformed the quality and performance of other large-scale complex systems and could be used to improve health care systems [40]. Furthermore, the committee recognized that an engineering–health care partnership could transform a fragmented health care delivery system comprised of independent groups (e.g., individual or small group practices, hospitals, supported living centers, allied health practices, etc.) into an integrated, high-performance system. For example, inefficiencies and problems in health care often arise from conflicting, incomplete, or suboptimal elements which adversely affect other components and individuals, including physicians, survivors, and co-survivors (e.g., family members) [40].

## HFE Application for Improving Patient Safety in Health Care Systems

To date, HFE has been most widely applied in health care in an effort to reduce medical errors that threaten patient safety as well as to enhance quality of care and patient outcomes. Errors are commonly defined as "… occasions in which a planned sequence of mental or physical activities fails to achieve its intended outcome and when these failures cannot be attributed to the intervention of some chance agency" [41]. Errors can be in the form of either omissions or commissions. Omission errors occur when someone forgets to do something that needs to be done, such as a physician forgetting to change a medication dosage for a patient or a nurse forgetting to provide a patient with their prescribed medication. Errors of commission occur when a person performs the wrong action in a given situation. Examples of commission errors might be a physician who prescribes the wrong medication for patient, or a nurse who provides a medication to the wrong patient.

Traditionally, poor patient outcomes due to such medical errors or "oversights" in patient care have been attributed primarily to the technical skills or competency of an individual health care provider (HCP). Specifically, the culture within most health care settings has been one of censuring individuals for the errors they make. This situation is not too surprising given that the culture of medicine has long focused on perfection and individual accountability for one's actions. For example, within surgical specialties, the primacy of technical skills is the underlying assumption driving rankings of surgical performance across institutions or among one's surgical colleagues. "Once outcomes (usually mortality) have been correctly adjusted for patient risk factors, the remaining variance is presumed to be explained by individual surgical skill" (p. 476) [33]. Hence, when the patient does not do well or surgical errors are made, it is logical from this perspective to question the involved surgeon's skill or aptitude. Resultant safety interventions, therefore, often take the form of "blame you, shame you, train you" programs that are rarely effective in preventing recurrence, because they fail to focus on the underlying systemic problems that cause errors or impact quality of care and outcomes [33, 42].

Contrary to this traditional perspective, research in other complex settings (e.g., nuclear power and aviation industries) *suggests that human error is caused often by a combination of active and latent failures*, only the last of which is an unsafe act of an individual [16, 43]. Therefore, interventions targeting underlying system factors are often more efficacious than approaches focusing exclusively on individual characteristics. For example, the Systems Engineering Initiative to Patient Safety (SEIPS) model [30] (Fig. 16.1), a commonly used HFE model, indicates that understanding why errors occur, and how they can be prevented, requires the consideration of the entire organizational system in which health care is provided. According to SEIPS, several other variables beyond individual skills of the provider and the condition of the patient need to be examined:

- Environmental factors – equipment design and/or environmental distractions
- Social factors – teamwork and communication
- Supervisory issues – training, staffing, and scheduling
- Organizational variables – procedures, policies, and resources [16, 33, 42]

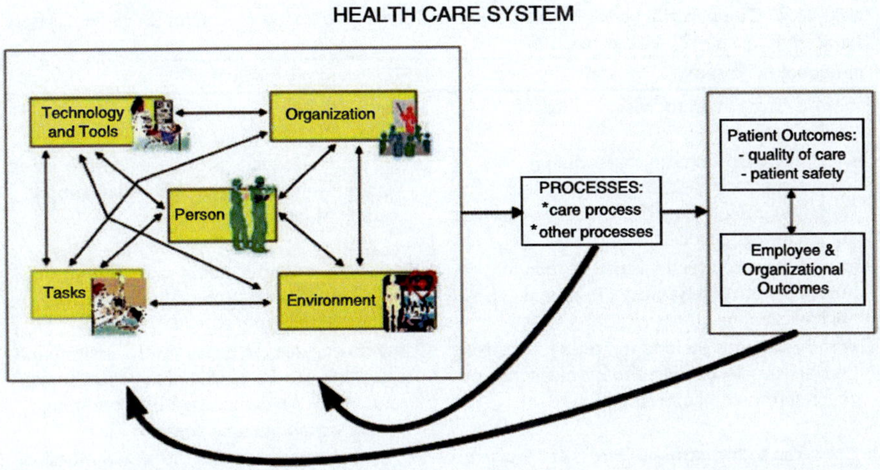


**Fig. 16.1** Modified Systems Engineering Initiative for Patient Safety (SEIPS) model (Reproduced from [Work system design for patient safety: the SEIPS model, Carayon P, Schoofs Hundt A, Karsh BT, Gurses AP, Alvarado CJ, Smith M et al., 15, i50–8, Copyright 2006] with permission from BMJ Publishing Group Ltd.) [30]

According to this perspective, errors are the natural consequences (not causes) of the systemic breakdown among these factors impacting performance. *Health care quality improvement programs are likely to be most effective when they intervene at specific failure points within the system rather than focusing solely on the individual who committed the error.*

Table 16.2 provides a more complete and direct comparison between the traditional view and the HFE systems perspective. Of particular importance is the focus of safety interventions that result from each approach. The traditional approach of "blame the individual" generally concentrates on the errors made by the HCP, blaming them for inattentiveness, forgetfulness, or even incompetence. As would be expected, the traditional approach focuses on changing the individual through remedial training, awareness campaigns, incentives to perform safety, and even punishment, none of which are very effective in reducing errors or improving patient care and outcomes. In contrast, the HFE system approach focuses on the contextual and situational factors that impact HCP behavior and performance. The essence of this approach is captured in the adage "you can't change the human condition but you can change the condition under which humans work" [43].

As an example in cancer survivorship, adherence to 5 or more years of endocrine therapy is emerging as a significant problem in breast cancer treatment. Endocrine therapy significantly decreases the risk of breast cancer recurrence and improves survival [44–46], yet a significant percentage of patients may prematurely discontinue therapy or miss doses [47]. Even a relatively modest degree of nonadherence (i.e., 90% vs. 80% of doses being taken) may impact breast cancer outcomes [48].

**Table 16.2** Comparison between the person and system focus perspectives to patient safety (Based on Reason [42] with permission)

| Traditional perspective | HFE system perspective |
|---|---|
| Focus on errors and procedural violations of individuals. | Humans are fallible and errors are to be expected, even in the best organizations. |
| Unsafe acts arise from aberrant mental processes such as inattentiveness, lack of good judgment, forgetfulness, recklessness, or even negligence. | Errors are consequences of deficient processes and/or system failures rather than simply causes of bad outcomes. |
| Interventions are directly aimed at reducing the "unwanted variability" in human behaviors. | Consistency in performance is important but flexibility is also invaluable during dynamic operations. |
| Common methods include retraining, recurrent proficiency tests, disciplinary measures, or even termination and litigation. | Countermeasures are based on the assumption that "though we cannot change the human condition, we can change the condition under which humans work." |
| When taken to the extreme, errors are viewed as a moral issue, with the notion that bad things (i.e., errors) happen to bad people. | The best people can make the worse mistakes. The important issue is not who blundered but how and why the defenses failed. |

Rather than blame the survivor or HCP for nonadherence, a HFE systems approach would evaluate factors that support the goal of medication adherence. No systematic approach exists for tackling this issue, and typically providers must remember to assess adherence for each patient. HFE analysis suggests a targeted approach would conserve valuable clinic time and provider resources. An HFE solution would have pharmacies automatically generate a reminder to both provider and survivor when refill frequency drops below a prespecified cutoff. This would provide redundancy within the system (both the patient and provider are notified), would target discussions regarding adherence to patients who most need it (efficiency), but still allow exploration of the reasons for nonadherence (patient-centered). Such a system would also remind busy clinics of the need to check for adherence, which might not consistently occur otherwise (safety).

Although the system-focused approach is relatively new to health care and the community-based health care system, there is an increasing awareness of the impact that systemic factors can have on shaping human performance. For example, the role that poorly designed medical devices can play in producing errors leading to patient harm is becoming increasingly apparent [49]. Roughly half of all medical device recalls result from design flaws, with specific types of devices being associated with unusually high use-error rates, such as infusion delivery devices. Social variables, such as teamwork and communication factors, are also of growing concern. The Joint Commission on Health Care Quality and Safety recently reported "communication" as the number one root cause (65%) of reported sentinel events between 1995 and 2004 [50]. Supervisory and organizational factors, such as shift work scheduling and unit staffing can impact errors such as medication errors within intensive care units [51]. These findings clearly indicate the importance of the system-focused approach to understanding how system design affects quality of care and patient outcomes across the health care system as a whole. We will demonstrate how the SEIPS model can be expanded to improve processes of care that affect care of survivors across multiple providers and organizations.

## Dimensions of Quality in Cancer Survivorship

The IOM described the crises in the American health care system [52] and identified six dimensions of quality requiring improvement in order for gains to be made in a complex health care system. These dimensions were initially envisioned for the health care delivery system in general. However, they are also applicable for improving systems of care for cancer survivors. Table 16.3 broadly defines each dimension alongside a specific example (Case 1) from the survivorship system. The remainder of the chapter (Cases 2 and 3) will explore various issues with survivorship care using a HFE systems-centered approach to analyze the contextual and situational factors that influence survivorship care.

**Case 1** D.J. is a 36-year-old female diagnosed with Stage IIa (T2N0cM0) HR+ HER2– breast cancer in January 2009. She underwent lumpectomy and sentinel node dissection, completed 4 cycles of TC and 6 weeks of whole breast radiotherapy. She was started on adjuvant tamoxifen in July 2009.

**Table 16.3** Dimensions for health care quality improvement and application to cancer survivorship

| Dimension | Definition and "cancer translation" | Examples from Case 1 |
|---|---|---|
| Safety | Avoid "injuries" to patients from the care that is intended to help them. "Improve patient awareness of late or long-term side effects of cancer." | D.J.'s menses stopped on chemotherapy, but resumed erratically in the following months. She experienced significant hot flashes and sleep disturbance. Her PCP (a nurse practitioner) considered starting her on an SSRI. Following discussion with her oncologist, D.J. elected to proceed with a brief trial of an SSRI with low potential for interaction with tamoxifen. |
| Effective | Provide services based on scientific knowledge to all who could benefit, and refrain from providing services to those not likely to benefit. "Provide care in an evidence-based fashion." | D.J. needs to be counseled regarding the need to report any change in vaginal discharge or new bleeding as a possible indicator of hyperplasia or endometrial cancer. However, her providers should refrain from screening transvaginal ultrasounds as these are an ineffective screening tool for endometrial cancer [53]. |

(continued)

**Table 16.3** (continued)

| Dimension | Definition and "cancer translation" | Examples from Case 1 |
|---|---|---|
| Patient-centered | Provide care that is respectful of and responsive to individual patient preferences, needs, and values, and ensure that patient values guide all clinical decisions.<br>"Provide care and resources that addresses the unique needs of each survivor." | D.J. is not interested in future pregnancy, but is sexually active. She was counseled regarding contraceptive options and elected to have a copper-IUD placed. For younger women such as D.J., future fertility is often an important issue. Women desiring future pregnancy may be concerned about the risk of chemotherapy-induced ammenorhea and the teratogenic effects of tamoxifen; concerns for relapse in the years post diagnosis may also complicate the timing of pregnancy.<br>Alternatively, some women who remain fertile may not immediately or ever desire future pregnancy. This can raise concerns about safely preventing pregnancy in women with HR+breast cancer. Providers must be responsive to both short-term and long-term patient goals. |
| Timely | Reduce waits and sometimes harmful delays for both those who receive and those who give care.<br>"Avoid delay in survivor care." | D.J. lives and works 40 min from her oncologist's office. She has difficulty attending her follow-up appointments, and questions the need for follow-up with both the medical and radiation oncologist. Her medical and radiation oncologist agreed to stagger visits every 6 months. Additionally, she will see her PCP locally every 6 months, and will have her mammogram locally. Because her PCP and oncologists are part of the same health care system and use an electronic medical record, they are all able to view her health care data. |
| Equitable | Provide care that does not vary in quality because of personal characteristics such as gender, ethnicity, geographic location, and socioeconomic status.<br>"Provide quality care regardless of individual characteristics of the survivor." | Because the primary clinic's NP was willing to perform part of her breast cancer care, D.J. is able to see at least one provider every 3 months. She admits that although she worries about breast cancer recurrence, she would likely have been able to keep only 1 or 2 appointments per year at a more distant location. |
| Efficient | Avoid waste, including waste of equipment, supplies, ideas, and energy.<br>"Provide organized, cost effective, and coordinated care to address the survivor's unique needs." | D.J.'s medical and radiation oncologists have successfully negotiated surveillance with each other and her PCP and established a plan of care. This improves access for new patients who may need chemotherapy or radiation, but does not leave either D.J. or her PCP without specialized guidance. Her oncologists also shared other patients with this PCP, and were motivated to shift some follow-up care for other patients with early stage breast cancer. |

These guiding factors can serve as a road map to better care for cancer survivors. However, in order to improve system performance and outcomes, analysis of system complexity is needed. For example, knowing that we need to "avoid delays in survivor care" or "provide organized, cost effective and coordinated care to address the survivor's unique needs" is only the first step. HFE methods can be used to redesign the system to effectively achieve these objectives. Some of these methods include failure-mode effects analysis (FMEA), critical incident methods, and process mapping that can all be used to assess various dimensions of system complexity. While the goal of this chapter is not to describe every HFE method available, we do want to emphasize that *regardless of the method used, identifying the various dimensions of system complexity is an important initial step.*

## System Complexity in Survivorship Care

Complexity often adversely affects systems performance and expected outcomes. This situation presents unique challenges to HFE in the design, implementation, and maintenance of systems [54]. For example, in the "health care cancer survivorship system," complexity can adversely affect communication among primary care providers, oncologists, and survivors [26]. Vicente [54] and Carayon [55] identified several interrelated characteristics that contribute to system complexity (Table 16.4). The survivorship system possesses many characteristics that impact complexity, thereby affecting outcomes. While these characteristics have been evaluated in the context of problems in health care in general, they have not been evaluated in the area of cancer survivorship health care.

**Table 16.4** Cancer survivorship health care system complexity (Adapted from Vincente [54] and Carayon [55] with permission)

| Factors affecting system complexity | Examples in breast cancer survivors |
|---|---|
| Social: Composed of many people who must work together. | Breast cancer is treated in a multidisciplinary fashion. A patient may see multiple HCPs (e.g., surgeon, medical oncologist radiation oncologist, nurse practitioners, oncology nurses, phlebotomists, radiotherapy technicians, etc.). The complexity of this provider network may be further complicated by other medical comorbidities (cardiac toxicity from an anthracycline) or preexisting conditions requiring the patient to see additional HCPs. |
| Heterogeneous perspectives: People with different backgrounds and different value structures need to be accounted for in the decision making process. | A variety of end users may exist within the survivorship system: survivor, co-survivor, PCP, oncologists, professional patient advocates, and other specialists. These groups will have different goals, needs, and as individuals, different values, cultures, and perspectives. |

(continued)

**Table 16.4** (continued)

| Factors affecting system complexity | Examples in breast cancer survivors |
|---|---|
| Dynamic system: Delay in effect of actions. No immediate change based on action taken today. | Monitoring factors affecting bone health in breast cancer often does not produce any immediate outcome. Encouraging adequate calcium and vitamin D in survivors to decrease the development of low bone density generally does not have an immediate impact on health outcomes. |
| Hazardous system: Hazards in the system that can affect the individual or groups, or have economic, social, public, or environmental consequences. | Medical errors in oncology can have a broad range. In the survivorship setting, many errors may be omissions: failure to cross-check for medication interactions or delay in obtaining health care records. |
| Coupling: Complex systems are typically comprised of many subsystems that are highly coupled/interact. | Decisions made during active treatment by the oncology team may dictate need for future follow-up and surveillance by the PCP. |
| Automation: Highly automated system. | Automation in survivorship care often occurs with scheduling, pharmacies, and routine blood panels. Problems may occur when the existing automation process does not have sufficient flexibility to address the survivor's needs. |
| Uncertainty: Uncertainty in available information. | Treatment recommendations may diverge wildly in areas where little data exists to guide decision-making (e.g., treatment of small HER2+ breast cancers). |
| Disturbances: Individuals responsible for dealing with unanticipated events. | Unanticipated changes in patient status due to an adverse event may occur (e.g., adverse drug reaction) or there may be a disruption in survivor–physician relationship due to retirement of the HCP or change in health insurance (USA). |
| Working across boundaries: Work may occur across organizational, geographical, and temporal boundaries. | A cancer survivor will likely see numerous HCPs, from different organizations, all of whom directly influence the survivor's care. Therefore, reporting of treatment histories, plans and follow up care must be coordinated [55, 56]. |
| Role of the end users: Increased demands are placed on patients and their families to be actively involved and to co-manage their own care. | There are multiple types of end users in the cancer survivorship system: HCPs, cancer survivors, co-survivors, employers, and patient advocates. As increased demands are placed on survivors to be actively involved in their care, resources are needed to support decision-making and long-term needs [26, 57]. |

## Application of HFE to Elements of Health Care in Cancer Survivorship

A quality survivorship health care system needs to provide effective and timely care for survivors, some with chronic conditions, to optimize quality of life. In general, health care systems have been slow to recognize that those with chronic health conditions, including cancer survivors, are often the primary managers of their health [58]. Cancer survivors must manage long-term or late-term effects through prescribed medications, therapy, diet, and exercise. Therefore, a critical role of the survivorship system is to support HCP, survivors, their families, and the community in working toward optimizing health and quality of life.

The Chronic Care Model (CCM) [59] emphasizes patient-centered care and incorporates both community and health care systems to improve quality of life and health outcomes in individuals with chronic disease [60, 61]. The focus of the CCM (Fig. 16.2) is to improve self-efficacy and empower individuals with chronic conditions so that they are able to take responsibility for self-management. Cancer, similar to other chronic conditions, involves management by multiple specialists, often practicing in different organizations or locations. An important factor in this model is that resources from both the health care and community systems are likely needed to optimize patient outcomes.

In comparison, the Systems Engineering Initiative for Patient Safety (SEIPS) HFE model, has been geared toward the HCP and understanding factors contributing to medical errors and patient outcomes. The focus has been on describing the relationship between the work system, individual performance, and patient safety. Thus far, the community system has not been an integrated piece in the SEIPS model. While SEIPS has primarily focused on improving patient safety, it can be readily applied to improving other health care outcomes, including cancer survivor outcomes.

By using a survivor-centered approach and incorporating the community system, similar to the CCM, the SEIPS – Survivor Centered model (Fig. 16.3)

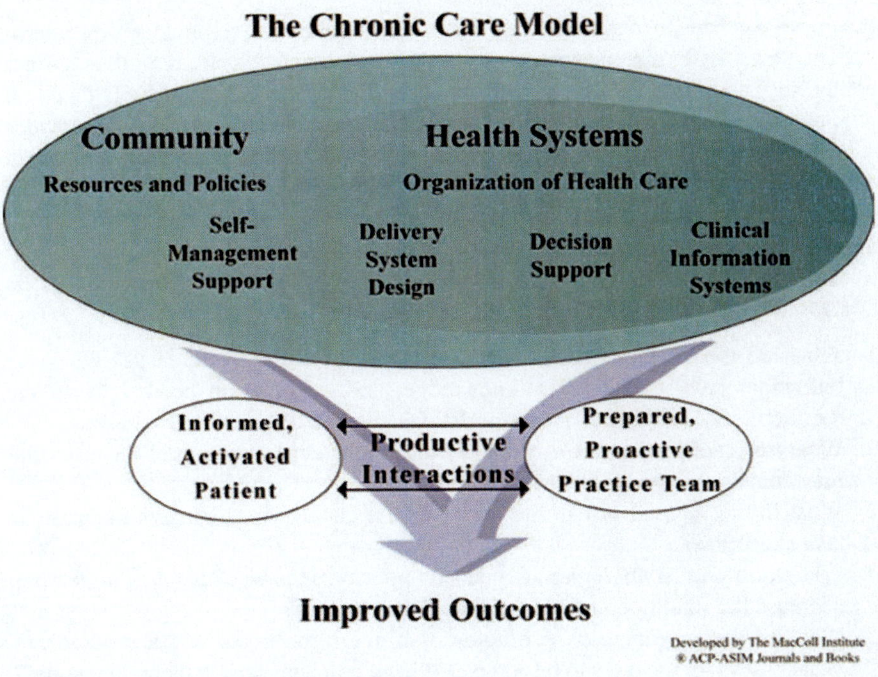


Fig. 16.2 The Chronic Care Model (with permission)

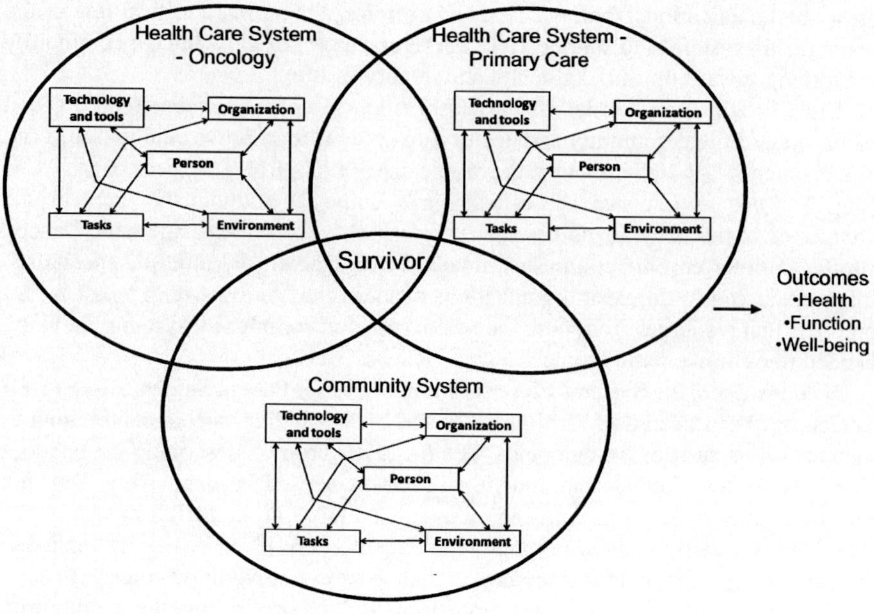


**Fig. 16.3** SEIPS – Survivor Centered model (with permission)

provides a mechanism to evaluate the systems (e.g., health care, community), the microsystems (e.g., HCP, screening program) and their interrelatedness as well as system complexity, all of which affect survivor outcomes. Furthermore, the HFE focus on human-centered design is analogous to the focus on patient-centered care, and provides a method for evaluating complex system issues. As described previously, the human element is central to system performance and the system is evaluated in terms of the interaction between the person and various components of the system as well as the interaction among system components that affect human performance.

Based on the domains in the SEIPS model, the following questions should be addressed when performing a HFE analysis of the system [31].

1. What are the characteristics of the *individual* performing the tasks? Does the individual have the abilities, knowledge, and information needed to do the required task? If not, can accommodations/support be provided?
2. What *tasks* need to be performed and what are the characteristics of the tasks that may contribute to poor outcomes?
3. What in the internal or external *environment* can serve as barriers or facilitate task execution?
4. What *tools and technologies* are needed to perform the task? Do they increase or decrease the likelihood of a high-performing system?
5. What in the *organization* promotes or hinders the tasks and the outcomes. What allows for the tasks to be completed in an efficient, safe, and timely manner?

These questions provide a framework to evaluate organizational and group-level interactions, use of technology, and optimal communication methods in order to improve survivor outcomes. We will use Case Examples 2 and 3 to illustrate how the SEIPS – Survivor Centered model can be used to evaluate factors that affect behavior, performance, and survivor outcomes.

## *Case 2 Using the SEIPS model to analyze a survivorship care plan to improve survivor outcomes*

Ms. M is a 66-year-old female originally diagnosed in 1993 with left Stage II infiltrating ductal carcinoma, ER+/PR-/HER2 unknown. She underwent a mastectomy and axillary dissection and then received adjuvant chemotherapy (AC × 4 cycles). She did not receive adjuvant tamoxifen. Fourteen years later, she was found to have recurrent disease in her mastectomy scar (biopsied January 2007). This was excised and pathology revealed infiltrating carcinoma, modified Bloom-Richardson grade 2, ER+ PR-HER2+. She declined further chemotherapy or trastuzumab. She received definitive radiotherapy, completed in March 2007, and then started anastrozole. The patient's oncologist retired in May 2008, and she was not seen in oncologic follow-up until Summer 2008. At that time, her new oncologist noted that Ms. M had never had a DEXA (she was at increased risk for low bone density based on age >65, use of anastrozole and premature ovarian failure due to chemotherapy in 1993). Ms. M preferred to have her DEXA locally due to the distance from her treating oncologist (120 mile round trip). She was given a referral and her DEXA was completed 3 months later (Fall 2008). Ms. M brought the report to her next oncology visit (2 months later in Winter 2009). Her DEXA revealed osteoporosis at the femoral neck (t-score –2.6) and osteopenia at the spine (t-score –1.9). Ms. M's risk factors were assessed: she was not taking any calcium supplementation and had a vitamin D deficiency at 10 ng/mL (25,OH Vitamin D range 30–50 ng/mL). In Spring of 2009 (2 months after starting regular calcium, vitamin D and an oral bisphosphonate) Ms. M sustained a hip fracture requiring hospitalization and surgery[1].

### HFE Analysis – Case 2

Ms. M's case exemplifies problems that occur in a fragmented health care system traditionally focused on reactionary versus chronic care management. It is recognized that many survivors do not receive routine or necessary primary care after active treatment. Data are limited, but this likely stems from inadequate provider-to-provider and provider-to-patient communication. Consequently, survivor care plans have been suggested to facilitate communication between oncology, PCPs and survivors, with an ultimate goal of improving follow-up care [3]. The overall

[1] We acknowledge that even an intravenous bisphosphonate immediately following her DEXA might not have prevented her fracture. However, her osteoporosis could clearly have been identified earlier by her PCP or oncologists based on her multiple risk factors. Earlier intervention could have impacted the outcome.

purpose of the survivor care plan is to inform survivors and PCPs about the rendered oncologic care and describe the anticipated medical and psychosocial aspects of oncologic care [62–64].

To date, little research has been conducted to validate the content and evaluate effectiveness in communicating necessary information across organizations and providers. The IOM report [3] details suggested elements of the care plan, and additional literature has addressed the elements for specific disease groups, particularly breast cancer [65]. However, the majority of survivors report never receiving either a treatment summary or survivor care plan (SCP) [66, 67]. Importantly, a number of factors, many of which are influenced by system complexity, will affect the implementation and effectiveness of SCPs. We will analyze factors that may affect successful implementation of an SCP and identify possible solutions to these problems. The analysis addresses the five elements of the SEIPS – Survivor Centered model: individuals, tasks, environment, organization, tools/technologies, and organization. We will reference Ms. M's case as a discrete, hands-on example.

1. At an *individual level*, there is uncertainty as to the roles and responsibilities of the oncologist and PCP. In Ms. M's case, she had largely been transitioned to follow-up with her PCP until her recurrence in 2007 (14 years after primary diagnosis). Following her recurrence, her PCP assumed that oncology was resuming primary management of her medical care. However, Ms. M's oncology care was fragmented by the retirement of her previous oncologist. Additionally, much of the time that Ms. M spent with her first oncologist in 2007 (the time of recurrence) was devoted to discussion of prognosis and benefit of further chemotherapy versus endocrine therapy alone. Such transitions of care present unique communication challenges for the HCP and the cancer survivor.

   Survivor-related information may not be delivered in a timely manner or be incomplete. In Ms. M's case, she was initially diagnosed in 1993, long before the era of SCPs. A new SCP could have been created in 2007, at the time of her recurrence. However, Ms. M's example points to a number of issues that need to be addressed with SCPs:

   (a) Will they be useful as static documents (i.e., could a document created and unaltered since 1993 have meaning in 2007)? If no, how can they be updated? How often should they be updated? Who is responsible for updating the SCP?
   (b) If recommendations for follow-up care are made in an SCP, who will ensure that care occurs? Will the appropriate HCPs (e.g., oncologist, PCP) and survivor be notified if recommended follow-up does not occur?
   (c) Should the oncology community "retroactively" create SCPs for a large number of survivors? If so, how and who will do this?
   (d) Is the SCP written in a manner to be useful to multiple end users of the document?

   PCPs may lack confidence in their skills and knowledge in cancer survivorship. In Ms. M's case, her PCP was not aware that anastrozole could exacerbate bone density loss. He recognized that she should have had a DEXA at age 65.

However, the PCP was reluctant to order one following her recurrence due to uncertainty regarding her life expectancy. For an SCP to impact deficiencies such as these, they must be able to provide the necessary information in a timely manner during the transition of care. Furthermore, the SCP should contain sufficient evidence-based information to effectively manage survivorship care and guide a PCP.

Improper use of SCPs can be caused by lack of information and instructions. Do the PCP and survivor have the necessary information and judgment to use these documents as intended? As previously described, the end users may vary widely in terms of role and expected cancer literacy, as well as the purpose they expect these documents to fulfill. An oncologist seeing a patient following a transfer of care due to insurance change may desire very different information than a cardiologist, cancer genetics counselor, PCP, or survivor. Survivors, PCPs, and even oncologists, may not be aware of the recommendations for receiving treatment summaries or care plans, or of resources for creating these documents, and guidelines may be lacking on which to base follow-up recommendations (e.g., for disease types less common than breast or colon). Therefore, the needs of the end users must be carefully assessed: otherwise the SCP may fail to prove effective. End users may require training, adequate instruction, and ongoing support to effectively use the SCPs. In Ms. M's case, she had difficulty functioning as an advocate for her own care. Even after zoledronic acid was initiated post fracture, Ms. M remained unclear about when and why she had last had a DEXA. In order to make SCPs useful documents for patients like Ms. M, accompanying education and emphasis on self-advocacy is needed.

2. At the *task* level, the necessary tasks must be executable in a timely manner to complete an SCP. Questions to be addressed:

    (a) What are the tasks involved in the creation and management of SCPs?
    (b) What integration across departments or organizations is needed for successful task execution?
    (c) What tasks need to be completed in order for the SCP to be updated efficiently and effectively?

    In Ms. M's case, creating even an accurate treatment summary was not easy. Her records spanned multiple years (1993–2010) and many of the old pathology details are unavailable. Records regarding total doses of chemotherapy drugs given are also no longer available, as is the reason why she was not prescribed tamoxifen following initial diagnosis. This limited the future accuracy of her SCP.

3. At the *environmental* level, there is currently no reimbursement offered to incentivize oncologists, nor is there any clear penalty for failing to provide these documents. Are there environmental factors, such as local, state, or federal laws that influence the development and use of the SCP? Furthermore, environmental change empowering, perhaps even expecting, survivors to act as health-care advocates also needs to occur. In addition, environmental change may be needed to empower PCPs to act as the gatekeepers of quality survivor care.

4. At the *technology level*, does the technology support use and updates of the SCP? Or, is the information static? In this case example, an SCP may have been useful if it had been created anew following her recurrence. However, a static document created at the time of diagnosis could not possibly have reflected the up-to-date surveillance needs or long-term treatment effects. Assuming the SCP is not a static document, how will it be updated in a timely manner based on new evidence-based information pertaining to survivor care?

   The use of technology (electronic medical records or ehealth systems) to update the SCP may be a method to meet survivor and provider needs while providing up-to-date information. There is an increasing recognition that technology, including information and communication technology and decision support systems, may be key to improving quality of care and patient outcomes [25, 28, 52]. In fact, the use of health information technology to address communication challenges inherent within a fragmented heath service is a priority for the Department of Health and Human Services [26]. Some critical questions to be addressed concerning the SCP include:

   (a) What technology is needed to support the format and maintenance of the SCP?
   (b) How can information in the SCP be automatically updated in a timely manner?
   (c) Can the technology notify end users (e.g., oncologists, PCPs, survivors) when critical changes are made to the SCP?
   (d) Does the technology support transfer of information from an existing medical record or chart?
   (e) Will end users (e.g., oncologists, PCPs, survivors) have access to the various technologies and tools needed to complete tasks related to the SCP?

5. At the *organizational level*, SCPs may be difficult to implement and use effectively under existing organizational structure, policies, and procedures.

   (a) Can information from multiple health care organizations (or possibly community organizations, such as advocacy groups) be included in the SCP?
   (b) Can the SCPs be shared with end users that may work at different organizations or practice groups?
   (c) Do organizations have a systematic plan that supports the cross-organizational use of SCP by multiple end users?
   (d) Do organizations have the processes and procedures in place to ensure accuracy of the SCP?

An SCP would not have addressed one of the most significant difficulties encountered in Ms. M's case: documents were not reliably tracked or transmitted between health care systems. Indeed, an SCP may have been one more document to lose in the shuffle. SCPs are time-consuming to create, and often paper-based, minimizing the ability to distribute the document. The most common disease types, such as breast and colon cancer, have disease-specific forms readily available from ASCO. However, it has not been feasible for less common disease types. At the organizational level, a systematic plan that supports the cross-organizational use of SCP by multiple end users is needed. Health care organizations must promote and encourage the use of SCPs while ensuring accuracy and timeliness of updates.

Looking at follow-up, the organization must have the processes and procedures in place to ensure accuracy of the SCP. SCPs can be created by either HCP staff (such as in the ASCO model) or be maintained by a cancer survivor (such as in the LIVESTRONG model). Currently, many SCPs are being created by manually transferring information from an existing medical record or chart. As with any system where data is not automatically imported and a method for data verification does not exist, the possibility of data corruption exists.

### HFE Summary – Case 2

A major concern with current SCPs is that they are potentially static, unless some method is developed for repeatedly updating the plan. An SCP likely needs to be modified over time, in order to ensure survivor care continues to reflect the evolving knowledge base. The type (e.g., pen/paper, computer, internet, electronic medical record), the quality, and the availability need to be evaluated. In addition, the usability, responsiveness, and integration with other technologies will need to be assessed.

## *Case 3* ***Using the SEIPS model to analyze use of a survivorship clinic to improve survivor outcomes.***

Ms. T is a 35-year-old female recently diagnosed with a ER+ PR-HER2+ Stage IIa breast cancer (T1N1cM0). She initially presented for medical care in fall 2008 after episodes of dyspnea and dizziness. She was 6 months postpartum at that time, and was found to have a significant postpartum cardiomyopathy with an EF of 35% and runs of ventricular tachycardia. She was started on carvedilol, lisinopril, and had an AICD placed. During the examination for AICD placement, a mass was found in her left breast and axilla. Mammogram and eventual biopsy confirmed an invasive ductal carcinoma; she underwent a lumpectomy and axillary dissection revealing a 1.8 cm primary, and two positive lymph nodes. Repeat ECHO revealed that her EF had normalized to 55%, and she received 6 cycles of TCH, breast irradiation, and adjuvant tamoxifen as well as completing trastuzumab. In fall 2009, her medical oncologist began discussing the plan for surveillance; R.T. had no PCP at this time (like many women her age, she was only seeing an OB/Gyn.) Issues for follow-up include:

1. Cardiac follow-up and evaluation, in light of her postpartum CM, trastuzumab, and left-sided radiation.
2. *Endocrine issues*. Significant hot flashes, vaginal dryness; low libido; her menses had not stopped during chemotherapy and she was interested in a second child; bone health.
3. *Genetic testing*. She had elected not to proceed with testing prior to surgery, as she felt overwhelmed with the multiple medical issues.
4. Lymphedema.
5. *Insurance and work*. She had been finishing a graduate degree at the time of diagnosis, and was just about to begin the search for a postdoc when her career was derailed by the diagnosis.

## HFE Analysis – Case 3

Ms. T's case example exemplifies the potentially very complex problems that breast cancer survivors, particularly those who are very young at diagnosis, may encounter. Like many younger patients, Ms. T was not accustomed to seeing a PCP on a routine basis, having had virtually no health care needs aside from pregnancy until 2008. Not surprisingly, Ms. T's OB/Gyn was not comfortable addressing her complex, multifactorial health care issues and her new PCP was also reluctant and felt challenged by these issues.

Survivorship clinics have been suggested as a method to address the complex issues facing cancer survivors and their need for multidisciplinary care [3]. Similar to other chronic illnesses, such as diabetes, stroke, TBI, asthma, and cardiac, which often have specialty clinics, cancer survivors may benefit from the comprehensive care offered by experts in specialty survivorship clinics. While no definitive model exists, survivorship clinics include specialists who focus on managing, educating, and counseling survivors on the potential late effects of treatment and healthy lifestyle practices. Survivorship clinics may also provide referrals to specialists and community resources for management of specific issues.

A number of factors, many of which are influenced by system complexity, will affect the implementation and effectiveness of these clinics. We will analyze factors that may affect successful implementation of a survivorship clinic and identify possible solutions to these problems. Similar to the HFE analysis of the prior case study, we will use the five elements of the SEIPS – Survivor Centered model: individuals, tasks, environment, organization, tools/technologies, and organization. We will reference Ms. T's case as a discrete, hands-on example.

1. At an *individual level*, young female cancer survivors may not have a PCP and if they do, the PCP may be reluctant to assume primary management of survivors with complex issues. In Ms. T's case, she had only been seen by an OB/Gyn and did not have a PCP. She found it difficult to find a PCP willing to manage the complex issues she was experiencing. Importantly, Ms. T *also* did not feel comfortable with a PCP managing her care. This is not uncommon: breast cancer survivors, while confident in the general care provided by their PCPs, are not as confident with their PCPs' cancer-specific survivorship care [68]. Survivors often do not regard the PCPs as having an integral role in their survivorship care [69]. Furthermore, PCPs have expressed uncertainty about assuming greater responsibility for survivors' cancer-related care with many lacking confidence in their skills and knowledge in cancer survivorship. PCPs may feel ill-prepared for the many issues that may emerge and their lack of access to information about evidence-based practice for survivors [69].

   In this case, both Ms. T and her PCP were reluctant to have the PCP assume primary responsibility for Ms. T's care. Therefore, Ms. T decided to proceed with follow-up care at a survivorship clinic. However, the nearest survivorship clinic was more than 3 h away. This distance limited the trips she could easily make to the clinic. Therefore, communication between the survivorship clinic,

Ms. T, and her PCP is critical. Some critical questions to be addressed concerning the survivorship clinic include:

(a) At the survivorship clinic, who is responsible for providing the end users (e.g., oncologist, PCP, community services, and survivor) information in a timely manner? This may be especially challenging if multiple specialists at the clinic see the survivor.
(b) If recommendations for follow-up care are made at the clinic, who will ensure that care occurs? Will the appropriate HCPs (e.g., oncologist, PCP) and survivor be notified if recommended follow-up does not occur?
(c) What if there are questions or changes in survivor status? Who will the PCP or survivor contact at the clinic? What mechanisms are in place to facilitate communication among the end users?
(d) How will communication within the survivorship clinic be timely and complete? Who will be responsible for coordination of care and information within the clinic?
(e) Is information communicated in a manner that is useful to multiple end users?

2. At the *task* level, can the necessary tasks be executed in a timely and efficient manner? Questions to be addressed include:

(a) Is the survivor able to be seen on a timely basis in the clinic?
(b) How are health care tasks across various specialists within the clinic integrated?
(c) What tasks need to be completed in order for information from the survivor clinic to be efficiently and effectively communicated to the PCP?
(d) What mechanisms are in place to monitor follow-up?

In Ms. T's case, communication between the clinic, PCP, and additional HCPs was not easy given the geographic distance and different health care systems. It is critical to identify who is responsible for information sharing and how to manage incoming questions and requests from HCPs outside the survivorship clinic.

3. At the *environmental* level, reimbursement for survivor education, coordination of care, and evaluation for referral to ancillary services is often lacking. Are there environmental factors, such as local, state, or federal laws or insurance payment that affect reimbursement for these services?
4. At the *technology level*, does the technology support communication of information among HCPs within the survivor clinic and among those outside the survivor clinic? In the case example, how is information communicated to Ms. T's PCP and OB/Gyn, both of which operate in small clinics not affiliated with the survivorship clinic. While both (PCP and OB/Gyn clinics) use electronic medical records, their systems are not compatible or integrated with the survivorship clinic. As discussed previously, the use of electronic medical records or ehealth systems has been identified as a method to meet both survivor and provider needs while providing timely and accurate information. However, some critical questions to be addressed include:

(a) How can technology be used to integrate health care information across varying health care organizations?
(b) How does the technology ensure confidentiality?
(c) How does the technology ensure that appropriate prompts or warnings occur?
(d) Is information readily updated and requests identified across varying organizations?
(e) Will individuals (e.g., oncologists, PCPs, survivors) have access to the various technologies and tools needed to complete tasks related to management of care?

For example, Ms. T mentioned some vague but persistent abdominal bloating and distension at a visit to her PCP. While the PCP was not overly concerned, this could be a problem warranting further workup, as a possible sign of peritoneal recurrence or development of a new primary (ovarian cancer). Additionally, Ms. T mentions that a paternal cousin has just been diagnosed with breast cancer at 41 (no genetic testing was done at diagnosis). These data need to be communicated automatically and not wait for Ms. T's annual visit to her oncologist or the survivorship clinic.

5. At the *organizational level*, survivor clinics are resource-intensive and may be difficult to implement and use effectively under existing organizational structure, policies, and procedures.

   (a) Can information from multiple health care organizations (or possibly community organizations, such as advocacy groups) be integrated into care at the survivorship clinic?
   (b) Can medical information be shared with end users that may work in multiple organizations or practice groups?
   (c) Do organizations have a systematic plan that supports the cross-organizational use of information from survivorship clinics by multiple end users?
   (d) Will organizations be able to deliver the educational and counseling services with existing reimbursement models?

Survivorship clinics will likely adopt a Chronic Care Model with active treatment interventions being only part, and potentially a small part, of the survivor's care. Additional care management strategies may include promotion of healthy lifestyles, referral to ancillary services, such as social and vocational services, and referral to patient advocacy and support groups. Historically these services are not reimbursable, or if they are, reimbursement levels are low.

From an HFE standpoint, a major concern of survivorship clinics is that they are resource-intensive and may operate in isolation of other health care and community systems, unless some method is developed for integrating care. Looking at follow-up, the organization must have the processes and procedures in place to ensure that accurate information is communicated and received in a timely manner.

**HFE Summary – Case 3**

Basic challenges associated with the delivery of care in cancer survivorship clinics are patient tracking and case management. HFE tools could be used to develop an information system for tracking, monitoring, and cueing care delivery for survivors seen at specialty clinics. It is important to integrate information and communication systems to provide access to and disseminate information to appropriate end users. Ideally, the architecture of the resulting system would be flexible and compatible with multiple clinic and organizational electronic medical record systems. Minimizing miscommunication, confusion, delays, and/or variations in the quality of care during transition points is a key area in which HFE techniques may be helpful.

## Conclusion

"Health care is on a collision course with patient needs and economic reality" [70]. The economic reality of the large number of survivors and the varying survivor needs is already stressing a system with limited resources. Without careful planning, the survivorship "system" will follow a similar path and encounter comparable problems as the health care in general. The survivorship system needs to support the long-term demands of numbers of survivors, attention to cost effect approaches, surveillance of a number of cancer, medical status, health behavior, function and well being, and the specific needs of patients, families, and caregivers. HFE models and methods can be used to optimize the balance and needs among survivors, other health care users, health care providers, policies, procedures, and technologies. As an example, the SEIPS – Survivor Centered model provides a framework to evaluate the varying aspects of the survivorship system and their respective interactions, ultimately improving survivor outcomes.

## References

1. Erikson C, Salsberg E, Forte G, Bruinooge S, Goldstein M. Future supply and demand for oncologists: challenges to assuring access to oncology services. J Oncol Pract. 2007;3(2):79–86.
2. Yabroff K, Lawrence W, Clauser S, Davis W, Brown M. Burden of illness in cancer survivors: findings from a population-based national sample. J Natl Cancer Inst. 2004;96(17):1322–30.
3. Hewitt M, Greenfield S, Stovall E. From cancer patient to cancer survivor: lost in transition. Washington, DC: National Academies Press; 2006.
4. Miedema B, MacDonald I, Tatemichi S. Cancer follow-up care. Patients' perspectives. Can Fam Physician. 2003;49:890–5.
5. Nissen M, Beran M, Lee M, Mehta S, Pine D, Swenson K. Views of primary care providers on follow-up care of cancer patients. Fam Med. 2007;39(7):477–82.
6. Wilson JR. Fundamentals of ergonomics in theory and practice. Appl Ergon. 2000;31(6):557–67.
7. Salvendy G, editor. Hand book of human factors and ergonomics. 3rd ed. Hoboken: Wiley; 2006.

8. Wickens C, Gordons S, Liu Y. An introduction to human factors engineering. New York: Addison-Wesley; 1998.
9. Kirwan B. An overview of a nuclear reprocessing plant Human Factors programme. Appl Ergon. 2003;34(5):441–52.
10. Baker K, Olson J, Morisseau D. Work practices, fatigue, and nuclear power plant safety performance. Hum Factors. 1994;36(2):244–57.
11. Kleiner BM. Macroergonomic analysis and design for improved safety and quality performance. Int J Occup Saf Ergon. 1999;5(2):217–45.
12. Shappell S, Detwiler C, Holcomb K, Hackworth C, Boquet A, Wiegmann DA. Human error and commercial aviation accidents: an analysis using the human factors analysis and classification system. Hum Factors. 2007;49(2):227–42.
13. Tvaryanas AP, Thompson WT, Constable SH. Human factors in remotely piloted aircraft operations: HFACS analysis of 221 mishaps over 10 years. Aviat Space Environ Med. 2006;77(7):724–32.
14. Wiegmann DA, Shappell SA. Human error and crew resource management failures in Naval aviation mishaps: a review of U.S. Naval Safety Center data, 1990–96. Aviat Space Environ Med. 1999;70(12):1147–51.
15. Wiegmann DA, Shappell SA. Human error analysis of commercial aviation accidents: application of the Human Factors Analysis and Classification system (HFACS). Aviat Space Environ Med. 2001;72(11):1006–16.
16. Wiegmann DA, Shappell SA. A human error approach to aviation accident analysis: the human factors analysis and classification system. Aldershot; Burlington: Ashgate; 2003.
17. van Erp JB, Eriksson L, Levin B, Carlander O, Veltman JA, Vos WK. Tactile cueing effects on performance in simulated aerial combat with high acceleration. Aviat Space Environ Med. 2007;78(12):1128–34.
18. Stanton N. Human factors in nuclear safety. Bristol: Taylor & Francis; 1996.
19. Sanders MS, McCormick EJ. Human factors in engineering and design. 7th ed. New York: McGraw-Hill; 1993.
20. Giuliano KK. Basic strategies for reviewing medical device research. AACN Adv Crit Care. 2008;19(3):258–60.
21. Hallbeck MS, Koneczny S, Buchel D, Matern U. Ergonomic usability testing of operating room devices. Stud Health Technol Inform. 2008;132:147–52.
22. Pattison M, McQuaid H, Wilcox A. Incorporating human factors in product design and development. Med Device Technol. 2007;18(7):28. 30, 23.
23. Perry SJ. An overlooked alliance: using human factors engineering to reduce patient harm. Jt Comm J Qual Saf. 2004;30(8):455–9.
24. Privitera MB, Design M, Murray DL. Applied ergonomics: determining user needs in medical device design. Conf Proc IEEE Eng Med Biol Soc. 2009;2009:5606–8.
25. Bates D, Gawande A. Improving safety with information technology. N Engl J Med. 2003;348(25):2526–34.
26. Hesse BW, Hanna C, Massett HA, Hesse NK. Outside the box: will information technology be a viable intervention to improve the quality of cancer care? J Natl Cancer Inst Monogr. 2010;2010(40):81–9.
27. Walker JM, Carayon P. From tasks to processes: the case for changing health information technology to improve health care. Health Aff. 2009;28(2):467–77.
28. Karsh B. Beyond usability: designing effective technology implementation systems to promote patient safety. Qual Saf Health Care. 2004;13(5):388–94.
29. Karsh BT, Holden RJ, Alper SJ, Or CK. A human factors engineering paradigm for patient safety: designing to support the performance of the healthcare professional. Qual Saf Health Care. 2006;15 Suppl 1:i59–65.
30. Carayon P, Schoofs Hundt A, Karsh BT, Gurses AP, Alvarado CJ, Smith M, et al. Work system design for patient safety: the SEIPS model. Qual Saf Health Care. 2006;15 Suppl 1:i50–8.
31. Carayon P. Handbook of human factors and ergonomics in health care and patient safety. Mahwah: Lawrence Erlbaum Associates; 2007.

32. Singh H, Thomas EJ, Mani S, Sittig D, Arora H, Espadas D, et al. Timely follow-up of abnormal diagnostic imaging test results in an outpatient setting: are electronic medical records achieving their potential? Arch Intern Med. 2009;169(17):1578–86.
33. Vincent C, Moorthy K, Sarker S, Chang A, Darzi A. Systems approaches to surgical quality and safety: from concept to measurement. Ann Surg. 2004;239(4):475–82.
34. Karsh BT, Brown R. Macroergonomics and patient safety: the impact of levels on theory, measurement, analysis and intervention in patient safety research. Appl Ergon. 2010;41(5):674–81.
35. Karsh BT, Escoto KH, Beasley JW, Holden RJ. Toward a theoretical approach to medical error reporting system research and design. Appl Ergon. 2006;37(3):283–95.
36. Silver MP, Geis MS, Bateman KA. Improving health care systems performance: a human factors approach. Am J Med Qual. 2004;19(3):93–102.
37. Cacciabue PC, Vella G. Human factors engineering in healthcare systems: the problem of human error and accident management. Int J Med Inform. 2010;79(4):e1–17.
38. Gustafson DH, Hawkins R, Pingree S, McTavish F, Arora NK, Mendenhall J, et al. Effect of computer support on younger women with breast cancer. J Gen Intern Med. 2001;16(7):435–45.
39. Owens BH, Robbins KC. CHESS: comprehensive health enhancement support system for women with breast cancer. Plast Surg Nurs. 1996;16(3):172–5. 82.
40. Reid PR, Compton WD, Grossman JH, Fanjiang G, National Academy of Engineering., Institute of Medicine, et al. Building a better delivery system: a new engineering/health care partnership. Washington, DC: National Academies Press; 2005.
41. Reason JT. Human error. London: Cambridge University Press; 1990.
42. Reason J. Human error: models and management. BMJ. 2000;320(7237):768–70.
43. Reason J. Heroic compensations: the benign face of the human factor. Flight Safety Australia. 2001;28–31.
44. Clarke M, Collins R, Darby S, Davies C, Elphinstone P, Evans E, et al. Effects of radiotherapy and of differences in the extent of surgery for early breast cancer on local recurrence and 15-year survival: an overview of the randomised trials. Lancet. 2005;366(9503):2087–106.
45. Forbes JF, Cuzick J, Buzdar A, Howell A, Tobias JS, Baum M. Effect of anastrozole and tamoxifen as adjuvant treatment for early-stage breast cancer: 100-month analysis of the ATAC trial. Lancet Oncol. 2008;9(1):45–53.
46. Coombes RC, Kilburn LS, Snowdon CF, Paridaens R, Coleman RE, Jones SE, et al. Survival and safety of exemestane versus tamoxifen after 2–3 years' tamoxifen treatment (Intergroup Exemestane Study): a randomised controlled trial. Lancet. 2007;369(9561):559–70.
47. Chlebowski RT, Geller ML. Adherence to endocrine therapy for breast cancer. Oncology. 2006;71(1–2):1–9.
48. Dezentje VO, van Blijderveen NJ, Gelderblom H, Putter H, van Herk-Sukel MP, Casparie MK, et al. Effect of concomitant CYP2D6 inhibitor use and tamoxifen adherence on breast cancer recurrence in early-stage breast cancer. J Clin Oncol. 2010;28(14):2423–9.
49. Kaye R, Crowley J. Medical device use safety: incorporating human factors engineering into risk management. Guidance for industry and FDA premarked and design control reviewers. US Department of Health and Human Services, Food and Drug Administration, Center for Devices and Radiological Health, Division of Device User Programs and Systems Analysis, Office of Health Industry Program. Rockville; 2000.
50. Joint Commission on Healthcare Quality and Safety. Sentinel event statistics, 2006. Retrieved from http://www.jointcommission.org/sentinel_event.aspx.
51. Carlton G, Blegen MA. Medication-related errors: a literature review of incidence and antecedents. Annu Rev Nurs Res. 2006;24:19–38.
52. Institute of Medicine. Committee on Quality of Health Care in America. Crossing the quality chasm: a new health system for the 21st century. Washington, DC: National Academy Press; 2001.
53. Weaver J, McHugo JM, Clark TJ. Accuracy of transvaginal ultrasound in diagnosing endometrial pathology in women with post-menopausal bleeding on tamoxifen. Br J Radiol. 2005;78(929):394–7.

54. Vicente KJ. Cognitive work analysis: toward safe, productive, and healthy computer-based work. Mahwah: Lawrence Erlbaum Associates; 1999.
55. Carayon P. Human factors of complex sociotechnical systems. Appl Ergon. 2006;37(4):525–35.
56. Friedman TL. The world is flat: a brief history of the twenty-first century. 1st ed. New York: Farrar, Straus and Giroux; 2005.
57. O'Hair D, Villagran MM, Wittenberg E, Brown K, Ferguson M, Hall HT, et al. Cancer survivorship and agency model: implications for patient choice, decision making, and influence. Health Commun. 2003;15(2):193–202.
58. Wagner E, Davis C, Schaefer J, Von Korff M, Austin B. A survey of leading chronic disease management programs: are they consistent with the literature? Manag Care Q. 1999;7(3):56–66.
59. Wagner E, Austin B, Von Korff M. Improving outcomes in chronic illness. Manag Care Q. 1996;4(2):12–25.
60. Bodenheimer T, Wagner E, Grumbach K. Improving primary care for patients with chronic illness: the chronic care model, Part 2. JAMA. 2002;288(15):1909–14.
61. Bodenheimer T, Wagner E, Grumbach K. Improving primary care for patients with chronic illness. JAMA. 2002;288(14):1775–9.
62. Hewitt ME, Ganz P, National Coalition for Cancer Survivorship, National Cancer Policy Forum, National Cancer Institute, Lance Armstrong Foundation, et al. Implementing cancer survivorship care planning: workshop summary. Washington, DC: National Academies Press; 2007.
63. Ganz P. Survivorship: adult cancer survivors. Prim Care. 2009;36(4):721–41.
64. Ganz PA, Hahn EE. Implementing a survivorship care plan for patients with breast cancer. J Clin Oncol. 2008;26(5):759–67.
65. American Society of Clinical Oncology – Breast Cancer Survivorship Care Plan 2009. Retrieved from http://www.jointcommission.org/sentinel_event.aspx.
66. Hill-Kayser C, Vachani C, Hampshire M, Jacobs L, Metz J. An internet tool for creation of cancer survivorship care plans for survivors and health care providers: design, implementation, use and user satisfaction. J Med Internet Res. 2009;11(3):e39.
67. Ganz P. Monitoring the physical health of cancer survivors: a survivorship-focused medical history. J Clin Oncol. 2006;24(32):5105–11.
68. Mao JJ, Bowman MA, Stricker CT, DeMichele A, Jacobs L, Chan D, et al. Delivery of survivorship care by primary care physicians: the perspective of breast cancer patients. J Clin Oncol. 2009;27(6):933–8.
69. Kantsiper M, McDonald EL, Geller G, Shockney L, Snyder C, Wolff AC. Transitioning to breast cancer survivorship: perspectives of patients, cancer specialists, and primary care providers. J Gen Intern Med. 2009;24 Suppl 2:S459–66.
70. Porter ME, Teisberg EO. Redefining health care: creating value-based competition on results. Boston: Harvard Business School Press; 2006.

# Part V
# The Future is Now

# Chapter 17
# Cancer Survivorship and National Health Reform

Sara Rosenbaum, Jennifer Lee, Mandi Pratt Chapman, and Steven R. Patierno

## Introduction

There is no more compelling case for national health reform than cancer treatment and survivorship. Half of all men and more than one-third of all women will be diagnosed with cancer during their lifetimes [1]. There are more than 13 million cancer survivors in the USA with approximately 1.4 million new cases of cancer diagnosed annually [2]. As a result of earlier detection, improved therapies, and increased attention to treatment sequelae, more patients are in need of cancer treatment and follow-up care than ever before. Five-year survival rates for all cancers diagnosed between 1999 and 2005 reached 68%, up from 50% during the 1975–1977 time period [1]. In addition to an ever-increasing patient pool, cancer survivors are living longer and in need of more comprehensive follow-up care over a longer period of time.

This chapter reviews the evidence regarding health-care access and quality in the case of cancer and assesses the implications of the Patient Protection and Affordable Care Act [3], as amended by the Health Care and Education Reconciliation Act of 2010 [4].

## Policy Context

In the complex US health-care system, patients face an ever-increasing risk of losing the ability to negotiate their care in the face of critical illness. Well-educated patients with access to resources struggle to maximize the quality of their treatment. As with many serious health conditions, cancer care is characterized by fragmentation flowing from the multidisciplinary nature of cancer treatment, which spans both inpatient and outpatient care across the clinical care enterprise.

S. Rosenbaum (✉)
Department of Health Policy, The George Washington University School of Public Health and Health Services
e-mail: sara.rosenbaum@gwumc.edu

M. Feuerstein and P.A. Ganz (eds.), *Health Services for Cancer Survivors*,
DOI 10.1007/978-1-4419-1348-7_17, © Springer Science+Business Media, LLC 2011

Communication among and within the members of this enterprise is not standardized and is frequently incomplete and imperfect. These challenges intensify for those who are uneducated, poor, uninsured or underinsured, or who face language barriers. Systemic barriers inherent in the US health-care system create significant health-care disparities and exacerbate the unequal burden of disease borne by minorities and the medically underserved. Studies show that the quality of cancer care provided to individual patients varies greatly; the poor as well as racial, linguistic, and cultural minorities often receive the most disconnected, untimely, and ill-managed care, with health outcomes substantially worse than those experienced by their more affluent, white counterparts [5–7].

The physical, psychological, emotional, spiritual, functional, and economic impact of cancer and its treatment can be difficult even for those with reasonable financial means and a strong support network. For those without strong financial and social support, the impact of cancer can be completely devastating. Indeed, cancer's broader economic and social costs are enormous. Approximately 11% of all cancer patients are uninsured, with higher figures among persons who are members of racial and ethnic minority groups [8]. The high cost of cancer's primary treatment and survivorship phases means that more than one in four people with cancer are exposed to the problem of underinsurance [9], defined by one leading study as out-of-pocket cost exposure for medically necessary care that exceeds 10% of annual family income (5% in the case of low-income adults) [10]. Total costs associated with cancer are expected to surpass $260 billion in 2010, with $102 million in direct medical costs and the remainder in costs attributable to lost productivity and premature death [1]. Between 1990 and 2008, spending on cancer treatment increased more than twofold, even adjusting for inflation [11]. Nearly 20% of cancer survivors failed to receive one or more needed medical services in the previous year because of cost concerns; care missed included 7.8% for medical care, nearly 10% for prescription drugs; 11.3% for dental care, and 2.7% for mental health care [12].

Insurance status, perhaps more than any other economic factor, determines the timeliness and quality of health care, if it is received at all [7]. Lack of adequate and affordable health insurance to cover cancer-related care has serious negative consequences including sometimes debilitating debt for the uninsured and their caregivers. Quality of life may also be impaired by lack of access to supportive care services due to out-of-pocket expenses and transportation costs.

Furthermore, the quality of cancer treatment both during the primary and survivorship phases raises serious issues, particularly for those most vulnerable. The evidence suggests a lack of adherence to clinical standards across numerous domains of screening, diagnosis, treatment, and aftercare, including diagnostic procedures, patient counseling, therapy and treatment, and treatment of conditions associated with cancer such as depression and anxiety [13–16]. Disparities in quality are notable for minority patients and patients who depend on Medicaid. Lack of standardization is in part due to the low percentage of adult cancer patients (only 3–5%) who participate in the clinical trials that form the evidence base needed to develop clinical care guidelines. Even fewer minority, low income, uninsured, and underinsured patients participate in clinical trials, reducing generalizability of trial results [17–19]. In the post-treatment period, the Institute of Medicine (IOM) has found a serious lack of evidence-based guidelines for survivorship care; lack of integration of survivor care into treatment planning; poor coordination of care; and an absence of a locus of responsibility for follow-up care [20].

Finally, there is evidence of a lag between the demand for oncology services and the supply of care. Demand is expected to rise by nearly half between 2005 and 2020, with supply of care rising by only 14% over the same time period [21].

In its 2006 report, *From Cancer Patient to Cancer Survivor: Lost in Transition* [20], the IOM issued sweeping recommendations related to treatment and survivorship. Recommendations related to health-care access and quality include the elimination of barriers to health insurance during treatment and survivorship, benefit, coverage, and payment design that incorporates evidence on appropriate treatment, the development of quality survivorship treatment measures, and comprehensive survivorship planning as an integral part of treatment. These recommendations stem from what the IOM identified as the "four essential components of survivorship care": (1) prevention of recurrent and new cancers and of other late effects; (2) surveillance for cancer spread, recurrence or second cancers, and assessment of medical and psychological effects; (3) interventions for consequences of cancer and its treatment; and (4) coordination between primary and specialty care. The IOM also called for a public health response, including survivorship surveillance, community resources for survivorship, educational clearinghouses for health-care professionals, primary and secondary prevention such as smoking cessation and cancer screening, and program evaluation and identification of best practices.

## The Patient Protection and Affordable Care Act

The Patient Protection and Affordable Care Act (hereinafter referred to as the Affordable Care Act), was enacted into law on March 23, 2010. Full implementation occurs on January 1, 2014, with numerous intermediate stages. The Act represents a public policy watershed, revising and extending the existing web of laws that together form the federal legal framework of the US health-care system in order to establish what has, until now, been fundamentally absent from the American health-care system: a near-universal guarantee of access to affordable health insurance coverage, from birth through retirement. When fully implemented, the Act will reduce the number of uninsured Americans by more than half. The law will result in health insurance coverage for about 94% of the American population, reducing the uninsured by 31 million persons, and increasing Medicaid enrollment by 15 million beneficiaries. As stated in the letter from Douglas W. Elmendorf to the Honorable Harry Reid in March 2010, approximately 24 million persons are expected to remain without coverage.

At the same time, the Act leaves much US health law untouched. Laws that establish licensure standards for health professionals and health-care institutions – a uniquely state-based body of law under the American legal system – remain unaffected. Similarly, the Act makes no fundamental changes in medical liability law, also a key aspect of state law, both common law and statutory law. Furthermore, the Affordable Care Act does not alter the powers and duties of public health agencies, also a dimension of state law under federal Constitutional principles [22]. In a similar vein, in accordance with the overarching principle that people should be able to keep the coverage they have, the Act preserves the major laws governing public and private health insurance, including Medicare, Medicaid, state health insurance laws, and federal laws applicable to employee health benefit plans under the Employee Retirement Income Security Act of 1974 (ERISA).

The Affordable Care Act's major contribution is to revise existing laws to strengthen and extend existing forms coverage, while simultaneously introducing a new legal structure – the health insurance Exchange – whose purpose is to provide an additional and powerful pathway to accessible, nondiscriminatory coverage. Together these reforms are aimed at assuring that regardless of financial, health, family, or work-related circumstances, American citizens and individuals legally present in the USA are no longer without a pathway to coverage. This multilayered legal approach is accompanied by a new system of tax-supported subsidies designed to make coverage affordable to millions of people whose incomes exceed Medicaid eligibility standards but are inadequate to reasonably cover the cost of coverage.

The Act goes beyond coverage, employing financial incentives to address the deeper challenges associated with improving the quality of health care and holding down health-care costs. Moreover, the legislation lays the groundwork for addressing certain underlying issues of provider supply and health-care access (particularly in the case of primary health care) while also establishing a framework for strengthening public health and the relationship between community health and individual patient care.

These efforts are contained in a law that spans over 1,000 pages in its officially printed form and consists of 10 separate legislative Titles addressing issues of coverage, access, quality, workforce, public health, and other matters. A search of the Act reveals that the word "cancer" is explicitly referenced in 14 separate sections of the law and in numerous contexts: coverage of clinical preventive and treatment services including clinical trials, health-care quality, oral health promotion, cost containment, community health interventions, quality improvement, patient care improvement, and research innovation [3]. Because the Act is designed to broadly address the accessibility, quality, and cost of health care across all conditions, the limited references to cancer should come as no surprise; at the same time, the presence of cancer as an identified condition at numerous points in the law underscores the extent to which cancer and cancer survivorship are paradigms of the types of serious and potentially long-lasting health conditions whose treatment the Act was designed to address.

The Act's provisions reflect certain fundamental aims: The first and most prominent aim is to achieve near-universal coverage through a body of restructured health insurance law and financial subsidies combined with shared responsibility among government, individuals, and employers. A second aim is to improve the fairness, quality, and affordability of health insurance coverage. A third aim is to improve health-care value, quality and efficiency while reducing wasteful spending and making the health-care system more accountable to a diverse patient population.

A fourth is to strengthen primary health-care access while bringing about longer-term changes in the availability of primary and preventive health care. A fifth and final aim is to make strategic investments in the public's health, through both an expansion of clinical preventive care and community investments.

## *Coverage*

### Universal and Mandatory Coverage

By establishing premium and cost-sharing subsidies, new fairness rules for the health insurance industry, and a new market for health insurance purchasing, the Affordable Care Act positions the nation for a near-universal expectation of access to affordable coverage [3]. The Act strengthens public and private health insurance coverage while building a new health insurance market for individuals and families who do not have affordable employer coverage or another form of "minimum essential coverage" such as Medicare or Medicaid [3].

The *quid pro quo* for this near-universal guarantee is the duty to secure it, a duty that extends to all US taxpayers while excluding individuals not legally present in the USA. The Act contains certain exemptions for persons for whom enrollment is contrary to religious belief or remains unaffordable or a hardship [3]. But otherwise the mandate covers all persons. Indeed, it is the legal mandate to acquire insurance that makes universal coverage feasible, since healthy individuals are essential to formation of a risk pool, and without a mandate, large numbers of healthy persons would fail to enroll. Without the mandate, the health insurance industry would not – and indeed, could not – eliminate discriminatory pricing and coverage practices, since such exclusionary practices represent the means by which insurers protect themselves against adverse risk selection. Without the mandate, universal coverage is virtually impossible, as is stabilization of the insurance foundation on which the entire health-care system rests.

The Affordable Care Act in essence represents an effort to reframe the economic relationship between Americans and the health-care system, introducing a universal system of prepayment in order to stem the health insurance crisis that has enveloped individuals, families, communities, the health-care system, and the national economy as a whole [3]. It is also this basic effort to reinvent Americans' relationship to health insurance that lies at the epicenter of the legal battle over the law's constitutionality, which began with passage of the law and which inevitably will culminate in a landmark decision by the US Supreme Court.

The core of the law – the mandate – rests for its legal validity on a determination by the courts that Congress possesses the constitutional power to regulate how Americans buy health care and economically interact with the health-care system. Those who view the legislation first and foremost as a means to financially right the health-care ship consider the legislation to be a fundamental intervention into economic matters and thus an exercise of Congressional power that lies well within the constraints of the Constitution's Commerce Clause [23]. Those who oppose the law label it as one that forces individuals to engage in economic activity in the first instance – that is, as a law that forces economic activity on noneconomic actors who wish to remain outside of health-care commerce. Under this opposing view, the law exceeds Congress' power to act because unlike state governments, which possess police powers, Congress cannot regulate noneconomic conduct. Proponents of the law argue that contrary to this view, the law simply changes the financial basis of our relationship to the health-care system, requiring us to prepay for much of the health care that we all use over the course of our lives [24].

## Health Insurance Reforms

In addition to establishing universal coverage and shared responsibility, the Affordable Care Act sets federal standards for health insurance and employer-sponsored health benefit plans [3]. These requirements considerably expand on previous federal standards first introduced into the Public Health Service Act (with parallel amendments to ERISA and the Internal Revenue Code in order to reach self-insured plans) as part of the Health Insurance Portability and Accountability Act of 1996 (HIPAA) [25]. Some of the requirements take effect prior to 2014 while others become effective on January 1, 2014, when the obligation to enroll in coverage commences. The changes are broad and are intended to make coverage fairer and more accessible, as well as less discriminatory against the sick. With the exception of "grandfathered" health plans (i.e., health plans in effect on March 23, 2010, so long as the plans do not make significant changes in eligibility, benefits and coverage, premiums, and cost sharing) [3] several of the federal reforms take effect in the near term [3]: prohibition of rescissions (i.e., cancelations); a ban on exclusion of children under 19 with preexisting conditions; extension of dependent coverage to age 26; the use of uniform coverage documents; expanded appeals rights in the case of adverse claims determinations; the development and use of uniform explanation of coverage documents and standardized definitions; quality reporting; clear accounting for costs including standards for "medical loss" ratios in order to assure minimum expenditures on health care; a ban on lifetime and certain annual coverage limits, and certain patient protections such as coverage of emergency care without prior authorization and access to pediatric and obstetrical and gynecology care.

The broader reforms aimed at preventing discrimination on a broad scale take effect January 2014 [3]: a prohibition against pricing discrimination and a requirement that insurers use "modified community rating" pricing structures that take into account only age, family status, and tobacco use (a reinsurance system is put into place as well in order to assure stabilization during the financial transition to modified community rating); a prohibition against preexisting condition exclusions and discrimination based on health status (with an exception for certain employer-sponsored "wellness programs" that will be allowed to tie premiums to participation in wellness activities as well as actual health outcomes); guaranteed availability and renewability of coverage; nondiscrimination against health-care providers; coverage of "essential benefits" in the case of insurance products sold in the individual and "small group" markets; prohibition of excessive waiting periods (over 90 days) before coverage begins; and coverage of routine medical costs for "qualified" individuals (including individuals with cancer) participating in certain "approved" clinical trials, including federally funded trials.

Taken together, the Act's expanded insurance standards are designed to set a federal minimum; it is the expectation under the Affordable Care Act that state insurance departments will implement and enforce these federal standards as part of their insurance oversight powers. As stated in a letter from Jane Cline to Honorable Kathleen Sebelius in August 2010, as of August 5, 2010, the National Association of Insurance Commissioners reported that half the states have concluded that their insurance departments have the power to implement the federal standards either as a result of explicit legislation or under general administrative powers, and furthermore, that nearly all states had the power to directly enforce federal standards.

At the same time, the federal government cannot force states to oversee and enforce federal laws without running afoul of the US Constitution's Tenth Amendment protection against the commandeering of state law enforcement resources [26]. Thus, the Affordable Care Act provides that the federal government will oversee and enforce all federal standards against state-regulated insurers if states are unable to do so [3].

Several provisions are of particular note in the context of cancer. The first is coverage – without patient cost-sharing (deductibles, coinsurance, and copayments) – for preventive services with an "A" or "B" rating from US Preventive Services Task Force, immunizations recommended by the Advisory Committee on Immunization Practices (ACIP), and other preventive services for children, adolescents, and women identified by the Health Resources and Services Administration [3]. This requirement begins with the first plan year that occurs after September 23, 2010 (6 months after the date of enactment) [3]. This provision is important for cancer prevention through access to appropriate primary care that can identify and intervene when risk factors for cancer are evident (e.g., obesity, tobacco use, alcohol abuse). Coverage for appropriate screenings and vaccinations can also detect cancer at earlier, more manageable stages (e.g., breast, cervical, colorectal screening) or may considerably decrease cancer incidence rates (e.g., HPV vaccine).

The second is the prohibition against discrimination based on preexisting condition and health status. This prohibition existed under HIPAA; the Affordable Care Act extends the prohibition to the individual market and bars eligibility factors based on health status, medical condition (both physical and mental), claims experience, receipt of health care, medical history, genetic information, or evidence of insurability. This ban against eligibility restrictions based on health status reaches both current and new enrollees. This ban is especially important for pediatric cancer survivors who often experience a gap in coverage when they age out of their parent's insurance and have not yet secured their own employer-based coverage. Preexisting condition exclusions have historically made it difficult for some survivors to obtain affordable, quality insurance coverage. This ban also protects individuals who have a family history of cancer as well as those who may have comorbidities or sequelae resulting from cancer or its treatment who require ongoing care.

The discrimination ban does, however, permit the use of employee wellness programs that tie premiums to health status factors as long as the wellness program is "reasonably designed" to promote health or prevent disease and the incentive does not amount to more than discrimination based on health status. Wellness programs tied to health outcomes must have reasonable alternative standards for individuals whose medical conditions make it "unreasonably difficult" to attain a particular result. In the case of cancer, physical or functional late effects of treatment could potentially qualify individuals for alternative standards.

The third provision is the ban on lifetime and certain annual coverage limits. Caps on coverage are one prominent reason for underinsurance, which can seriously impact health outcomes of cancer survivors who require lifelong follow-up care. Those without adequate coverage are more likely to forgo recommended tests and treatments and less likely to visit a physician when sick. By delaying or forgoing care, diagnosis of recurrent or new cancers may be delayed, comorbidities may become exacerbated, quality of life declines, and years of survival may decrease. Serious late effects of treatment or a new cancer diagnosis could mean financial devastation for a patient with such coverage limitations [27].

The fourth provision is the requirement that insurers in the individual and small group markets cover an "essential benefit package" which consists of 10 broad benefit classes (ambulatory patient services, emergency services, hospitalization, maternity and newborn care, mental health and substance abuse disorder services, prescription drugs, rehabilitative and habilitative services and devices, laboratory services, preventive and wellness services and chronic disease management, pediatric services including oral and vision care) [3]. In defining the meaning of essential benefit classes, the Secretary is directed to utilize coverage designs applicable to employer sponsored plans, but at the same time is barred from making coverage decisions, determining reimbursement rates, establishing incentive programs, or designing benefits in ways that "discriminate against individuals because of their age, disability, or expected length of life." The importance of an essential benefit package for cancer patients and survivors cannot be overstated given the multidisciplinary nature of cancer care – which (in addition to standard preventive care) can include inpatient stays, visits to the emergency department, outpatient treatments, mental health counseling, chemotherapy and prescription drugs, rehabilitative services (physical, occupational, and speech), as well as ongoing disease management and survivorship care.

The final coverage provision of particular note is coverage of routine care costs associated with clinical trials as an element of all individual and group health plans whether insured by an issuer or self-insured by an employer. Under the law, cancer is sufficient to make an individual "qualified" for purpose of clinical trial participation, and an "approved clinical trial" includes FDA approved drug trials (as well as trials that are exempt from FDA approval), federally funded trials involving the NIH, the CDC, the Agency for Health Care Research and Quality (AHRQ), the Centers for Medicare and Medicaid Services (CMS), the Departments of Defense or Veterans Affairs (assuming that NIH guidelines for research are met), and qualified nongovernmental research entities identified in NIH guidelines. This provision is of critical importance to cancer patients. Historically, the lack of coverage for routine care costs prevented some patients from enrolling in clinical trials that could be their best chance for survival and could contribute to increased knowledge to improve therapies for future generations of patients. Coverage of routine care costs removes a financial barrier for patients and incentivizes greater participation in trials, which is particularly important for minority populations who are underrepresented in already abysmally low cancer trial participation rates.

### Health Insurance Exchanges

Beyond subsidizing coverage and regulating the insurance and group health plan markets, the Affordable Care Act (ACA) creates state health insurance Exchanges for both individuals and small businesses [3]. Exchanges are meant to simplify and ease health insurance purchasing by creating a one-stop shopping market for insurance products that qualify for federal tax subsidies and that meet federal and state standards and thus are certified as "qualified health benefit plans." Exchanges are also expected to assure the quality of coverage through the selection of qualified health plans, provide information and enrollment assistance, coordinate enrollment with state Medicaid programs, calculate subsidy eligibility, oversee plan performance, and provide information to the federal government regarding subsidy eligibility and plan performance [3].

Qualified health benefit plans, whether sold inside or outside Exchanges, will be required to meet a series of federal requirements including coverage of "essential benefits" (with special rules for abortion coverage) [3] defined under the Act to include both preventive services as well as a range of benefit classes that reflect a standard employer-sponsored plan. Qualified health plans also will be required to meet federal standards related to provider network sufficiency (including contracts with "essential community providers") and health-care quality. In addition, qualified health benefit plans will be required to make performance information conforming to national quality measurement benchmarks available to patients and consumers [3].

### Medicaid

In expanding existing coverage, the Act fundamentally restructures Medicaid to cover all citizens and legal US residents with family incomes below 133% of the federal poverty level (as measured through a new "modified adjusted gross income" test) and to streamline enrollment [3]. (Medicaid's 5-year waiting period for legal residents will continue to apply to recently arrived persons, who during this time will qualify for tax subsidies and enrollment through a health insurance Exchange.) The principal group of individuals assisted as a result of this change are adults who are not caretakers of minor children nor disabled within the meaning of the Social Security Act. That is, they are adults who either never had children or whose children are grown. These newly eligible adults also include adults who fall into a "traditional" category (e.g., a parent of a minor child) but whose income exceeds a state's eligibility standard (which can be as low as 20% of the federal poverty level) [28].

Newly eligible Medicaid beneficiaries will be entitled to "benchmark" coverage consisting of plans that resemble those that are considered qualified benefit plans in their approximation of employer coverage (including coverage of preventive services). State Medicaid programs also will be expected to raise primary care payments to Medicare levels, with financial incentives included in the legislation to make payment reform feasible. At the same time, the Medicaid reforms lack certain elements found in the insurance reforms. For example, the clinical trials coverage requirement applicable to state-regulated insurance and employer-sponsored plans is not applicable to Medicaid, although states may cover the routine costs of clinical trials as a coverage option. Neither do the ACA Medicaid amendments require coverage of preventive screening benefits for adults who fall into "traditional" Medicaid eligibility categories, predominantly the very poorest women who are caretakers of minor children, as well as disabled nonelderly adults. It is not yet clear how this might affect cancer survivors who seek preventative screening services for potential second cancers (e.g., a Hodgkin's Lymphoma survivor seeking screening mammography). At present the benchmark-equivalent coverage says only "other appropriate preventative services as designated by the Secretary…." This issue will likely need to be further clarified.

The importance of preventive care access and coverage for cancer survivors cannot be overstated. In many ways, survivorship is a period of new prevention in which monitoring for potential late effects, surveillance for recurrent and new cancers, and health education to optimize wellness and quality of life are paramount. While the requirement for preventive service coverage has a critical and beneficial impact on cancer patients, the lack of coverage for preventive screening benefits for "traditional" Medicaid recipients creates a gap in coverage for those most at risk for developing cancer due to environmental risk-factors – the very poor. Additionally, the lack of coverage of routine care costs in clinical trials for Medicaid recipients places limits on those who could, arguably, most benefit from expanded access to clinical trials.

## Medicare

The Act amends Medicare to entitle beneficiaries to annualized wellness visits, the development of a personal prevention plan, and expanded coverage for preventive services classified as A or B by the US Preventive Services Task Force, as well as colorectal cancer screening [3].

Given that 60% of cancer diagnoses occur among individuals age 65 or older, the impact of health reform on Medicare coverage directly affects a large number of cancer patients [29]. Depending on how it is implemented, the law's addition of coverage for annualized wellness visits can provide a critical source of ongoing survivorship monitoring through primary care providers for Medicare beneficiaries who are cancer patients, particularly as coverage reforms begin to interact with the broader use of electronic health records as a result of the health information technology adoption incentives under the HITECH Act, which became law in 2009 as part of the economic stimulus legislation [30]. An interesting area for future discussion is that there are no specific provisions that broaden Medicare's coverage in area of incentives for improved communications with providers in the context of care coordination, patient navigation, survivorship care planning, or demonstration projects to create an evidence base for reimbursement.

### Coverage Reforms in Advance of January 1, 2014

In advance of the 2014 effective date for the mandate, the subsidies and the Exchanges, the Act permits states to expand Medicaid for low-income adults as a state option. The Act also creates high-risk health insurance pools (known as preexisting condition health plans) that are meant to provide affordable coverage on an interim basis for several hundred thousand people whose preexisting health conditions make coverage unavailable, uninsurable, or both [3].

## *Improving Health-Care Quality, Efficiency, and Accountability*

Beyond insurance, the ACA begins the job of realigning the health-care system for long-term changes in health-care quality, the organization and design of health-care practice, and health information transparency. It does so by introducing broad changes into Medicare and Medicaid that empower both the HHS Secretary and state Medicaid programs to test new modes of payment and service delivery, such as medical homes (termed health-care homes in Medicaid), clinically integrated "accountable care organizations," payments for episodes of care, and bundled payments [3]. Cancer is specifically identified as a candidate quality improvement model to be tested by the newly established Center for Medicare and Medicaid innovation in the case of Medicare. Specifically the law provides, as a candidate test model, "aligning nationally recognized, evidence-based guidelines of cancer care with payment incentives in areas of treatment planning and follow-up care planning" for individuals eligible for Medicare, as well as those eligible for both Medicare and Medicaid [3]. This aspect of reform has implications for cancer care coordination as well as the provision of survivorship care plans for patients completing cancer treatment, which is one of the ten recommendations issued by the IOM in its 2006 *Lost in Transition* report [20].

These changes are intended to allow public payers to slowly but decisively begin to nudge the health-care system into behaving in different ways in terms of how health professionals work in a more clinically integrated fashion, measure the quality of their care and report on their performance, and target for quality improvement serious and chronic health conditions, including conditions that result in frequent hospital admissions and readmissions. HHS and states are expected to test payment and delivery system reforms that also attract private payer involvement in order to maximize the potential for cross-payer reforms that can in turn exert additional pressure on health-care providers and institutions.

The Act also invests in the development of a multi-payer National Quality Strategy whose purpose is to generate multi-payer quality and efficiency measures to promote value purchasing, greater safety, and far more extensive health information across public and private insurers [3]. In this regard, the Act will attempt to build on the HITECH Act, enacted into law in 2009 as part of the American Recovery and Reinvestment Act (ARRA) [30], and further lay the groundwork for performance reporting on a system-wide basis so that patients can more readily get information about their own health care and how their health-care providers perform. In addition, the Act establishes the Patient-Centered Outcomes Research Institute in order to promote the type of research essential to identifying the most appropriate and efficient means of delivering health care for diverse patient populations [3]. Throughout these initiatives to improve quality and information, the Act attempts to emphasize efforts to collect information about health and health-care disparities in order to allow the nation to better assess progress not only for the population as a whole but for patient subpopulations at elevated risk for poor health outcomes.

Even as the legislation invests nearly $1 trillion over the 2010–2019 time period aimed at make coverage affordable, the Act proposes to offset these expenditures through curbs on Medicare and Medicaid spending, new taxes on high cost plans, and tax shelters used most heavily by affluent families. In addition, and of particular note to public health policy and practice, the Act significantly alters the obligations and reporting rules for nonprofit hospitals by imposing new conduct and reporting obligations on hospitals as a condition of maintaining their federal nonprofit status (a tax exemption worth more than $100 billion annually; states also provide parallel exemptions). The changes include requiring hospitals to undertake ongoing community health needs assessments, furnish emergency care in a nondiscriminatory fashion (a requirement already applicable under the Emergency Treatment and Active Labor Act (EMTALA), which is unaltered by the ACA), alter their billing and collection practices, and maintain widely publicized written financial assistance policies that provide information about eligibility, how the assistance is calculated, and how to apply for assistance [3].

## Making Primary Health Care More Accessible to Medically Underserved Populations

An estimated 60 million individuals are considered medically underserved as a result of a combination of elevated health risks and a shortage of primary health-care professionals [31]. To begin to more rapidly alleviate this shortage in advance of the implementation of the health insurance coverage requirements, the Act invests in a major expansion of community health centers and the National Health Service Corps. Over the FY 2011–FY 2015 time periods the Act invests $11 billion in health centers and $1.5 billion in the National Health Service Corps. Together these expansions are expected to result in a doubling of the number of patients served, raising the total number of health center patients from 20 million in 2010 to approximately 40 million by 2015 [32].

The expansion of access to primary care has important implications for cancer prevention and survivorship care. A full one-third of cancers are preventable through healthy diet, physical activity, and maintaining a healthy weight. Another one-third is susceptible to prevention through tobacco cessation [33]. Primary care providers can educate at-risk populations on appropriate behavior changes to minimize their risk for cancer. Cancer survivors can also reduce their chances of recurrence and second malignancies as well as optimize their overall wellness through primary care monitoring and surveillance, particularly when primary care providers are in communication with the patient's oncology team about that individual's risk profile for late effects or recurrence. Finally, models of shared survivorship care between oncologists and primary care providers can only be effective if an adequate supply of primary care providers are available and trained to care for cancer survivors.

### Improving the Public's Health and Training Health Professionals

In addition to insuring most Americans, making an effort to rationalize health care, investing in primary health care in medically underserved communities, and broadening coverage for effective clinical preventive health services, the ACA is intended to make direct public health investments. Part of these investments come in the form of new regulatory requirements related to coverage of clinical preventive services without cost sharing, a fundamental shift in the relationship between health insurance and clinical preventive care. In addition, the Act provides for the development of a national prevention plan and the establishment of a Prevention and Public Health Trust Fund to finance community investments that will improve public health [3]. The Fund, whose value is set at $15 billion, will provide additional funding for prevention activities beginning in FY 2010 and continuing annually.

The Act also authorizes new investments in training primary care health professionals [3]. With the exception of new investments in establishing "teaching health centers," these changes are authorized but not funded as part of the Act and will need separate appropriated funding.

## Conclusion and Implications

As a major shift in public policy, the Affordable Care Act opens a significant window of opportunity to improve the accessibility and quality of cancer treatment in both its primary and survivorship phases. What is made of this window of opportunity will depend in great measure on the policy presence of the cancer community itself.

The Act is intended to extend, stabilize, and improve coverage, lays the groundwork for long-term quality improvement, and takes important steps toward public health and workforce training. At the same time, implementation presents unprecedented challenges at the federal and state levels of policymaking, and much rides on the ability of the cancer policy community to recognize and respond creatively to these challenges. Some of the most important are discussed below.

*Enrolling all eligible people.* When the mandate, subsidies, health insurance Exchanges, and Medicaid expansions go live on January 1, 2014, the Act will be positioned to achieve its central aims: stabilizing coverage for nearly all Americans and assuring that health insurance coverage is available, accessible, and affordable. The task involved in enrolling more than 30 million people, including some of the poorest and hardest to serve, is immense. Outreach will need to be extensive and involvement will be essential on the part of community health-care providers, public health agencies, and nonprofit organizations serving the poor and underserved. In the runup period to 2014 states will be putting Medicaid expansions, insurance reforms, and Exchanges into place, developing streamlined enrollment procedures, and seeking outreach partners. The lack of health insurance coverage remains the single greatest barrier to high-quality affordable health care, including cancer care.

*Transitioning among sources of coverage.* Even when the expanded insurance system is fully operational, a major challenge remains the multi-payer nature of the health insurance system. As income and employment status fluctuate, and as employer behavior changes in the face of the options available to the workforce, transitioning among payers can be expected, particularly for individuals with lower incomes. In the modern world of insurance, this transitioning phenomenon is not just about transitioning among payers, but among care systems as well as a result of networked health plans. Of crucial importance is the development of cross-payer markets in order to minimize breaks in coverage and care. This means alignment whenever possible among insurance products sold to Medicaid programs, Exchanges, and directly to employers and individuals who elect to continue to purchase coverage outside the Exchange. (Premium subsidies for individuals are available only inside the Exchange system, which may help minimize the number of individuals who purchase coverage directly). Of central importance to continuity of care – an essential aspect of health-care quality for persons with chronic conditions – will be incentives for plans to serve multiple markets, as well as strong standards for provider networks where cancer treatment and survivorship care are concerned, so that the transition across care systems does not result in a loss of quality. Cancer treatment and survivorship care represent key issues of focus, including both standards for patients who face transition across payer systems as well as multi-payer quality performance measures that establish accountability for cross-system patient management.

*Implementation of insurance reforms.* The implementation of reforms applicable to insurance coverage and group health plans is a basic component of the law. Of particular focus in a cancer policy context are implementation standards for the essential benefit package (particularly the meaning of case management for chronic conditions), permissible employer practices in the case of wellness programs to avert performance measures that discriminate against sick patients, implementation of the clinical trials coverage rules, and articulation of access standards for the provider networks established by qualified health plans.

*Improving the quality of care for Medicaid beneficiaries.* Medicaid becomes the linchpin of the entire new law, accounting for half of all new covered persons. When fully implemented, Medicaid will cover some 75 million persons. As crucial as Medicaid is, the evidence suggests that the quality and accessibility of care for Medicaid beneficiaries leaves a great deal to be desired. Areas of focus include implementation of payment reforms for primary care providers, payment improvements for specialty care – including oncology care, the recruitment of providers into networks, the development of quality of care standards that address the cultural and language needs of Medicaid beneficiaries and that are appropriate for a population with relatively low health literacy, assuring full coverage of clinical preventive care for all Medicaid-enrolled adults, and the adoption by states of coverage of routine costs associated with clinical trials. At the same time, the issue of how Medicaid pays for ongoing medical and surgical treatment remains unaddressed, leaving the problem of low payment rates that deter access to such treatments as chemotherapy still a distinct part of the Medicaid landscape.

*Testing quality improvement models.* The legislation places great emphasis on testing new care models in Medicare and Medicaid that are aimed at achieving greater quality of care and greater financial efficiencies. Cancer is explicitly identified as a condition that deserves focus as new models are tested. Much work needs to be done to design health homes for Medicaid beneficiaries (whether or not also eligible for Medicare) who are living with cancer and who are cancer survivors, and the incentive for such testing is inclusion in the Center for Medicare and Medicaid Innovation's list of fundable pilots. Patient navigation is one quality improvement that has increased access to cancer care by connecting Medicaid beneficiaries to medical homes [34–37].

*National quality strategy and comparative clinical effectiveness.* The legislation places special emphasis on the development of a national quality strategy applicable to all payers, and that can develop quality performance and reporting standards while making data on the quality of care available. Similarly, the law emphasizes the role of comparative clinical effectiveness research and the dissemination of findings, particularly research aimed at managing high cost and chronic health conditions. Comparative effectiveness research on models of survivorship care are critically needed to identify effective, efficient approaches to caring for survivors' long-term needs – particularly given that the projected number of cancer care and primary care providers cannot meet the demand for services for a growing population of cancer survivors.

The potential combined impact of a national quality strategy and comparative clinical effectiveness research cannot be underestimated. Together these two advances position health-care providers and policymakers to strive for system-wide quality improvement. The evidence regarding the value of cancer survivorship treatment presents an important opportunity to use the quality improvement tools embodied in the law to better assure that regardless of payer, the health-care system as a whole is held to consistent standards of performance and has equal access to information on clinical effectiveness and performance-linked health outcomes. This aspect of reform responds to the need for clinical practice guidelines for comprehensive cancer survivorship care that was highlighted by the IOM in its *Lost in Transition* report. The IOM noted that although some guidelines are currently available for certain aspects of care, most are incomplete. Specifically, the IOM recommended: "Health care providers should use systematically developed evidence-based clinical practice guidelines, assessment tools, and screening instruments to help identify and manage late effects of cancer and its treatment. Existing guidelines should be refined and new evidence-based guidelines should be developed through public and private-sector efforts [20]."

*National prevention strategy including oral health.* Finally, the ACA positions the country to engage in thoughtful and deliberate efforts to improve the health of the population as a strategy for bringing down health-care costs. Along with broad community efforts to reduce cancer risk, better management of cancer and cancer survivorship should be understood as measures of population health. How a nation responds to persons with chronic conditions is, under the terms of the Act, as key an indicator of public health responsiveness as the prevention of disease.

Additionally, the inclusion of oral health in the national prevention strategy has two significant implications for the cancer community – the detection and treatment of oral cancer and the monitoring of oral health problems resulting from cancer treatment modalities, such as radiotherapy, chemotherapy, or steroid therapy that may create heightened risks for dental problems or osteonecrosis. The need for coordinated oral health care for cancer survivors represents a major opportunity to inject cancer survivorship into the center of the national dialog on the management of chronic disease.

The ACA provides opportunities for improvements to access, affordability, and quality of care for cancer patients, but much remains to be done in terms of implementing reform and advocating for policies to optimize the quantity and quality of life of cancer survivors. Navigating patients to expanded Medicaid programs as well as Medicaid reforms (payment reforms for primary and specialty care providers, expansion of provider networks, preventive care for all Medicaid recipients, and clinical trial coverage); cultural competency standards; access to appropriate screening and care for undocumented residents; psychosocial support for all cancer patients and their families; creation of healthy environments and healthy behavior education for the poorest and most vulnerable cancer survivors; and efficient models of long-term comprehensive survivorship care for a growing population of cancer survivors continue to challenge our ability to provide equitable, quality, affordable, and timely cancer care to those in need.

## References


1. United States. American Cancer Society. American Cancer Society facts and figures 2010. Atlanta: American Cancer Society; 2010.
2. National Cancer Institute. Surveillance epidemiology and end results: cancer fact stats: all sites [document on the Internet]. Maryland: The Institute; 2010 [cited 2010 August 21]. Available from: http://seer.cancer.gov/statfacts/html/all.html#incidence-mortality.
3. United States Congress. Patient protection and affordable care act. Washington, DC: USC publication 111–148; 2010.
4. United States Congress. Health care and education reconciliation act. Washington, DC: USC publication 111–152; 2010.
5. United States National Cancer Institute. Presidents Cancer Panel. Bethesda: NCI; 1998.
6. Schwartz KL, Crossley-May H, Vigneau FD, Brown K, Bauerjee M. Socio economic status and stage at diagnosis for five common malignancies. Cancer Causes Control. 2003;14:761–6.
7. United States. Institute of Medicine. Unequal treatment: confronting racial and ethnic disparities in healthcare. Washington, DC: IOM; 2003.
8. Thorpe KE, Howard D. Health insurance and spending among cancer patients. Health Aff. 2003;W3:189–98.
9. Banthin JS, Bernard DM. Changes in financial burdens for healthcare: national estimates or the populations younger than 65 years. JAMA. 2006;296(22):2712–9.
10. Schoen C, Collins SR, Kriss JL, Doty M. How many are uninsured? Trends among U.S. adults 2003–2007. Health Aff (Milwood). 2008;4:298–309.
11. Elkin EB, Bach PB. Cancer's next frontier: addressing high and increasing cost. JAMA. 2010;303(11):1086–7.
12. Weaver KE, Rowland JH, Bellizzi KM, Asia NM. Foregoing medical care because of cost: assessing disparities in health care access among cancer survivors living in the United States. Cancer. 2010;116(14):3493–504.
13. Rabb SS, Gryzbicki DM. Quality in cancer diagnosis. CA Cancer J Clin. 2010;60(3):139–65.
14. United States. Institute of Medicine. Insuring quality cancer care. Washington, DC: IOM; 1999.
15. Foley K et al. Survival disadvantage among Medicaid-insured breast patients treated with breast conserving surgery with radiation therapy. Breast Cancer Res Treat. 2007;101(2):207–14.
16. Snyderman D, Wynn D. Depression in cancer patients. Prim Care. 2009;36(4):703–19.
17. Tornoux C, Katsahian S, Chevret S, Levy V. Factors influencing inclusion of patients with malignancies in clinical trials. Cancer. 2006;106(2):258–70.
18. Kolata G. Grant system leads cancer researchers to play it safe. The New York Times. 2009 June 27.
19. Gralow J et al. Clinical cancer advances 2007: major advances in cancer treatment, prevention, and screening. J Clin Oncol. 2008;26(2):403–11.
20. United States. Institute of Medicine. From cancer patient to cancer survivor: lost in transition. Washington, DC: IOM; 2006.
21. Association of American Medical Colleges, Center for Workforce Studies. Forecasting the supply of and demand for oncologists: a report to the American Society of Clinical Oncology (ASCO). Washington, DC: AAMC; 2006.
22. Gostin LO. Public health law: power, duty, restraint. California: University of California Press; 2008.
23. United States. U.S. Constitution. Article 1 §8. Washington, DC: U.S. Constitution; 2010.
24. Rosenbaum S, Gruber J. Buying health care, the individual mandate, and the constitution. N Eng J Med. 2010;363:401–3.

25. United States Congress. Health insurance portability and accountability act. Washington, DC: USC publication 104-191; 1996.
26. United States Congress. United vs. Lopez. Washington, DC: USC; 1996.
27. United States. National Cancer Institute. Presidents Cancer Panel. Bethesda: NCI; 2004.
28. Rosenbaum S. A customary and necessary program: Medicaid and health reform. N Eng J Med. 2010;362:1950–5.
29. Horner et al. SEER cancer statistics review, 1975–2006, National Cancer Institute [document on the internet]. NCI: 2006 [cited 2010 August 23]. Available from: http://seer.cancer.gov/csr/1975 2006/.
30. United States Congress. HITECH Act. Washington, DC: USC publication 111-5; 2010.
31. National Association of Community Health Centers. Access denied. Washington, DC: NACHC; 2008.
32. National Association of Community Health Centers. Expanding Health Centers under Health Care Reform. Washington, DC: NACHC; 2010.
33. World Cancer Research Fund/American Institute for Cancer Research. Food, nutrition, physical activity and the prevention of cancer: a global perspective. Washington, DC: WCRF/AICR; 2007.
34. Vargas RB, Ryan GW, Jackson CA, Rodriguez R, Freeman HP. Characteristics of the original patient navigation programs to reduce disparities in the diagnosis and treatment of breast cancer. Cancer [serial on the Internet]. 2008 [cited 2010 Aug 23]. Available from: http://dx.doi.org/10.1002/cncr.23547.
35. Battaglia CA, Roloff K, Posner MA, Freund KM. Improving follow-up to abnormal breast cancer screening in an urban populations: a patient navigation intervention. Cancer. 2007;109(supp):359–676.
36. Patierno SR, LaVerda N, Alexander L, Levine P, Young HA. Longitudinal network patient navigation: development of an integrative model to reduce breast cancer disparities in Washington, DC. Oncol Issues. 2010;25(2):28–36.
37. Freeman HP. Patient navigation: a community center approach to reducing mortality. J Can Educ. 2006;21(1 supp):S11–4.

# Chapter 18
# Quality Health Care for Cancer Survivors

**Michael Feuerstein and Patricia A. Ganz**

## Introduction

As the chapters in this book illustrate, the knowledge that forms the current fundamentals of quality care for cancer survivors is not the province of a few professions. This can be both a blessing and a curse. Interdisciplinary research and practice can be difficult and costly, but at this point such a diverse perspective is imperative. The chapters in this book clearly illustrate that many researchers and providers from multiple health professions are involved in designing, studying, and providing elements of health care to cancer survivors. Many not involved in cancer survivorship often ask the question, "Isn't quality care similar to that of any chronic illness such as patients post-bypass surgery or those with arthritis, diabetes or post stroke? What is so unique about cancer?" The answer to this question is that we really do not know at this point. Given the recent growth in numbers of cancer survivors and the projected rise in numbers of cancer survivors in the future, we must empirically determine similarities and differences among various chronic illnesses in terms of patterns of comorbidities, long-term and late effects, function, and well-being in order to provide the proper chronic health care management for these diverse illnesses. This is particularly the case because much has been learned about the long-term management of chronic disorders other than cancer. Since surviving cancer is now conceptualized as a chronic disease, one logical question is, "What does the current literature on evidence-based evaluation and management of chronic illness tell us that we might apply to cancer?"

Patients with very different chronic diseases often express similar challenges optimizing health, function, and well-being. These often include the management of comorbid illnesses; episodic fatigue, pain, dysphoria, and distress, problems with weight, diet, and activity level, and in some, returning to or sustaining a viable work life. There are certainly a range of long-term and late medical and nonmedical

M. Feuerstein (✉)
Department of Medical & Clinical Psychology, Preventive Medicine and Biometrics, Uniformed Services University of the Health Sciences, Bethesda, MD, USA
e-mail: mfeuerstein@usuhs.mil

M. Feuerstein and P.A. Ganz (eds.), *Health Services for Cancer Survivors*,
DOI 10.1007/978-1-4419-1348-7_18, © Springer Science+Business Media, LLC 2011

effects that can vary across and within different types of chronic illnesses as well but there are many commonalities. Research on the epidemiology, prevention, and management of these chronic illnesses will clarify differences and similarities among these illnesses, however, at this point in the evolution of this knowledge perhaps we can gain a better understanding of what needs to be considered in the long-term management of cancer survivors from the literature on chronic illness care in general.

We should be cautious not to blindly generalize all findings on chronic illness management to cancer survivorship care. Wholesale adoption of existing approaches to chronic illness in general is ill-advised. We may need to generate unique variations of current approaches to chronic care given what we now know about cancer survivors and their current care specific needs. However, chronic care has been operational in primary care for two decades. Many internists, family physicians, and nurse practitioners, have clinically valuable skills that can readily transfer to the management of cancer survivors as well. Chronic illness care has been evaluated as a topic of health services research for over a decade [1]. Many groups around the world have led efforts to improve chronic care within existing health care systems. We can learn from the knowledge they have accumulated.

## Chronic Care in Perspective

To date, the most well-studied approach to chronic care is based on the Chronic Care Model (CCM) first proposed by Wagner in the late 1990s [2]. This perspective came about based upon the assumption that the approach to acute care (detection, diagnosis, treatment, and recovery) did not fit diseases that were not "cured" but rather "managed" over time. This view was and remains applicable to cardiovascular illness, arthritis, diabetes, and various chronic pain conditions, to name but a few. In fact, the CCM was viewed as a useful way to conceptualize chronic illness where care requires: (1) a focus on continuity, (2) communication, (3) self-management of symptoms, and (4) attention to functional limitations that persist over time or are episodic but can be disruptive to patients over long periods of time.

The original components of the CCM include: (1) community resources and policies, (2) organization of health care within some type of health system, and (3) continuous productive interactions among an informed activated patient and a well-prepared proactive practice team [2]. A few years later, Barr and colleagues [3] expanded the model to include more detail on the role of the community (i.e., public policy, supportive health care, and community environment) in achieving such a practice model for essentially any chronic illness (refer to Fig. 18.1).

Over the decade from 2000 to 2010, health services research on the application of the CCM within a primary care setting was a major priority [4–7]. Both meta-analyses and systematic reviews of this research have been published [8, 9]. The research on this approach to care has generally targeted illnesses such as

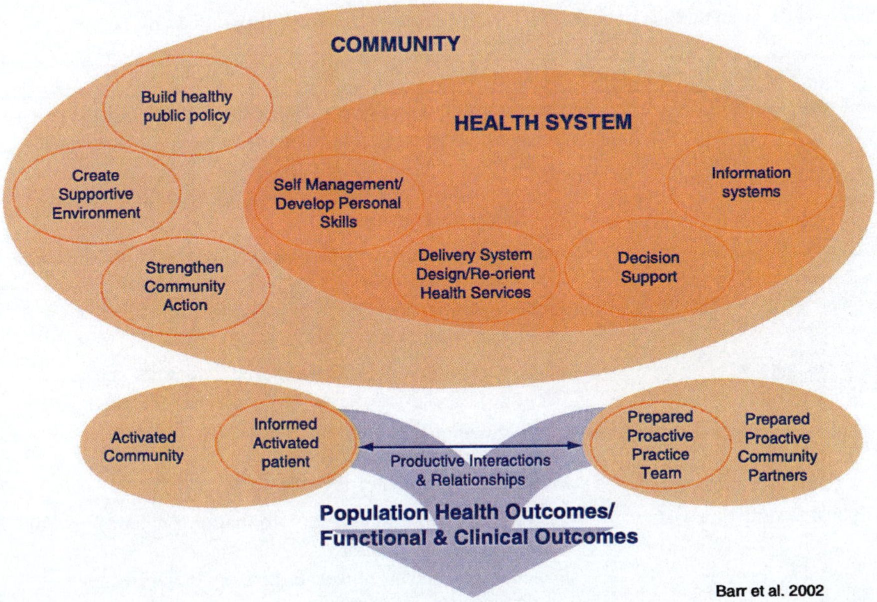


**Fig. 18.1** Expanded Chronic Care Model [3] with permission

asthma, congestive heart failure, depression, and diabetes. The research indicates that while the majority of studies did not implement all components of the CCM, when at least one aspect of care was implemented, self-rated health improved in all four of the chronic health problems studied [8]. Another major review of the application of the CCM in chronic obstructive pulmonary disease also found no effect when only one CCM component was implemented, but that emergency visits and hospitalizations were significantly lower when two or more CCM components were implemented [10]. Another review found that when the CCM was operational, improvements in biomarkers in diabetes and a reduction in medical costs for patients with heart failure, asthma, and diabetes were observed [9]. A description of the elements of Wagner's CCM is described in Table 18.1. As you can see from the table, this type of health care often requires an overall redesign of the delivery of health care.

## Evidence-Based Health Care

The CCM highlights the role health care providers can play in decision support. While many chronic disorders have a more established evidence base for long-term disease management, as time goes on it is expected that cancer survivor-specific

**Table 18.1** Interventions components of the Chronic Care Mod (Reprinted by permission of publisher)

| Chronic Care Model component | Intervention |
|---|---|
| Self-management | Education (giving information alone) and/or<br>Behavioral support (providing tools to modify behaviors ) and/or<br>Motivational (linking specific goals for behavioral changes to clinical information |
| Delivery system design | Interventions that provided "advanced access" to medical care (24 h/day, 7 days/week) for partcipants and/or<br>Implemented practice teams to coordinate preventative measures for chronic care |
| Decision support | Used or implemented evidence-based guidelines and/or<br>Integrated specialty expertise (e.g., referrals for management of comorbidities) and/or<br>Identified barriers to care and/or<br>Performed performance reviews |
| Clinical information system | Clinical registries (population information databases) and/or<br>Clinical reminders and/or<br>Provider (physicians, nurses, respiratory therapists, pharmacists, etc.) feedback |

guidelines will emerge and form much of the basis for decisions regarding evidence based approaches to manage the problems that cancer survivors experience [11].

Health care services research informs us that even when evidence-based guidelines are available, it is not atypical that nearly half of providers studied do not adhere to them. For example, one study of adherence to pneumonia prevention guidelines found that 44% of physicians did not adhere to guidelines [12]. A review of barriers to guideline adherence includes lack of awareness of guidelines, familiarity, agreement, self-efficacy, outcome expectancy, inertia, and external barriers such as inconvenience and time constraints [13].

In another area of health care that requires the integration of medical, physical therapy, psychological evaluation, and management, investigators [14] evaluated a newly developed integrated evidence-based guideline for acute low back pain in a large HMO with over 9 million subscribers. The authors found that despite extensive implementation efforts including extensive training of health care providers, the use of facility-based champions to assist with guideline adoption, management structure where adherence to policy among military physicians was likely (TriCare, Department of Defense), and a tightly regulated and monitored health care system were not necessary or sufficient factors to ensure adherence. The provider adherence rate to the guidelines was only about 40% across 4 years of observation in over 250,000 low back pain cases. However it was observed that as primary care provider adherence to the evidence based guidelines improved, patients' perceived health and physician rating of function was also improved. As illustrated in this study and many others over the past decade [13], the adoption of guidelines by both providers and consumers represents a formidable challenge.

## Integrated Care

As commented on throughout this book the integration of different specialties represents an important feature of cancer survivor chronic care. The development of a network of referral sources with health care professionals that may not currently be on a list of referrals for cancer patients (e.g., physical therapist, mental health provider, nutritionist, exercise specialist) may prove helpful in long term survivor care. What seems to be important in the literature reviewed in this area is indicates that the provision of follow-up health care by a multidisciplinary group of experienced professionals is preferred and may result in improved outcomes.

## Self-management

Self-management, or the empowerment of patients to monitor and employ various strategies (e.g., stress management, healthy diet, physical activity) to improve symptoms and lifestyle behaviors, is another important element of chronic care. While as providers we can offer treatment approaches (e.g., medications, psychosocial consultation, physical therapy), there are several elements of health promotion, physical function, and improving a sense of well-being that require a certain degree of self-management in order to optimize long term outcomes. Although much of the responsibility for this element of care rests on the shoulders of cancer survivors themselves, providers can help facilitate and maintain these health behaviors, particularly during a follow-up visit where there may be a need for a renewed emphasis on these behaviors. The chapters on health behavior change, emotional distress or well-being, and other symptoms indicate that while this seems like a simple effort, healthy lifestyle and symptom management in those with a chronic health problem is difficult to maintain over time. Integration of self-management, provider support, specific intervention, and referral can be helpful when problems are reported or observed.

## Clinical Information System

The final element of the CCM is the use of some type of clinical information system. While there has been much attention paid to the electronic medical record over the past decade and more recently as a means for better documentation of health care over a lifetime, the electronic medical record represents only one element of health care to facilitate care. The electronic medical record can provide useful information to mitigate unnecessary and unsafe duplication of care and reduce the need for retrospective recall of provider and survivor. However, information systems can also be created to address many of the current barriers to providing the quality of care cancer survivors need.

User-friendly clinical information systems have also been developed to track the process and outcome of health behavior changes [15, 16], and these tracking systems are often a necessary step to achieve long-term behavior change, functional improvement, and well-being. Such systems have evolved that allow for real time or home monitoring of blood glucose in diabetes; pain frequency and severity in arthritis; physical deconditioning in chronic pain; diet and physical activity in weight management; and work absence and distress levels over time in a number of chronic illnesses [15, 16]. Patients can now Tw self-monitor and track their actions and symptoms using cell phones, PDAs, other electronic devices, and specialized web sites on the Internet [15–17]. This continuous monitoring of progress in many outcomes can provide useful feedback regarding trends to the provider and survivor on a real-time basis that might justify a course correction in behavior change.

## What Have We Learned About Chronic Health Care?

A review of over 100 studies of chronic illness management programs that used the CCM as a framework for delivery of care indicated that inclusion of EACH element discussed above was infrequent [8]. This was the case in highly managed care settings where systems can be put in place relatively easier than in certain types of health care settings, and where incentives for service provision and reimbursement were aligned. Only one study in the review included all six elements proposed by CCM. The table also indicates that none of the studies that met the rigorous inclusion criteria investigated the self-management–motivation component of the CCM. This latter finding supports the well-known observation that the behavior change process in contrast to the other elements of the CCM continues to be poorly understood in terms of how to implement, who will implement, and the cost of implementing self management efforts to help change health status in order to achieve clinically meaningful long-term change. As with the study of evidence-based guidelines for low back pain [14] discussed earlier in this chapter, patient reports of health were related to the number of components of the Chronic Care Model implemented (Table 18.2) [7]. Upon close scrutiny of the data, behavior change, multispecialty use of a PDA, patient information system, multispecialty practice, group/individual planned visits, and practice champions were all related to better general health status in CCM. The research on CCM indicates that some elements of care were more likely to be implemented than others. However, as the number of elements of care increased, outcome was also improved. Overall, this approach seems promising for some aspects of cancer survivor care and should be investigated specifically in relation to improve systems of care in cancer survivors. Table 18.2 below provides a summary of the effect sizes observed for each of the major elements of the chronic health care model and the specific clinical outcomes, quality of life outcomes, and process of care outcomes [8].

**Table 18.2** CCM elements and clinical, quality of life, and health care outcomes (Reprinted by permission of publisher [8])

| | Clinical outcome | | | | | | | |
|---|---|---|---|---|---|---|---|---|
| | Continuous variable[a] (lower is better) | | Dichotomous variable (lower is better) | | Quality of life (higher is better) | | Process of care (higher is better) | |
| Element present | Effect size (95% CI) | No. | Relative risk (95% CI) | No. | Effect size (95% CI) | No. | Relative risk (95% CI) | No. |
| Delivery system | −0.21 (−0.40, −0.02) | 33 | 0.77 (0.62, 0.96) | 30 | 0.33 (−0.10, 0.76) | 12 | 1.16 (1.01, 1.34) | 21 |
| Self-management support | −0.22 (−0.38, −0.05) | 35 | 0.81 (0.66, 0.99) | 36 | −0.33 (−0.25, 0.19) | 22 | 1.31 (1.00, 1.71) | 15 |
| Decision support | −0.14 (−0.33, 0.05) | 24 | 0.87 (0.69, 1.09) | 17 | 0.04 (−0.36, 0.45) | 7 | 1.29 (1.08, 1.54) | 18 |
| Clinical information systems | −0.06 (−0.27, 0.15) | 13 | 0.83 (0.64, 1.07) | 10 | −0.28 (−1.08, 0.51) | 2[b] | 1.08 (0.91, 1.28) | 9 |
| Community resources | −0.11 (−0.41, 0.19) | 4[b] | NE | 0 | NE | 1 | NE | 0 |
| Health care organization | −0.02 (−0.33, 0.29) | 4[b] | 0.82 (0.56, 1.20) | 3[b] | −0.38 (−1.26, 0.49) | 3[b] | 0.88 (0.67, 1.16) | 5 |

*CI* indicates confidence interval, *NE* not estimable

[a]Includes data only on studies related to depression and diabetes

[b]Pooled estimates based on fewer than five studies should be interpreted with caution

## Chronic Care and Cancer Survivorship Health Care

### *The Process of Chronic Care Management*

The key findings based on health services research aspects on the chronic care approach are listed in Table 18.3. There are some general observations from this literature that can guide efforts to improve the quality of survivorship health care. Below is a top line summary of the highlights of this past research and the implications for optimizing cancer survivor health care in the near future.

1. Education is simple to add to chronic care programs and is a very common element of chronic care. There is much information available to cancer survivors. However, survivors of cancer still face challenges in determining where to locate specific information and how to determine its accuracy. Also, survivors need different information at varying points in the natural history of survivorship that are based on the problems presented at that time. What specific information and how and when to deliver this information remains unclear. The goals or expected outcomes of providing this information need to be better defined as well.
2. Chronic care practice teams of providers are often used for clinical decision making in the CCM. Chapters in this book highlighted the use of teams including oncologists, oncology nurses, internists, psychologists, social workers, physical therapists, and rehabilitation medicine specialists. This team approach can also provide a focus on preventive health. Currently, there is mixed evidence about the delivery of preventive health services to cancer survivors; Studies of Medicare claims have found that breast cancer survivors receive more preventive health services than controls, however colorectal cancer survivors receive fewer services [18, 19]. This aspect of cancer survivor care needs to be carefully evaluated by cancer type and the most cost-effective models of care for achieving patient-tailored integrated care empirically determined.
3. Self-managed care has proven to be difficult to implement in chronic care efforts. While teams of providers aid in decision making, the CCM of chronic care has not been able to provide the self-management element that is needed to initiate and maintain behavior change and recover from relapses in behavior change or lifestyle change efforts. Research in this area has identified some major advances (e.g., change efforts that are ore responsive to cultural barriers and the importance of conceptualizing health behavior change as a process with stages rather than a simple go/no go effort) [20, 21]. Despite such advances, this is an area in need of much work in general and in the translation to cancer survivorship care.
4. Symptom burden (e.g., fatigue, distress, cognitive limitations, pain) can be better managed through self-management and appropriate use of medications, but also is one that often requires the attention of professionals familiar with problems associated with these problems. While symptom management is clearly an

**Table 18.3** Highlights from health services research on the Chronic Care Model for non cancer related chronic illness

| | |
|---|---|
| 1. | Each element of the CCM is not consistently included in all clinical programs. |
| 2. | Education is the most frequently implemented self-management component. |
| 3. | Efforts to enhance motivation and change behavior were the elements that were least often represented. |
| 4. | The use of practice teams to provide preventive care was the most commonly used element. |
| 5. | Provision of multidisciplinary support teams to make decisions regarding care was the second most common system innovation. It too fell short in terms of frequency of use when considering the number of studies that did not include this element of care. |

element of chronic care management in general, with cancer there appears to be qualitative differences (e.g., subthreshold levels of depression and anxiety) that require greater attention in both research and clinical application. High levels of various symptoms or clusters of symptoms are observed in 30–50% of cancer survivors [22]. This burden can impact heath, function, and overall sense of well-being. It usually is something that wanes as time from primary cancer treatment increases. Time following treatment however, it can persist at some level and can also reoccur over a lifetime. These symptoms often do not reach clinical levels, can be misdiagnosed as depression or anxiety, or can be missed altogether during clinic visits. There is a major need to recognize the existence of symptom burden and develop and implement brief tools to monitor it over time. The need to develop innovative approaches to prevent or manage symptoms requires an integrative perspective. Attention to this problem it is not simply for those survivors experiencing severe symptoms or for those with the resources to seek help.

5. Information technology, while rapidly advancing, is still in its infancy as a means of accelerating health quality and cost reduction [23]. Interesting the health services literature on the CCM has indicated that this component of the CCM approach was the least commonly found in what was operationally defined as well-designed chronic care systems. Of all the other elements, which included change in provider practice or something the patient was required to act on, enhancements in information technology require a high level of capital investment. While the development of this technology has progressed since the major meta-analysis on the CCM was published in 2005 [8], it is time to explore its use in other applications of the CCM to cancer survivorship. Real time monitoring of many targeted outcomes (e.g., activity levels) is an area ripe for further development, evaluation, and application. We must not lose sight of the fact that economic incentives need to be better aligned with desired outcomes in this area of health care. For years in the area of cancer, program development and implementation has been significantly financed through donations. While these donations currently represent a critical aspect of the development and implementation of survivor care, viable financial models in order for services to continue, improve and expand need to be developed and implemented.

## The Future

Cancer survivorship is a major public health problem that is projected to grow significantly over the next 40 years particularly as the world population ages. The chapters in this book provide a first hand account of cancer survivor health services that have evolved since I (MF) was diagnosed with brain cancer eight years ago. Over these years we have witnessed the efforts of many to achieve these improvements. As you can see there is still so much more to accomplish.

Quality health care for cancer survivors will continue to improve as we learn more about their unique and common challenges with other chronic diseases. Indeed, there will come a time when quality care for cancer survivors is simply an element of good health care in general. Presently, this is clearly not the case and efforts at multiple levels (medical school, continuing education, health care education in general, reform of heath care systems and daily practice, advocacy, legal reform, and societal expectations and goals) need to be revamped and move at a steady but never-ending pace until all cancer survivors can expect and receive the care they truly need throughout their life in order to optimize their health, function, and well-being. We must settle for nothing less.

## References

1. Epping-Jordan J, Pruitt S, Bengoa R, Wagner E. Improving the quality of health care for chronic conditions. Qual Saf Health Care. 2004;13:299–305.
2. Wagner E. Chronic disease management: what will it take to improve care for chronic illness? Eff Clin Pract. 1998;1:2–4.
3. Barr V, Robinson S, Marin-Link B, Underhill L, Dotts A, Ravensdale D, et al. The expanded chronic care model: an integration of concepts and strategies from population health promotion and the Chronic Care Model. Hosp Q. 2003;7(1):73–82.
4. Ohman-Strickland P, Hudson S, Piasecki A, Hahn K, Cohen D, Orzano J, et al. Features of the chronic care model (CCM) associated with behavioral counseling and diabetes care in community primary care. J Am Board Fam Med. 2010;23(3):295–305.
5. Pearson M, Wu S, Schaefer J, Bonomi A, Shortell S, Mendel P, et al. Assessing the implementation of the chronic care model in quality improvement collaboratives. Health Serv Res. 2005;40(4):978–96.
6. Dorr D, Wilcox A, Burns L, Brunker C, Narus S, Clayton P. Implementing a multidisease chronic care model in primary care using people and technology. Dis Manage. 2006;9(1):1–15.
7. Hung D, Glasgow R, Dickinson M, Froshaug D, Fernald D, Balasubramanian B, et al. The chronic care model and relationships to patient health status and health-related quality of life. Am J Prev Med. 2008;35(5S):S398–406.
8. Tsai A, Morton S, Mangione C, Keeler E. A meta-analysis of interventions to improve care for chronic illnesses. Am J Manage Care. 2005;11(8):478–88.
9. Bodenheimer T, Wagner E, Grumbach K. Improving primary care for patients with chronic illness: the chronic care model, part 2. JAMA. 2002;288:1909–14.
10. Adams S, Smith P, Allan P, Anzueto A, Pugh J, Cornell J. Systematic review of the chronic care model in chronic obstructive pulmonary disease prevention and management. Arch Intern Med. 2007;167(6):551–61.

11. Sackett D, Rosenberg W, Gray J, Haynes R, Richardson W. Evidence based medicine: what it is and what it isn't. BMJ. 1996;312:71–2.
12. Halm E, Atlas S, Borowsky L, Benzer T, Metlay J, Chang Y, et al. Understanding physician adherence with a pneumonia practice guideline. Arch Intern Med. 2000;160:98–104.
13. Cabana M, Rand C, Powe N. Why don't physicians follow clinical practice guidelines? A framework for improvement. JAMA. 1999;282(15):1458–65.
14. Feuerstein M, Hartzell M, Rogers H, Marcus S. Evidence-based practice for acute low back pain in primary care: patient outcomes and cost of care. Pain. 2006;124(1):140–9.
15. Jamison R, Raymond S, Levine J, Slawsby E, Nedeljkovic S, Katz N. Electronic diaries for monitoring chronic pain: 1-year validation study. Pain. 2001;91:277–85.
16. Tate D, Wing R, Winett R. Using internet technology to deliver a behavioral weight loss program. JAMA. 2001;285(9):1172–7.
17. Farmer A, Gibson O, Tarassenko L, Neil A. A systematic review of telemedicine interventions to support blood glucose self-monitoring in diabetes. Diabet Med. 2005;22(10):1372–8.
18. Earle C, Burstein H, Winer E, Weeks J. Quality of non-breast cancer health maintenance among elderly breast cancer survivors. J Clin Oncol. 2003;21(8):1447–51.
19. Earle C, Neville B. Under use of necessary care among cancer survivors. Cancer. 2004;101:1712–9.
20. Prochaska J, DiClemente C. Stages and processes of self-change of smoking: toward an integrative model of change. J Consult Clin Psychol. 1983;51:390–5.
21. Cassidy C. Using the Transtheoretical Model to facilitate behavior change in patients with chronic illness. J Am Acad Nurse Pract. 1999;11(7):281–6.
22. Cleeland C, Bennet G, Dantzer R, Doughtery P, Dunn A, Meyers C, et al. Are the symptoms of cancer and cancer treatment due to a shared biologic mechanism. Cancer. 2003;97(11): 2919–25.
23. Chaudhry B, Wang J, Wu S, Maglione M, Mojica W, Roth EM, et al. Systematic review: impact of health information technology on quality, efficiency, and costs of medical care. Ann Intern Med. 2006;144:742–52.

# Index



M. Feuerstein and P.A. Ganz (eds.), *Health Services for Cancer Survivors*,
DOI 10.1007/978-1-4419-1348-7, 

## D

## P